HUMANITY'S BURDEN

Humanity's Burden provides a panoramic overview of the history of malaria. It traces the long arc of malaria out of tropical Africa into Eurasia, its transfer to the Americas during the early years of the Columbian exchange, and its retraction from the middle latitudes into the tropics since the late nineteenth century. Adopting a broadly comparative approach to historical patterns and processes, it synthesizes research findings from the natural and social sciences and weaves these understandings into a narrative that reaches from the earliest evidence of malarial infections in tropical Africa up to the present. Written in a style that is easily accessible to nonspecialists, it considers the significance of genetic mutations, diet, lifestyle, migration, warfare, palliative and curative treatment, and efforts to interrupt transmission on the global distribution of malaria.

James L.A. Webb Jr. is professor of history at Colby College where he teaches courses in world history, African history, ecological history, and historical epidemiology. He is the author of *Desert Frontier: Ecological and Economic Change along the Western Sahel, 1600–1850*, and *Tropical Pioneers: Human Agency and Ecological Change in the Highlands of Sri Lanka, 1800–1900*.

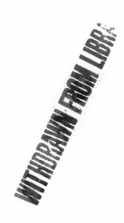

Studies in Environment and History

Editors
Donald Worster, University of Kansas
J.R. McNeill, Georgetown University

Humanity's Burden

A Global History of Malaria

JAMES L.A. WEBB Jr.

Colby College

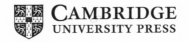

CAMBRIDGE
UNIVERSITY PRESS

CAMBRIDGE UNIVERSITY PRESS
Cambridge, New York, Melbourne, Madrid, Cape Town, Singapore, São Paulo, Delhi

Cambridge University Press
32 Avenue of the Americas, New York, NY 10013-2473, USA

www.cambridge.org
Information on this title: www.cambridge.org/9780521670128

First published 2009

Printed in the United States of America

A catalog record for this publication is available from the British Library.

Library of Congress Cataloging in Publication Data
Webb Jr., James L.A.
Humanity's burden : a global history of malaria / James L.A. Webb Jr.
p. ; cm. – (Studies in environment and history)
Includes bibliographical references and index.
ISBN 978-0-521-85418-4 (hardback) – ISBN 978-0-521-67012-8 (pbk.)
1. Malaria – History. I. Title. II. Series.
[DNLM: 1. Malaria – history. 2. Antimalarials – history.
3. Communicable Disease Control – history. 4. Disease Outbreaks – history.
5. Quinine – history. WC 750 W366h 2009]
RC160.W43 2009
614.5′32–dc22   2008021564

ISBN 978-0-521-85418-4 hardback
ISBN 978-0-521-67012-8 paperback

For James and Jeanne
and
Margaret and Eugene

"If we take as our standard of importance the greatest harm to the greatest number, then there is no question that malaria is the most important of all infectious diseases."

Sir Frank Macfarlane Burnet, *Natural History of Infectious Disease*, 3rd ed. (Cambridge: Cambridge University Press, 1962), 341.

"Just as the history of malarial disease shows it to have been a malady of all times, so the inquiry into its geography leads us to recognize in it a disease of all *races* and *nationalities*."

August Hirsch, *Handbook of Geographical and Historical Pathology*, vol. I (London: New Sydenham Society, 1883), 243.

"I do not know another disease that so mimics other disorders or that kills so rapidly that we can see the patient literally slipping away under our eyes. No matter how much experience we have had or how widely we read about the disease we cannot be certain that we have mastered its recognition."

Michael Gelfand, *Rivers of Death in Africa* (London: Oxford University Press, 1964), 3.

"The first axiom of malariology, that lessons learnt in one part of the world may not be applied to other parts of the world, without local verification, is as true as ever; it is unfortunately as often neglected as ever."

D. Bagster Wilson, "Malaria in the African," *Central African Journal of Medicine* vol. 4, no. 2 (1958), 73.

"Everything about malaria is so moulded and altered by local conditions that it becomes a thousand different diseases and epidemiological puzzles. Like chess, it is played with a few pieces, but is capable of an infinite variety of situations."

Lewis Hackett, *Malaria in Europe* (London: Oxford University Press, 1937), 266.

Contents

Figures and Maps

FIGURES

MAPS

Acknowledgments

Research for this book has taken me to a number of different archives and libraries, and I am grateful to the Social Science Grant Committee of Colby College for ongoing financial support for travel to the institutional collections. In the United States, I consulted the holdings of the Smithsonian Institution, the National Library of Medicine, and the National Museum of Health and Medicine in Washington, DC; Merck and Co. in White House, New Jersey; the Rockefeller Archive Center in Sleepy Hollow, New York; the New York Botanical Garden in the Bronx, New York; and the Historical Society of Pennsylvania in Philadelphia, Pennsylvania. In the United Kingdom, I consulted the archives of Howards and Sons, Ltd. (Ilford) at the London Borough of Redbridge Central Library; the London Metropolitan Archives; the National Science Museum; the British Library; the Public Record Office of the United Kingdom; the Wellcome Institute for the History and Understanding of Medicine in London; and the Wellcome Unit for the History of Medicine at the University of Oxford. In France, I consulted documents at the Archives du Pharo in Marseilles. In Switzerland, I carried out research in the archives of the World Health Organization in Geneva. Via the Internet, I have used the archival materials of the Historical Collection at the League of Nations.

This book is thus based in part on primary archival research on selected topics. But for the most part, owing to its scope as a global history, this is a project of synthesis. I have drawn on secondary literatures in regional histories and in world history and on scientific research articles and literature reviews for information about contemporary scientific knowledge. Most malaria research studies today are technical and disciplinarily bounded, and the volume of research is considerable. Over the years of researching and writing this book, the Institute for Scientific Information (ISI) Web of Science electronically forwarded to me abstracts for scores of scientific articles each week. This online access has been critical to this project.

I have presented versions of the first chapter of this book at the African Studies Seminar at Harvard University; the Science, Technology, and Society Colloquium and the Environmental Studies Colloquium at Colby College; the African Studies Seminar at Boston University; the History of Economic Development and Growth (HEDG) annual workshop at the School of Oriental and African Studies at the University of London; the biannual meetings of the Society for Africanist Archaeology in Bergen, Norway; the Health and Medicine in Africa Workshop at Bryn Mawr and Haverford Colleges; and at a seminar in the Department of Social Studies of Medicine at the University of McGill Medical School. An earlier version of chapter 1 was published in the *Journal of World History* and appears with the permission of the University of Hawai'i Press. I have presented versions of the third chapter at the York University conference on Disease and Global Environmental History and at an annual meeting of the American Society for Environmental History. I wish to thank Emmanuel Akyeampong, Jim Fleming, Tom Tietenberg, Jim McCann, Gareth Austin, Scott MacEachern, Paula Viterbo, Myron Echenberg, Richard Hoffman, and Stuart McCook for the invitations to make these presentations and for their stimulating conversations.

I am grateful to colleagues who have read one or more of the book chapters in various stages of development. I thank Jean-Paul Bado, Richard Hoffman, Mary Jackes, Stacey Lance, Socrates Litsios, David Lubell, Maureen Malowany, Louis Molineaux, Randy Packard, and Leo Slater for their insights and suggestions. Mark Harrison, John McNeill, José Nájera, and Don Worster read the entire book and offered incisive commentaries. My wife, Alison Jones Webb, critiqued in detail the entire work, offering vigorous challenges on points of syntax, style, meaning, and interpretation.

An Introduction to Malaria in Human History

Malaria, the oldest and cumulatively the deadliest of the human infectious diseases, seeped into our very earliest human history. It was a primordial companion of our distant protohuman ancestors and an even earlier companion of the chimpanzees from which we branched off six to seven million years ago. During the last one hundred thousand years, malaria began a new chapter in the human heartland of tropical Africa. As our ancestors clustered in seasonal settlements to fish and gather, mosquitoes found a temporarily less-mobile source of nourishment. This allowed the malaria parasites carried by mosquitoes to infect a growing number of human hosts. From these humble beginnings, malaria became more deeply integral to human history. Malaria eventually traveled with some of our ancestors out of Africa into Eurasia, where new infections took root, even as it percolated more deeply throughout the African continent.

Over tens of thousands of years, as early humanity expanded in tropical Africa and across tropical Eurasia, malaria parasites continued to take advantage of our human propensity to migrate and our social need to congregate. Eventually, the parasites moved with their human hosts into the nascent river-basin communities that would ultimately develop into permanent settlements. Malaria traveled with infected hunters and adventurers across mountain ranges and deserts, and after the domestication of animals, malaria traveled more quickly, galloping across grasslands and plains. It became the principal disease burden of Eurasia as well as tropical Africa. Much later, thanks to the technological ingenuity of human beings, malaria sailed with infected passengers on shipboard across the oceans, rode the rails across the continents, and then flew aboard aircraft from one hemisphere to the other. It became a global disease.

Malaria is thus an ancient and a modern scourge. For much of its career it left little trace. It sickened us in early epochs, long before we were able to record our experiences. Even in recent millennia, it has frequently lain silent in the diverse records of our pasts, too common a disease to claim much notice. At other times, epidemic malaria has careened violently across the landscapes of world history, leaving death and suffering in its wake.

THE PARADOXES OF MALARIA

Malaria has etched highly varied patterns into human history. In some times and places malaria has appeared as a seasonal affliction and in others as a year-round burden. It has been a debilitator of general populations and a killer that targets young children and nonimmunes. For these reasons, our cultural assessments of malaria's significance have been highly diverse, and different societies have "known" malaria in very different ways.

These different experiences with malarial infections in the past are nearly impossible to quantify. Even today, malaria remains such a common disease that only imprecise estimates of its impacts are possible. The broad and inexact contours, however, tell the big story. An estimated 2.4 billion people are at risk of infection. An estimated 300 to 500 million people suffer bouts of the disease each year. Perhaps 90 percent of these occur in tropical Africa. Malaria kills somewhere between 1.1 and 2.7 million people per year. Of these deaths, approximately one million are children in tropical Africa between the ages of eighteen months and five years.[1]

Malaria is violent and dismal, and in the past it was erratically distributed over humid and arid landscapes, along the coast and in the forest, across cityscapes and rural landscapes, in subarctic, temperate, subtropical, and tropical zones. Over the course of the twentieth century, however, malaria lost its hold on the northern temperate world, and across those liberated landscapes cultural knowledge about malaria slipped away. Today, malaria is an almost forgotten disease in much of the Western world. My uncle Gene, born in Indianola, Mississippi in 1913, is now part of the oldest generation who can recall the agony of malarial fever and still have the bitter taste of quinine flow from a reservoir of memory. What was once a global affliction – the primary public health disaster in the United States during the nineteenth century, the principal disease of British India, the core challenge of the modernizing Italian state in the twentieth century, and the elusive target of the first global eradication campaign of the World

---

[1] World Health Organization, *WHO Expert Committee on Malaria: Twentieth Report* (Geneva: World Health Organization, 2000), 3, 24.

Health Organization (WHO) – is now broadly regarded as a "tropical disease."

The Ecology of Malarial Infections

Malarial infections are one consequence of a complex series of ecological interactions between malaria parasites, mosquitoes, and humans. The female *Anopheles* mosquito is considered the "definitive host" for the malaria parasites because the sexual cycle of parasite reproduction takes place within the mosquito's gut. The human being who is injected with the parasites by an infected mosquito is considered the "intermediate host." In the human being, the parasites pass through a series of transformations before developing into the sexual forms known as gametocytes, which can then be drawn up when another mosquito takes her blood meal. Both humans and mosquitoes are essential for the parasite to complete its life cycle and to be able to cause malarial infections.[2]

The term *malaria* needs to be unpacked. A borrowing from the Italian *"mala aria"* meaning "foul air," the term *malaria* rather confusingly bundles together the disease consequences of four different parasites that have broad biological similarities.[3] All are plasmodia, a particular type of single-celled life form. All have multistage life cycles that are surprisingly complex. Two of the four parasites are by far the most important – that is, two of the four have caused the lion's share of infections in the past and continue to do so today. These two principal types are called *Plasmodium falciparum* and *Plasmodium vivax*. The two parasites that cause malarial infections of minor global importance are known as *Plasmodium malariae* and *Plasmodium ovale*.[4] The "minor two" have never been the dominant forms in any configuration of historical or contemporary

[2] Meta-analyses of mosquitoes with plasmodium infections suggest that infected mosquitoes suffer increased mortality compared to uninfected mosquitoes, although the reasons for the increased mortality are not established. See Heather M. Ferguson and Andrew F. Reid, "Why Is the Effect of Malaria Parasites on Mosquito Survival Still Unresolved?" *Trends in Parasitology*, vol. 18, no. 6 (2002), 256–261.

[3] Mike W. Service and Harold Townson, "The Anopheles Vector," in ed. David A. Warrell and Herbert M. Gilles, *Essential Malariology*, 4th ed. (London: Arnold, 2002), 59–84.

[4] The malaria parasites are protozoa of the genus *Plasmodium*. Falciparum is considered to belong to the subgenus *Laverania*; vivax, malariae, and ovale to the subgenus *Plasmodium*. Falciparum, vivax, and ovale malarias occur only in human beings. Malariae is found in both humans and African apes. Robert E. Sinden and Herbert M. Gilles, "The Malaria Parasites," in Warrell and Gilles, *Essential Malariology*, 8; for a full description of the biology of the parasites see pp. 8–34.

disease, and for this reason, this book concentrates on the "big two" and traces out the historical patterns and processes through which one can glimpse the major outlines of the disease in our human past.

The four malaria parasites all produce fevers and anemia, and, if untreated, can open up a Pandora's box of complications. Some fevers erupt and then disappear; others do not. Two of the malarial infections – vivax, the most common and most broadly distributed, and ovale, the rarest form and most narrowly distributed – have relapses as one of their signature dynamics. Many months or even years may pass after a sufferer has shaken off a bout with vivax or ovale malaria, only to be felled again. This is because both vivax and ovale parasites have a dormant liver stage that releases fresh waves of parasites months or even years after an apparent "cure." By contrast, both falciparum and malariae infections are incapable of relapse. If a sufferer is cleared of a falciparum or malariae infection, she or he is free of the disease unless and until reinfected by another parasite-laden mosquito. The incubation period for the parasite (the delay from infected bite to fever) within the human being varies greatly. Falciparum incubation periods average twelve days; ovale averages seventeen days; malariae between eighteen and forty days; and vivax incubations range an average of fifteen days but can be delayed up to six to twelve months.[5]

Three of the different forms of malaria share a fever rhythm. Human beings infected with vivax, falciparum, and ovale commonly undergo a sledgehammer attack of fever every forty-eight hours. Sufferers with malariae infections are pummeled every seventy-two hours. Ovale infections were (and are) rare or nonexistent outside of tropical West Africa. The different periodicities – either of forty-eight or seventy-two hours – are signs that allowed close observers in earlier millennia to distinguish between the types of infections. In the Western world, the forty-eight-hour rhythmic assaults were called tertian fevers – because they occurred every first and third day. The seventy-two-hour fevers were quartan, because they occurred every first and fourth day. Western observers generally distinguished between the relatively low mortality of vivax and the high mortality of falciparum by calling the fevers benign tertian and malignant tertian, respectively.

Fever signals, however, sometimes get crossed up, or come in confusing patterns. A common diagnostic rubric from the seventeenth century into

[5] David A. Warrell, "Clinical Features of Malaria," in Warrell and Gilles, *Essential Malariology*, 192.

the twentieth century was to distinguish between "intermittent" fevers, in which an interval of normal temperature followed a febrile period, and "remittent" fevers, in which higher and lower temperatures fluctuated without a return to normal body temperature. The rubric promised more precision than it delivered, because the individual idiosyncrasies of malaria sufferers are highly various. Many people who are infected with malaria parasites suffer fluctuating fevers that do not have a distinctive periodicity. It is also possible to suffer two or more types of parasitical malarial infections at the same time. (Western fever theorists, recognizing this bewildering diversity, believed that fevers could mutate into different forms.) The most common forms of multiple infections are when falciparum joins forces with vivax, or less frequently, with malariae, or ovale, in subtropical or tropical areas.

The disease consequences of the "big two" are markedly different. Falciparum frequently produces severe anemia. If untreated, falciparum can also produce cerebral malaria, a condition that may lead to dangerous sequelae such as epilepsy, blindness, cognitive impairments, and behavioral disturbances, or it may lead to coma and death. Falciparum malaria can also reach the infant *in utero* if the mother is infected.[6] If the mother has acquired immunity to falciparum, however, in the postpartum period she is able to transfer antibodies passively to her infant and confer protection for the first several months of life. The sum total of the disaster falciparum causes cannot be precisely quantified, but it is thought to range between 25 to 50 percent of infected nonimmunes who go untreated. It is responsible for almost all of the deaths from malaria in the world.

By contrast, the disease consequences for those with vivax infections appear relatively minor. They include temporary debilitation during the course of and in the aftermath of the fever paroxysms. A common result of vivax malaria is anemia that may turn increasingly severe after relapses.[7] Vivax can also reach the infant *in utero*. In the postpartum period, even if the mother has acquired immunity to vivax, she is unable to pass this protection on to her baby.[8] It is possible to die from vivax infections,

---

[6] For an overview, see Caroline Shulman and Edgar Dorman, "Clinical Features of Malaria in Pregnancy," in Warrell and Gilles, *Essential Malariology*, 219–235.

[7] For an overview, see David A. Warrell, "Clinical Features of Malaria," in Warrell and Gilles, *Essential Malariology*, 191–205.

[8] V.A. Snewin, S. Longacre, and P.H. David, "*Plasmodium Vivax*: Older and Wiser?" *Research in Immunology*, vol. 142 (1991), 632.

particularly if the sufferer is undernourished or has a compromised immune system. The death toll of vivax – estimated at perhaps 1 to 2 percent of those with severe untreated infections during epidemics – is high compared to that of many other human infectious diseases. These differences between the parasites and the differential biological responses of their human hosts to the different forms of malarial infection suggest that we can think of human malaria as a kaleidoscope of different infections, with different overlapping patterns, most of which have left little or no evidence behind.

The parasites have different temperature requirements for reproduction within the mosquito host. Little is known, however, about the temperature requirements of *P. ovale*. It is principally confined to tropical Africa, with only occasional reports (some unconfirmed) of its presence in the west Pacific region, southern China, Burma, and Southeast Asia.[9] *P. vivax* has adapted to the widest range of temperatures and can extend its seasonal reach into the Arctic, although temperatures must exceed 15 degrees Centigrade (C) for at least a month. *P. malariae* seems to have a similar minimum temperature requirement but requires a longer time of development within the mosquito. *P. falciparum* requires more warmth than the vivax or malariae parasites. It does not reproduce when the temperature drops below 19 degrees C.[10]

Falciparum malaria, like vivax and malariae, is a global disease. However, owing to the higher temperature requirements for reproduction, the falciparum parasite has been able to extend its range only fitfully into the temperate zone. A band of potential falciparum infections straddles the tropics and extends north, for example, only into the southern reaches of China and to the south only to the lower reaches of Brazil. Some expanses of the globe, including the southern reaches of South America, from northern Argentina down to Cape Horn, and the southernmost regions of Africa including much of what is today the Republic of South Africa are altogether free from all four forms of endemic malaria.

The ecological patterns and requirements of the anopheline mosquito species that transmit malaria vary greatly. Perhaps seventy species *can* transmit malaria, and of these, forty species are thought to be of major importance. All require water in which to lay eggs and for the larvae to

---

[9] Sinden and Gilles, "Malaria Parasites," 25.
[10] George MacDonald, *The Epidemiology and Control of Malaria* (London: Oxford University Press, 1957), 6–16, esp. 10–11.

develop into adults. The blood meal provides essential nutrients for the cycle of producing eggs, which varies from two to three days in the tropics to longer periods (up to several weeks) in colder climates. Most female mosquitoes will produce four or five batches of eggs before they die.

The species' preferences for breeding habitats vary considerably. Some species prefer salt water; others prefer fresh water. Some breed only in marshes; others breed at the edges of streams or in springs, in ponds, or in puddles. A few species breed in leaf axils that capture rainwater. Some species live in lowlands; others live in highlands. Some strongly prefer human blood to animal blood, others the converse, and yet others do not have much preference for one over the other. Some are exquisitely suited to tropical climates; others buzz across a surprisingly wide range of terrains. There are, however, some broadly common behaviors. Most species feed between dusk and dawn. The peak periods of biting, however, vary by species. Some feed earlier in the evening; others feed after midnight. Where the mosquitoes take their blood meals also varies. Some species feed mostly indoors and are termed *endophagic;* others feed mostly outside of buildings and are thus *exophagic.* Another important variation in behavior is where the mosquitoes like to take a break from flight. The exophilic mosquitoes rest mostly outdoors; the endophilic rest indoors.

These behavioral variations are critically important because in conjunction with a wide range of human cultural practices that influence the availability of blood meals (such as sleeping indoors or outdoors and near a smoking fire or not, and penning livestock near human habitations or at a distance) they can have a significant influence on the local epidemiology of malarial infections. These mosquito behaviors, some of which have changed over time to exploit new opportunities, have made the lessons learned in localized malaria control difficult to extend even within a subregion. Anopheline mosquitoes, thus, are key actors in the drama of human malaria, although their roles have begun to be understood only since the late nineteenth century.

The female anopheline mosquitoes find some people to be more attractive sources of blood meals than others. The attractions are stimulated by the exhalation of carbon dioxide and other human odors, as well as by warmth and moisture. Some researchers suggest that there are other determinants. Some studies indicate that the malaria parasites may trigger chemical reactions in humans that render them more attractive to mosquitoes. It seems possible that we will come to better understand these more subtle attractants, stimulated by biochemical interactions, as a result of this research.[11]

The parasites' life cycles involve incubation in both human and mosquito hosts, and thus the relationships between mosquito, parasite, and human host are best conceived of as a triad. These triadic relationships are very complex and incompletely understood by researchers, but it is clear that, in the temperate regions, the malaria plasmodia respond to biological and seasonal clues in the human host. In the tropics, where there are mosquitoes year round, it is thought that the plasmodia respond to other clues. There, bites from uninfected mosquitoes may stimulate the formation of gametocytes within the human host and thereby increase the human reservoir of infection at the beginning of the transmission season.[12]

Another set of complex and incompletely understood relationships exists between the human hosts, the plants that we eat, and the malaria parasites. These relationships are sometimes referred to as the Human-Plant-Parasite (H-P-P) complex. Some of the core tuberous foodstuffs in the tropics, such as yams and cassava, release chemicals into the human bloodstream that partially inhibit the reproduction of the parasites. In the Mediterranean region, the fava bean, a staple foodstuff, has the same effect. Some common tropical spices act as oxidants and similarly may depress the parasite load of an infected individual.[13]

Other complex relationships exist between malaria and other diseases. For example, throughout much of tropical Africa, the broad distribution of the fly vector for trypanosomiasis (sleeping sickness) prevented the introduction from southern Eurasia and northern Africa of large

[11] Children infected by falciparum malaria in the gametocyte stage of plasmodial development (postmalarial attack) attract about twice as many mosquitoes as children who were either uninfected or infected with the earlier (premalarial attack) stages of plasmodia. When the infection was cleared, the children who had been twice as attractive to mosquitoes returned to a neutral status, with the same level of attractiveness to mosquitoes as the other children. Renaud Lacroix et al., "Malaria Infection Increases Attractiveness of Humans to Mosquitoes," *PLoS Biology*, vol. 3, no. 9 (2005): 1590–1593.

[12] Richard E.L. Paul, Mawlouth Diallo, and Paul T. Brey, "Mosquitoes and Transmission of Malaria Parasites – Not Just Vectors," *Malaria Journal*, vol. 3, no. 1 (2004), 2–3. This can be found online at http://www.malariajournal.com/content/3/1/39.

[13] Fatimah Jackson, "Ecological Modeling of Human-Plant-Parasite Coevolutionary Triads: Theoretical Perspectives on the Interrelationships of Human HbβS, G6PD, *Manihot esculenta*, *Vicia faba*, and *Plasmodium falciparum*," in ed. L.S. Greene and M.E. Danubio, *Adaptation to Malaria: The Interaction of Biology and Culture* (Amsterdam: Gordon and Breach, 1997), 139–207; Nina L. Etkin, "Plants as Antimalarial Drugs: Relation to G6PD Deficiency and Evolutionary Implications," in Greene and Danubio, *Adaptation to Malaria*, 139–176; Stuart J. Edelstein, *The Sickled Cell: From Myths to Molecules* (Cambridge, MA: Harvard University Press, 1986), 60–63.

domesticated animals that were susceptible to the disease. Because of the general absence of an alternate blood source from domesticated livestock, the tropical African mosquito vectors developed a uniquely strong preference for human blood meals. This preference, in turn, greatly intensified the transmission of malaria. Other complex relationships exist between the malarial infections. One study in the Ivory Coast, for example, indicates that infection with malariae affords some protection against falciparum; another in Papua New Guinea indicates that vivax has a similar effect.[14] Other studies suggest that a balance between falciparum and vivax exists in parts of the world where both infections coexist.[15]

THE HISTORICAL EPIDEMIOLOGY OF MALARIA

Beginning in the early nineteenth century, European and North American medical writers began to describe the geographical distribution of malarial infections and to assess the impacts of malaria on their regions.[16] The authors of these studies wrote about malarial environments where the principal breeding grounds for the local anopheline vectors were swampy and where the principal infections were vivax. These two features were broadly characteristic of both the eastern North American malarial zone and the western European malarial zone. These authors drew on culturally specific regional knowledge to explain the relationship between swamps and fevers. By the middle of the nineteenth century, a wealth of empirical observation seemed to establish the link between the effluvia of the swamps – the miasmas – and malarial fever.[17]

---

[14] Robert Sallares, "Pathocoenoses Ancient and Modern," *History and Philosophy of the Life Sciences*, vol. 27 (2005), 210–212.

[15] Snewin et al., "*Plasmodium Vivax*: Older and Wiser?," 634.

[16] John MacCulloch, *An Essay on the Remittent and Intermittent Diseases* (Philadelphia: Carey and Lea, 1830); Oliver Wendell Holmes, "Dissertation on Intermittent Fevers in New England," *Boylston Prize Dissertations for the Years 1836 and 1837* (Boston: C.C. Little and J. Brown, 1838); Daniel Drake, *A Systematic Treatise, Historical, Etiological, and Practical, of the Principal Diseases of the Interior Valley of North America* (Cincinnati: W.B. Smith and Co., 1850).

[17] Consider, e.g., the summary in 1864 by William H. Van Buren, one of the founders of the U.S. Sanitary Commission, of contemporary understandings of malaria:

  a. Individuals undoubtedly differ in degree of susceptibility, or in their liability to be attacked by miasmatic disease, but there is no amount of natural vigor of constitution, or positive high health, which will confer immunity against the effects of the poison.

  b. The young are usually more liable to the disease than those of mature age.

  c. Poisoning from malaria is more liable to take place between the hours of sunset and sunrise, and in those who are fasting, fatigued, or deprived of sleep.

The miasmatic theory of malarial fever could explain a great deal across large stretches of North America and Western Europe. It was inapt in many other world regions, however, where the vector mosquitoes bred in mountain streams, tidal floodplains, or hoof-print-size puddles. Fever theorists, confronted with this confounding complexity, advanced a more complex geographically based approach, describing the different landscape configurations that were dangerous to human health. These European writers played a major role in the early conceptualization of medical topography, and they also noticed that Europeans during their first years in the tropics generally came down with devastating fevers, and that they also "acclimated" to the tropics during an extended stay. The breadth of malarial infections in tropical South Asia led to racial notions that some peoples were more susceptible to fever than others, and that malaria had broad, enervating effects throughout entire cultural zones.[18]

This book is concerned, in part, with the changing distribution of malarial infections – what is known in modern parlance as spatial epidemiology – and in this sense, it follows in the footsteps of some of these early medical writers. Unlike the early authors, this book is also concerned with the changing nature, significance, and distribution of these infections over time. In modern parlance, the field of study that integrates both spatial and temporal dimensions of the changing patterns of disease is known as historical epidemiology. On a global canvas, this book traces the movements of malarial infections – in deep time from tropical Africa into Eurasia; later from Afro-Eurasia to the Americas; and relatively

---

d. After exposure to malaria, the attack of disease is not necessarily immediate; a period of incubation, varying from six to twenty days, usually intervenes, and during this the individual may enjoy perfect health. The attack, when it occurs, may assume the form of intermittent or remittent fever, or any of the other forms of miasmatic disease, varying in nature and degree of severity according to the impressibility of the individual and the virulence of the poison; or, the amount of poison imbibed may not have been sufficient to cause an explosion of purely miasmatic disease, but only enough to impress the miasmatic or paroxysmal type upon some intercurrent malady occasioned by another exposure.

e. After long exposure to malaria, even though no actual attack of sickness may have occurred, a debilitated condition of health is liable to arise, characterized by a sallow complexion, diminished strength, and impoverished blood; this is known as malarial cachexia.

William H. Van Buren, "Quinine as a Prophylactic against Malarious Diseases," in ed. William A. Hammond, MD, *Military, Medical and Surgical Essays Prepared for the United States Sanitary Commission* (Philadelphia: J.B. Lippincott and Co., 1864), 95–96.

[18] Mark Harrison, *Climates and Constitutions: Health, Race, Environment, and British Imperialism in India, 1600–1850* (New Delhi: Oxford University Press, 1999).

recently the retreat of malaria from the temperate zones to the tropics. It sketches the profound impacts of malaria on the evolution of human history and shows that malaria has affected virtually the entire range of human societies – from gatherers and yam cultivators in tropical Africa with low levels of technological sophistication through a range of subjects and citizens in contemporary states.

The problem of the definitive identification of a specific disease in the past is one of the most problematic issues in historical epidemiology. A classic example is the bubonic or Black Plague said to have struck Europe in the fourteenth century. Over the past century, historians of medieval Europe built a powerful circumstantial case that the epidemic had been caused by the plague bacillus (*Yersinia pestis*) spread by the brown rat. This interpretation passed into our general knowledge about the European past. Recent research, however, based on microbiological evidence and the demographic analysis of death notices, has advanced a different understanding. It now appears that Black Plague was a filoviral infection that produced a haemorrhagic fever and may be genetically related to Ebola fever.[19]

These problems of identification are most vexing when the diseases appear in epidemic form. The health crisis can peak and recede in a relatively short period of time, leaving only inconclusive evidence in its wake as to its origin and its nature. Some diseases have severely trounced human populations, and historians still do not know what the disease was. One famous example is the English sweating disease that caused wide suffering among young adult males in the fifteenth and sixteenth centuries.[20]

The case of malaria is dramatically different. The burden of human malaria is ancient and ongoing, and it has left its signatures in the human genome. Most infections have occurred in endemic regions that developed through historical processes of human migration and settlement. Epidemics of malaria undoubtedly preceded the development of zones of endemic infection, and epidemics have continued to break out on the

---

[19] Susan Scott and Christopher J. Duncan, *Biology of Plagues: Evidence from Historical Populations* (New York: Cambridge University Press, 2001); Samuel K. Cohn Jr., "The Black Death: The End of a Paradigm," *American Historical Review*, vol. 107, no. 3 (2002), 703–738.

[20] Recent research has suggested that the English sweats were caused by an arbovirus that originated from a small-mammal population. See J.N. Hays, *The Burdens of Disease: Epidemics and Human Response in Western History* (New Brunswick, NJ: Rutgers University Press, 2000), 69–70.

edges of endemic zones, as a result of human migration, warfare, and fluctuations in climate. Before the seventeenth century CE, the broad patterns and processes of the history of endemic malaria can be described, but the details and particulars of the epidemic outbreaks of malaria are unrecoverable. After the seventeenth century CE, the limited use of cinchona bark – and from the nineteenth century, the wider use of quinine and other cinchona alkaloids – allows for the positive, retrospective identification of malarial infections; the cinchona alkaloids were the first disease-specific drugs in the Western *materia medica*, and the relief that they afforded malaria sufferers confirms the presence of malarial infections.

THE META-CONDITIONS OF MALARIA HISTORY

Humanity's Burden explores the global history of malaria from an ecological perspective. It considers three broad, distinctive requirements for the transmission of malaria as *meta-conditions* that provide a framework for understanding the deep history of the disease.

One meta-condition is a critical level of human population density required to continue the cycle of infection. This condition was initially satisfied by seasonal settlement along the banks of tropical African rivers and then extended into tropical Euroasia, long before the emergence of permanent settlement and seed agriculture.

A second meta-condition is the expansion of disease-experienced populations – that is, those who are already parasitized and who have achieved either an enhanced immunological status or who benefited from genetic mutations that emerged from generations of ancestral suffering – into contact with those who are immunologically naïve. This repetitive pattern established itself in early tropical Africa, and over many millennia this pattern extended out from the early river-basin communities.

A third meta-condition is the existence of extensive zones of endemic infection. Over time, these Afro-Eurasian zones extended around the world and were constrained principally by temperature, altitude, and presence of vector mosquitoes. In these zones of endemic infection, epidemics did erupt when new strains of malaria were introduced, nutritional status of the population was severely compromised, or new environmental interventions (such as irrigation technologies) dramatically increased both mosquito habitat and mosquito densities.

THREE GREAT ZONES OF MALARIAL INFECTION

There were three great zones of malarial infection: the falciparum zone (in which falciparum infections were predominant), the vivax zone (in which vivax infections were predominant), and the zone of mixed infections. The zone of predominantly falciparum infections developed in tropical Africa, where mosquito activity was significant year round.[21] There, the malaria burden was extremely heavy. It produced important genetic mutations (discussed in Chapter 1) that dramatically reduced the prevalence of vivax without negative consequences and provided some protection from falciparum at a high cost in chronic disability. The mortality from falciparum infections became concentrated in young children. After repeated infections, the survivors began to acquire a more robust immunological status. Although most children, young adults, and adults in the falciparum zone suffered relapses and some suffered complications, few older than the age of five died from falciparum, unless their immunological status deteriorated.

The zone of predominantly vivax infections developed in the northern reaches of Eurasia. There, vivax malaria was generally seasonal in its rhythms; it was linked to the annual cycle of greatest mosquito activity in the warm summer months. Vivax was the great debilitator, not the great killer. The death rate from infections was rarely greater than 1 percent. Although it was possible to achieve functional immunity to vivax infections, many adults in endemic regions did not do so because the northern mosquito vectors did not have a strong preference for human blood, and the infections were seasonal rather than year round. The suffering could be pervasive as it was often distributed across age groups.

The zone of mixed infections separated the great zones of falciparum and vivax. Located along the southern rim of Eurasia, the zone of mixed infections extended from southern China through India to the greater Mediterranean basin. Across the zone, falciparum infections were present but were never predominant. The transmission of malaria varied: in the subtropics it was seasonal rather than year round, and in the tropics it was year round. The toll from death and sickness could be gruesomely

[21] Even within the great falciparum zone of tropical Africa, there is considerable variation in the extent of inoculation with malaria parasites. In a zone of moderate endemicity, the average person receives at least 100 bites per year by infected mosquitoes; in some holoendemic zones, the average person can receive up to 150 or 175 infected bites per night (Louis F. Amoroso Jr., Gilberto Corbellini, and Mario Coluzzi, "Lessons Learned from Malaria: Italy's Past and Sub-Sahara's Future," *Health and Place*, vol. 11 [2005], 69).

high when malaria afflicted human communities whose members had not acquired functional immunities. However, in general the burden of malaria was far lower in the zone of mixed infections than in the zone of falciparum.

MALARIAL GEOGRAPHIES AND CULTURAL RESPONSES

Within the three great zones of malaria, one important set of cultural responses to malaria was inscribed in patterns of human land use. Mountainous regions everywhere have enjoyed low or even null rates of malarial infection, compared to the surrounding lowlands. This is because most anopheline mosquitoes prefer habitat at lower altitudes. Without understanding that mosquitoes transmit malaria, many peoples have associated malarial fevers with the marsh and lowlands, and many mountain dwellers avoided the lowlands during the season of transmission, thus limiting their exposure to infection.[22] This pattern of avoidance has helped to underscore the distinctiveness of the highland and lowland cultures in many world regions, and in this regard, local epidemiology has been interwoven in the tapestries of ethnicity. This has been the pattern in highland eastern Africa, along the mountainous rim of southern Eurasia, in South and Central America, and in New Guinea. In South and Southeast Asia, the fractured patterns of highlands with their distinctive disease environments underwrote the cultural differences between the more technologically primitive "hill peoples" and the "peoples of the plains."

Another geographical pattern has been inscribed across the zones of pastoral nomadism in Central Asia and Africa, where low levels of human population density and the high mobility of the pastoral nomadic way of life reduced the transmission of malaria to a minor problem. In these zones, the epidemiology of malaria has underwritten the logic of the pastoral nomads' seasonal avoidance of settled farmers and reinforced ethnic difference. This in turn has contributed to the differences in lifestyles and ethnic identities of nomadic pastoralists around the great Saharan and Central Asian basins from those of the farming peoples with whom they seasonally interacted.

Sometimes the concerns with disease were paramount to economic success. Along the West African Sahel during the precolonial centuries (1600–1850), for example, the pastoral nomads traded grain, salt, and

---

[22] Christopher Conte, *Highland Sanctuary* (Athens: Ohio University Press, 2004).

animal products to settled farmers only in the dry season, when malaria transmission was relatively low.[23] During the rest of the year, long-distance traders, who dealt in slaves and in higher value-to-bulk goods such as gold, moved between constellations of separate residential areas that were adjacent to the major towns. These "double towns" have generally been understood as an effort to reinforce the ethnic and religious identity of the Muslim long-distance traders.[24] It was likely also an attempt to exercise some control over their exposure to the local disease environments.

A third geographical pattern involved the conversion of the forest to agricultural use and the encroachment of malaria-ridden agriculturalists on the domain of forest peoples who had been free from malaria. In many areas of the world, including tropical Africa and the tropical Americas, anopheline vectors did not live within the full-canopy rainforests.[25] Malaria did not become established in these forests until malaria-infected cultivators began to burn holes in the canopies, opening the way for slash-and-burn agriculture – initially, yam cultivation in tropical Africa and maize and manioc cultivation in the Atlantic forest of Portuguese Brazil. Along these agricultural frontiers, the cultural strategies available to indigenous peoples who were exposed to this onslaught were meager. Their best strategy was to withdraw deeper into the forest. By the twentieth century, the phenomenon of the "primitive peoples" of the rainforests of Brazil and Central Africa had come to be misinterpreted as the result of pristine isolation rather than strategic retreat.

The cultural understandings of local disease ecologies everywhere helped to determine the social response to malaria. The political elite of many agricultural societies put low-status workers – slaves, serfs, or people of the lower castes – to labor in what were perceived to be the most dangerous and arduous environments. Sometimes this meant situating low-status workers' huts near the cultivated fields and the housing of the elite at some remove, or it meant the retreat of the elite to new environs during the "unhealthy seasons." These strategies underlined class and "racial" differences within many agricultural societies.

Another dimension of cultural response stretched from aggressive landscape engineering to passive avoidance. Around the Mediterranean

---

[23] James L.A. Webb Jr., *Desert Frontier: Ecological and Economic Change along the Western Sahel, 1600–1850* (Madison: University of Wisconsin Press, 1995).

[24] Philip D. Curtin, *Cross-Cultural Trade in World History* (New York: Cambridge University Press, 1984), 38–41.

[25] The major exception was Southeast Asia, one of the hearths of malaria infection outside of tropical Africa.

basin and in southwest Asia, where the major anopheline vectors bred in lowlands and swamps, some cultures made the link between malaria and these environments. The ancient Romans, for example, experimented with swamp drainage, although apparently without much success.[26] The Abbasid Caliphate (750–1258) drained the region around Baghdad and reduced malaria transmission in the city. By contrast, in coastal and riverine regions of mainland and island Southeast Asia, where drainage was infeasible, avoidance was the mainstay approach. There, coastal peoples built their housing on stilts, above the flight patterns of the mosquitoes, and sometimes they draped cloth over frames around their sleeping areas.

Perhaps the most universal of mosquito control practices has been the use of repellents to deter nuisance bites. The repellents have ranged from animal fat, rancid butter, and vinegar to more pleasant odors such as the contemporary citronella candle that graces the outdoor evening party. The use of smoke has also been a near universal in societies that have had ready access to combustible materials. The efficacy of these repellents and the range of their employments undoubtedly varied a great deal, and it is not possible to make a summary judgment about them.

EXPLAINING MALARIA

Human beings everywhere developed cultural explanations of how, when, and why we get sick from malaria. Many societies evolved multiple ways to explain the suffering. One mode was religious, invoking visitations by demons, deities, or the wrath of a spiteful almighty. Another mode was "practical," stressing, for example, avoidance behaviors and the health consequences of traversing malarial lowlands during the warm seasons of the year. There was also the "metaphysical" mode; across much of Eurasia, societies employed the metaphor of "balance" and noted the occurrence of "unusual events" to explain human disease as the result of a disturbance in the natural environmental order.[27]

In the late nineteenth and early twentieth centuries, a new approach to explaining disease – that had some roots in both the older practical and metaphysical traditions – was born from the biological sciences. The

[26] The early Roman experience seems to have been largely unsuccessful and may have even increased the incidence of infection. Robert Sallares, *Malaria and Rome: A History of Malaria in Ancient Italy* (Oxford: Oxford University Press, 2002), 74–76.

[27] Gregg Mitman, "In Search of Health: Landscape and Disease," *Environmental History*, vol. 10, no. 2 (2005), 184–210.

plant ecologist Frederic Clements developed the idea of the biological community known as the ecosystem, and the ecological theorist Charles Elton – who gave us such important concepts as the "food chain" and "the ecological niche" – pioneered the idea that disease was the result of a disturbance in the functioning of the ecosystem, which was brought about by invasive species, the anthropogenic transformation of the biome, or unregulated population growth.[28] A corollary axiomatic belief was that disturbances would ultimately resolve in the direction of a new balance. The logic was extended to understand the relationship between parasitic diseases and their hosts. The assumption was that, over time, parasites would reach stable accommodations with their hosts. Virulence would evolve toward attenuation. A balance would be restored.

By the early twenty-first century, new understandings and evidence from the natural sciences, particularly from microbiology and evolutionary epidemiology, have suggested different approaches to the history of malaria. It is now clear that genetic mutations and immunological responses to malarial infections have played major roles in the human history of malaria. The persistent virulence of malaria – rather than its evolution toward attenuation – can be explained by new understandings of host-parasite relations that highlight the differences in biological dynamics between vector-borne and non-vector-borne diseases. New research in the social sciences, particularly from ecological history and the history of medicine, have allowed for a new appreciation of the range and diverse impacts of human interventions to control malaria. These new natural science and social science perspectives are critical to the global history of malaria that unfolds in the following chapters.

Humanity's Burden synthesizes an array of academic literatures from both the natural sciences and the social sciences. It explores the global history of malarial infections as a set of profound ecological problems that have changed over time – and thus as an epidemiological portal that allows us some glimpses into disease patterns and processes over the entire course of our human past.

---

[28] For insightful studies of the ecosystem idea, see Donald Worster, *Nature's Economy: A History of Ecological Ideas*, 2nd ed. (New York: Cambridge University Press, 1994) and Joel B. Hagen, *An Entangled Bank: The Origins of Ecosystem Ecology* (New Brunswick, NJ: Rutgers University Press, 1992).

I

Early Tropical Africa

An immensely long time ago, somewhere between two and three million years in the past, some of our earliest hominid ancestors, known as *Homo erectus*, began to explore new foraging grounds far beyond the savannas of tropical eastern Africa. Some of these explorations may have been driven by simple curiosity, others perhaps by population pressure that stretched resources too thin in the familiar home territory. Others may have been propelled by the desire to escape conflicts. If *Homo erectus* had much in common with modern human beings, a complex range of economic and sociocultural motivations may well have propelled the early explorations.

Some groups dispersed widely into the vast expanses of Afro-Eurasia. There they made tools and clothing and colonized a surprisingly wide swath of tropical and subtropical landscapes. These early migrants had extremely modest and primitive technologies, and it is remarkable that any of their remains and artifacts have survived. Much later, around 300,000 to 200,000 years ago – at roughly the same time that modern *Homo sapiens* emerged in tropical Africa – one of our hominid cousins, *Homo neanderthalis*, was colonizing parts of western Eurasia. Over time, across broad reaches of Eurasia, *Homo erectus* and *Homo neanderthalis* both succeeded in a widening array of physical environments and climatic conditions. Surprisingly, these broadening experiences were not to be the root source of the accelerated cultural and physical evolution that distinguishes modern humankind.

Our more recent evolution to *Homo sapiens* took place over the past two or three hundred thousand years only in tropical Africa. In the great heartland of our common African past, modern humankind gradually developed tools, adapted to new environments, and created a more complex material culture. The internal dynamics of these early epochs of modern humanity, however, remain obscure, and our early experiences that make up the bulk of time that we have been on the planet are generally considered as our "prehistory." In our two or three hundred millennia in Africa, we left little evidence behind. This long apprenticeship contrasts sharply with the rapid advances of humanity in regions outside of tropical Africa. The extended "Neolithic agricultural revolution" – with its gradual transitions to permanent settlement, seed agriculture, and the domestication of animals – is generally agreed to mark a revolutionary break with the early epochs. For this reason, it is customary for world historians, after acknowledging a long history of human foraging, to begin the teaching of world history with the agrarian era, some ten or eleven thousand years ago.[1]

Recent research findings in the fields of microbiology, archaeology, and archaeobotany, however, allow us new windows into the far-distant human past. These findings suggest new ways of understanding some of our earliest experiences that blur the sharp division between prehistory and history and suggest a different periodization of the deep past. Evidence about malaria has an important role to play in forging these perspectives. Malaria first emerged as a significant human disease in tropical Africa, and, over the long run of humankind on earth, it has likely killed more Africans than any other disease. This "malarial pressure" has left some genetic evidence in its wake.

THE GENOMES OF THE MALARIA PARASITES

Over the past several years, microbiologists have decoded the genomes for two of the principal malaria parasites – *Plasmodium vivax* and *Plasmodium falciparum* – that have played such an enormous role in world history.[2] Some of the initial interpretations of the microbiological evidence

---

[1] For a recent effort to bring early epochs into world history, see David Christian, *Maps of Time: An Introduction to Big History* (Berkeley: University of California Press, 2005).

[2] There are two other human malaria parasites: *Plasmodium ovale* and *Plasmodium malariae*. Both are far less lethal than *P. falciparum*, and they have received less attention from researchers.

  Other malaria-protective genetic mutations have emerged within African populations, such as thalassemias, Glucose-6-Phosphate Dehydrogenase deficiency (also known as G6PD deficiency) and Hemoglobin C (a genetic variation that is allelic with that for sickle cell but that does not impose as severe costs for individuals who are homozygous for this variation). These polymorphisms are not as protective as Duffy negativity and the sickle cell mutation discussed in this book. The historical issues concerning the emergence of these polymorphisms have not received as much scientific attention from the molecular biological community.

were highly divergent, in part because regular DNA and mitochondrial DNA produce different kinds of evidence.[3] In the past few years, some elements of general agreement about the early history of the parasites have begun to emerge.[4]

PLASMODIUM VIVAX

DNA evidence indicates that *P. vivax* is quite ancient, and that it diverged from an earlier malaria parasite that infected both apes and early hominids

The G6PD variant that is common in tropical Africa arose sometime between 10,000 and 2,000 BCE. A Mediterranean variant is more recent, dated to between 7,000 and 0 BCE. See Sarah A. Tishkoff et al., "Haoplotype Diversity and Linkage Disequilibrium at Human G6PD: Recent Origin of Alleles That Confer Malarial Resistance," *Science*, vol. 293 (2001), 455–462.

[3] The deep geographical origin of *P. vivax* is contested. One view holds that vivax malaria may have been present in the New World prior to European contact in the late fifteenth and early sixteenth centuries. Although most of the evidence suggests that this was not the case, recently scholars have called for biomolecular analysis of existing skeletal remains in the Amazon to reach a definitive conclusion. See Marcia Caldas de Castro and Burton H. Singer, "Was Malaria Present in the Amazon before European Conquest? Available Evidence and Future Research Agenda," *Journal of Archaeological Science*, vol. 32 (2005), 337–340.

The two principal views are that *P. vivax* originated either in Africa or in Southeast Asia. Because of the large number of variables and the nature of the evidence, at present there is considerable latitude for diverse interpretations, and it seems unlikely that the issue will be definitively settled. For recent evidence that *P. vivax* originated in Southeast Asia approximately 60,000 years ago, see Ananias A. Escalante et al., "A Monkey's Tale: The Origin of *Plasmodium Vivax* as a Human Malaria Parasite," *Proceedings of the National Academy of Sciences*, vol. 102, no. 6 (February 8, 2005), 1980–1985. In their view, *P. vivax* never was present in Africa; Duffy antigen negativity is either the result of a genetic accommodation to another, unknown agent or a random genetic variation that became fixed. Other microbiologists argue that *H. erectus* became parasitized by a "modern" form of *P. vivax* approximately one million years ago and introduced *P. vivax* into tropical Africa in a period before the emergence of *H. sapiens*.

For a fascinating article on the African origins of vivax, see Richard Carter, "Speculations on the Origins of *Plasmodium Vivax* Malaria," *Trends in Parasitology*, vol. 19, no. 5 (May 2003), 214–219. For an overview of some of the complications in unraveling the history of vivax, see Stephen M. Rich, "The Unpredictable Past of *Plasmodium Vivax* Revealed in Its Genome," *Proceedings of the National Academy of Sciences*, vol. 101, no. 44 (November 2, 2004), 15547–15548.

[4] In 2002, Richard Carter and Kamimi N. Mendis skillfully assayed the microbiological research literature and other natural science and historical literatures on malaria. See R. Carter and K.N. Mendis, "Evolutionary and Historical Aspects of the Burden of Malaria," *Clinical Microbiology Reviews*, vol. 15 (2002), 564–594. For a recent overview of the microbiological literature, see Aparup Das et al., "Genetic Diversity and Evolutionary History of *Plasmodium Falciparum* and *P. Vivax*," *Current Science*, vol. 92, no. 11 (2007), 1516–1524.

approximately two to three million years ago. Recent research on regular DNA evidence suggests that the most recent common ancestor (MRCA) of the contemporary forms of *P. vivax* is a malaria parasite that today infects a primate in Southeast Asia. The mitochondrial DNA evidence suggests that the MRCA of modern *P. vivax* can be dated to approximately 200,000 to 300,000 BP, about the same time that modern humans evolved into our present form. Just when and how the parasite became ensconced in tropical Africa has yet to be fully worked out. One possibility is that vivax-infected *Homo erectus* may have acquired the ancestral vivax parasite in Southeast Asia as far back as one million years ago, and then at some later point introduced it into tropical Africa.[5]

There is still much that remains unknown about the very early history of vivax infections in tropical Africa. At present, it is not possible to estimate the morbidity or mortality costs of the increasing malarial burden. It is possible that the virulence of early vivax in tropical Africa was greater than that of contemporary vivax, which generally sickens rather than kills.[6]

THE SPREAD OF DUFFY NEGATIVITY

At some point in the tropical African past, a random genetic mutation that protected the carrier from vivax infection emerged. In an environment rife with vivax infections, those who carried the mutation were healthier than those who did not. This genetic mutation is known as Red Blood Cell Duffy antigen negativity (hereafter, "Duffy negativity"). It occurs on an antigen receptor on the hemoglobin molecule, the portal that is normally invaded by the vivax parasite. Duffy negativity closes the portal, which shuts the parasite out. It renders the carrier completely unable to contract vivax malaria and, fortunately, produces no negative consequences for the carrier.[7] Today, this mutation is widely expressed in tropical Africa. An

---

[5] Somchai Jongwutiwes et al., "Mitochondrial Genome Sequences Support Ancient Population Expansion in *Plasmodium Vivax*," *Molecular Biology and Evolution*, vol. 8, no. 22 (2005), 1733–1739.

[6] The issue of the evolution of virulence is complex and unresolved. For an introduction, see Alison P. Galvani, "Epidemiology Meets Evolutionary Ecology," *Trends in Ecology and Evolution*, vol. 18, no. 3 (2003), 132–139. See also Margaret J. Mackinnon and Andrew F. Read, "Virulence in Malaria: An Evolutionary Viewpoint," *Philosophical Transactions of the Royal Society of London*, Series B, Biological Sciences, vol. 359, no. 1446 (2004), 965–986.

[7] Duffy antigen negativity (FY*o) is one of three forms of mutation on the Duffy antigen receptor. Duffy A (FY*A) and Duffy B (FY*B) confer limited immunity to malaria. Neither FY*A or FY*B occur in tropical Africa. For more on Duffy mutations, see

extraordinary 97 percent of contemporary West and Central African populations carry the mutation for Duffy negativity and thus are unable to contract vivax malaria (see Map 1.1).[8]

At some point in time our African ancestors largely succeeded in throwing off the burden of vivax malaria that would later torment populations in other parts of the world.[9] Where and when did Duffy negativity spread? Here, too, there is much that is currently unknown. It is not possible to determine where Duffy negativity first arose or if it arose independently in more than one population. It seems likely that this mutation became fixed at some point after the migrations of *Homo sapiens* out of tropical Africa that are dated to approximately 100,000 to 50,000 BP.[10]

A recent microbiological analysis has suggested that vivax pressure began to select for Duffy negativity somewhere between 97,200 and 6,500 BP. One view is that the selection began at the very end of this period. Here there are two strands of reasoning: (1) Climate change – the rapid warming of the planet at the end of the last glacial period – was responsible for more

---

Martha T. Hamblin and Anna Di Rienzo, "Detection of the Signature of Natural Selection in Humans: Evidence from the Duffy Blood Group Locus," *American Journal of Human Genetics*, vol. 66 (2000), 1669–1679; Martha T. Hamblin, Emma E. Thompson, and Anna Di Rienzo, "Complex Signatures of Natural Selection at the Duffy Blood Group Locus," *American Journal of Human Genetics*, vol. 70 (2002), 369–383.

    The biological process is termed *complement fixation*. It involves the binding of a complement (a heat-sensitive, complex system in fresh human and other sera) to an antigen-antibody complex so that the complement is unavailable for subsequent reaction.

[8] For a survey of genetic responses to malarial pressure, including sickle cell discussed later in this book, see Carter and Mendis, "Evolutionary and Historical Aspects," 570–573.

[9] Hamblin and Di Rienzo, the authors of a recent genetic analysis, have proposed that a "selective sweep" toward the fixation of Duffy negativity in Sub-Saharan populations began between 97,200 and 6,500 years ago. See their "Detection of the Signature of Natural Selection in Humans," 1669–1679.

[10] Human populations apparently were greatly reduced in number, perhaps to as few as 5,000 females, approximately 70,000 BP. This "population bottleneck" coincides with a cataclysmic eruption of the Toba volcano in Sumatra that produced a series of volcanic winters. See Stanley H. Ambrose, "Late Pleistocene Human Population Bottlenecks, Volcanic Winter, and Differentiation of Modern Humans," *Journal of Human Evolution*, vol. 34 (1998), 623–651; Michael R. Rampino and Stanley H. Ambrose, "Volcanic Winter in the Garden of Eden: The Toba Supereruption and the Late Pleistocene Human Population Crash," in ed. F.W. McCoy and G. Heiken, *Volcanic Hazards and Disasters in Human Antiquity* (Boulder, CO: Geological Society of America, 2000), 71–82. For critical interpretations of the Toba eruption and a rejoinder, see F.J. Gathorne-Hardy and W.E.H. Harcourt-Smith, "The Super-Eruption of Toba, Did It Cause a Human Bottleneck?" *Journal of Human Evolution*, vol. 45 (2003), 227–230 and Stanley H. Ambrose, "Did the Super-Eruption of Toba Cause a Human Population Bottleneck? Reply to Gathorne-Hardy and Harcourt Smith," *Journal of Human Evolution*, vol. 45 (2003), 231–237.

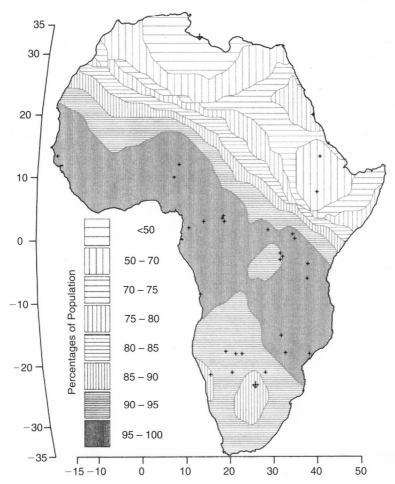

MAP 1.1. Distribution of Duffy Antigen Negativity (FY*o) in Africa
Source: L. Luca Cavalli-Sforza, Paolo Menozzi, and Alberto Piazza, *The History and Geography of Human Genes* (Princeton: Princeton University Press, 1994), Genetic Maps, 160.

mosquitoes and thus an increase in the malarial burden.[11] This increased burden was unstable and became amplified as the climate warmed. (2) This warming was coincident with the beginnings of African tropical

---

[11] Carter and Mendis, "Evolutionary and Historical Aspects," 577–578.
    The last glacial maxima in tropical Africa have been estimated at between 22,000–12,000 BP. See A.S. Brooks and P.T. Robertshaw, "The Glacial Maxima in Tropical Africa: 22,000–12,000 BP," in ed. O. Soffer and C. Gamble, *The World at 18,000 BP, Vol. 2: Low Latitudes* (London: Unwin Hyman, 1990), 121–169.

agriculture, which was stimulated by the arrival of seeds and new technologies from the early river-basin civilizations. According to this view, the arrival of the "Neolithic agricultural revolution" provoked a vigorous biological response – progress toward the fixation of the gene for Duffy negativity in the West and Central African populations, so that nearly all the individuals became carriers – that blunted the force of vivax malaria.[12] According to this view of world history, human populations in humid tropical Africa did not begin to enjoy an increase in their rates of population growth and cultural development until the introduction of new seeds and technologies that emerged from the river-basin civilizations and then diffused south.[13]

From the standpoint of recent Africanist archaeology, this interpretation of the history of Duffy negativity is somewhat problematic. If the selective fixation of the gene for Duffy negativity took place in the period beginning circa 3,000 to 2,000 BCE this adaptive genetic mutation would have required a high level of integration among disparate populations during a relatively brief period of several thousand years in order to be transmitted extensively throughout West and Central African populations to produce the near-universal present-day distribution. Cultural and linguistic evidence do not support this view; they indicate an increasing differentiation, rather than integration, among tropical African populations.

The archaeological record does, however, suggest other possibilities for understanding the emergence and fixation of the Duffy negativity gene that are consonant with a new appreciation of Africa's role in early human history. In recent years, archaeologists who specialize in tropical Africa have revised the chronologies of human evolution that were developed based on the European archaeological record, in light of the longer African archaeological sequences. In the broadest sense, their work shows

---

[12] The thesis that resistance to malaria is tied to the "agricultural revolution" in Africa is broadly accepted. See, e.g., Nina L. Etkin, "The Co-Evolution of People, Plants, and Parasites: Biological and Cultural Adaptations to Malaria," *Proceedings of the Nutrition Society*, vol. 62 (2003), 311–317; J.C.C. Hume, J. Lyons, and K.P. Day, "Human Migration, Mosquitoes and the Evolution of *Plasmodium Falciparum*," *Trends in Parasitology*, vol. 19, no. 3 (2003), 144–149.

[13] This argument was first advanced by F.B. Livingstone in his classic article "Anthropological Implications of Sickle Cell Gene Distribution in West Africa," *American Anthropologist*, vol. 60 (1958), 533–562. Recently, M. Coluzzi has written in support of this thesis in "The Clay Feet of the Malaria Giant and Its African Roots: Hypotheses and Influences about the Origin, Spread, and Control of *Plasmodium Falciparum*," *Parassitologia*, vol. 41 (1999), 277–283.

that not only did *Homo sapiens* emerge in Africa, but that very early processes of human cultural evolution took place in tropical Africa.

The findings of Africanist archaeologists have overturned the "human revolution" model of development that held that "modern" behavior of human beings gained first expression in Eurasia, in a burst of evolutionary change. Instead, the Africanist findings have located the origins of modern human behavior where one might have suspected – in Africa – and revised the basic chronology of early human history. The discovery of an early "middle stone age worked bone industry" – thought to represent large-scale seasonal fishing expeditions that would have necessitated seasonal settlement – located the early origins of complex thinking and behavior necessary for major cultural changes in east-central Africa rather than in Europe. This discovery also pushed back the temporal horizon of these cultural changes from circa 35,000 BP to circa 89,000 BP.[14] It now appears that the transition from the Middle Stone Age to the Late Stone Age in tropical Africa was an extremely gradual process that took place over perhaps two hundred thousand years.

These new interpretations of the African archaeological evidence thus argue for an African origin of new human cultural behaviors that arose at varying times and places across the African continent, and that these behaviors were exported with the African migrants who left to populate other regions of Eurasia. The archaeological record of these cultural achievements, although interrupted during the coolest millennia of the global glacial periods (known as "glacial maxima") in some parts of Africa such as the Sahara and the interior of Cape Province in South Africa, is sufficiently represented in other African biomes, including the expanses of steppe, savanna, and woodland, to support the idea of the continuous presence of probably widely dispersed human populations across these diverse environments.[15]

Africanist archaeologists have also documented the intensification of African cultural practices after about 50,000 BP, including novel technologies such as new projectiles that increased the productivity of hunting

[14] John E. Yellen et al., "A Middle Stone Age Worked Bone Industry from Katanda, Upper Semliki Valley, Zaire," *Science*, vol. 268, no. 5210 (1995), 553–556. For the interpretive comparison with Europe, see B. Bower, "African Finds Revise Cultural Roots," *Science News*, vol. 147, no. 17 (April 29, 1995), 260.

[15] Sally McBrearty and Alison S. Brooks, "The Revolution That Wasn't: A New Interpretation of the Origin of Modern Human Behavior," *Journal of Human Evolution*, vol. 39 (2000), 458.

and new fishing methods that allowed for the more efficient exploitation of a vast resource. The newly available technologies could support larger populations in a given territory. Moreover, these technologies apparently allowed for human groups to expand from the savanna into new habitats such as the tropical forest.[16] For the study of early malaria, the cumulative significance of these archaeological findings is that they make the point that human communities living in tropical Africa did not wait until the arrival of a Neolithic "development package" circa 3,000 BCE to expand their exploitation of new environments – including those that were ideal for the transmission of malarial infections.

These very early patterns of seasonal migration and riverbank settlement – tens of thousands of years before the last glacial maximum – would have provided ideal conditions for seasonal malarial infection. This seasonal infection – with elevated infant mortality – would have produced selection pressures that strongly favored the spread of Duffy negativity.[17] (Today, untreated vivax malaria in regions outside of Africa is associated with levels of mortality below 5 percent, and often in the range of 1–2 percent). The upshot is that it is no longer necessary to propose a dramatic "malaria revolution" in early tropical Africa that is a product of the introduction of a "Neolithic agricultural revolution," or to link the genetic inability to contract vivax malaria exclusively to a cycle of climate change. It appears far more likely that Duffy negativity emerged across the long process of human cultural evolution, in which human beings entered into new biomes and practiced seasonal settlement over a period of many tens of thousands of years.

This gradualist model of the spread of Duffy negativity is necessarily speculative. Its strengths are (1) that it is consonant with the microbiologists' broad time estimate for the emergence of Duffy negativity, and (2) that it fits well with the archaeologists' interpretations of their data. The implications of the gradualist model are that the emergence of Duffy negativity appears to be the very earliest known chapter in human beings' genetic adaptation to vector-borne infectious disease and the very earliest known chapter in humanity's long struggle with parasitic disease. This genetic adaptation appears to have occurred well before Eurasian populations domesticated livestock and thereby gained limited immunities to the parasites that were attached to the domesticated animals of the

---

[16] Ibid., 532.
[17] Carter and Mendis, "Evolutionary and Historical Aspects," 573.

Eurasian steppe – the horse, cow, goat, sheep, camel, and yak – or, for that matter, the donkey of the Nilotic steppe.[18] The demographic consequence of the emergence of Duffy negativity was likely significant. Its fixation reduced the disease burden for the communities who inherited the mutation and contributed thereby to an increase in their population. New technologies and strategies that human communities developed in the post–50,000 BP period also facilitated ongoing population growth. On this basis alone, all other things being equal, it seems probable that an accelerated process of population growth among some populations in Sub-Saharan Africa began to occur in an early period – well before the arrival of seeds and new technologies from the early river-basin civilizations. It is possible that this population pressure was in part responsible for increasing forays into the rainforests.[19] It is likely that Duffy negativity became even more widely expressed during the processes of more intensive rainforest exploitation that occurred in more recent millennia and that are discussed later in this chapter.

PLASMODIUM FALCIPARUM

The DNA evidence concerning the emergence of modern *P. falciparum* points to the very deep origin of the parasite. A simian ancestral parasite of *P. falciparum* diverged from the even older parasite of bird malaria approximately 130 million years ago, and *P. falciparum* diverged from an ancestral form that was common to both apes and protohumans approximately four to ten million years ago, very roughly coincident with the epoch during which the humanoid line diverged from the line of the African great apes.[20] Other aspects of the parasite genome, however, suggest more recent developments. One line of investigation suggests that the modern form of *P. falciparum* diverged from a protofalciparum parasite in the period 8,000 to 3,000 BCE.[21] In addition, a comparison of

---

[18] For an ambitious, brilliant interpretation of the period 9,000–1,000 BCE, see Christopher Ehret, *The Civilizations of Africa: A History to 1800* (Charlottesville: University of Virginia Press, 2002), 59–158.

[19] For the argument that population pressure played a major role in prehistory, see Mark Nathan Cohen, *The Food Crisis in Prehistory: Overpopulation and the Origins of Agriculture* (New Haven: Yale University Press, 1977).

[20] Some scholars estimate the period at five to seven million years ago for the divergence of modern falciparum malaria. A.A. Escalante and F.J. Ayala, "Phylogeny of the Malarial Genus Plasmodium, Derived from rRNA Gene Sequences," *Proceedings of the National Academy of Sciences USA* vol. 91 (1994), 11373–11377.

[21] Carter and Mendis, "Evolutionary and Historical Aspects," 564–594, esp. 572 and 578. See also Xin-zhuan Su, Jianbing Mu, and Dierdre Joy, "The 'Malaria's Eve' Hypothesis and

mitochondrial genome sequences has found evidence of an increase in human infections in the period 13,000 to 8,000 BCE.[22] Collectively, these findings indicate that human beings in Africa experienced a marked increase in *P. falciparum* infections many millennia before the earliest adoption of the package of Neolithic tools and seed agriculture by tropical African communities circa 3,000 BCE.[23]

The DNA evidence suggests that large-scale falciparum infections may have occurred tens of thousands of years later than vivax infections. This is probably owing to the differences in parasites' life cycles: chains of vivax infection are easier to sustain among hunters and gatherers and in groups that practice seasonal settlement because vivax parasites can relapse for up to three years after the initial infection. Vivax parasites could travel with the seasonal settler back into the rainforest or woodland or savanna, and carriers would remain able to infect mosquitoes and continue the chain long after leaving the settlement site. By contrast, falciparum sufferers remain infectious for a far shorter period of time, and thus the transmission of falciparum malaria is far more dependent on continuous high host density.[24]

The genetic mutations that helped carriers cope with falciparum infections arose much later than Duffy negativity. Unfortunately, those genetic mutations caused other serious health problems. Many individuals in tropical African communities came to carry a mutated hemoglobin molecule known as sickle cell hemoglobin, or hemoglobin S. In some tropical African communities today, up to 25 or 30 percent of the population have inherited the sickle cell gene from one of their parents and a normal hemoglobin gene from the other parent. Children who have one normal and one sickle cell gene have only one-tenth the risk of death from falciparum as do those who inherit the normal gene from both parents.[25]

---

the Debate Concerning the Origin of the Human Malaria Parasite *Plasmodium Falciparum*," *Microbes and Infection*, vol. 5 (2003), 891–896; Daniel L. Hartl, "The Origin of Malaria: Mixed Messages from Genetic Diversity," *Nature Reviews Microbiology*, vol. 2 (2004), 15–22.

[22] David J. Conway, "Tracing the Dawn of *Plasmodium Falciparum* with Mitochondrial Genome Sequences," *Trends in Genetics*, vol. 19, no, 12 (2003), 671–674. See also David J. Conway et al., "Origin of *Plasmodium Falciparum* Malaria Is Traced by Mitochondrial DNA," *Molecular and Biochemical Parasitology*, vol. 111 (2000), 163–171.

[23] David J. Conway and Jake Baum issue a cautionary note on the problems of dating the recent emergence of modern falciparum. See their essay "In the Blood – The Remarkable Ancestry of *Plasmodium Falciparum*," *Trends in Parasitology*, vol. 18, no. 8 (2002), 351–355.

[24] Hamblin, Thompson, and Di Rienzo, "Detection of the Signature of Natural Selection," 1677.

[25] Carter and Mendis, "Evolutionary and Historical Aspects," 571.

There is, however, a high price to be paid. Those carriers who inherit the sickled gene from both parents develop sickle cell anemia and die before the age of reproduction. The sickle cell mutation thus conveys both major costs and benefits to the human communities in which it becomes established.[26]

EARLY PROCESSES OF RAINFOREST EXPLOITATION

Archaeologists and archaeobotanists have developed new understandings of early human exploitation of the African tropical rainforest environments. Their findings have complicated the simple, familiar model of the development of human societies that postulated that early (modern) human groups in tropical Africa were hunters, gatherers, and fishers; that after the introduction of seed agriculture, human groups settled, multiplied more rapidly; and that, thereafter, human societies became complex. Recent research in archaeology and historical linguistics has upended a long-standing view that the introduction of agriculture from the early river-basin societies triggered a revolutionary advance in tropical African societies. This older view can be thought of as the "diffusionist" model of development.

Africanist scholars who have investigated human development in humid tropical Africa in the Late Stone Age have challenged the diffusionist model. One part of their challenge involves a revision of our understanding of just when human groups began to exploit the rainforest resources more fully. The history of the oil palm (*Elaeis guineensis* Jacq.) and the West African white and yellow Guinea yams (*Dioscoreae cayenensis* and *Dioscoreae rotundata*, respectively), all of which occurred naturally in the West African transitional biome between the woodlands and the forest, have been of particular research interest.[27]

The oil palm today is found in both West and West Central Africa. Specialists think that the presence of the oil palm is older in West Africa than in West Central Africa. Some specialists hold that human beings

---

[26] In genetic terms, the distribution of the sickle cell is thought to increase to the point where the aggregate survival advantages for heterozygous carriers balance the costs of sickle cell anemia to these communities. At this point is it considered to be in equilibrium, as a "balanced polymorphism." Frank B. Livingstone, "Malaria and Human Polymorphisms," *Annual Review of Genetics*, vol. 5 (1971), 33–64.

[27] For an overview of the ecological history of West Africa, see James L.A. Webb Jr., "Ecology and Society in West Africa," in ed. Emmanuel Akyeampong, *Major Themes in West Africa's History* (London: James Currey, 2005), 33–51.

probably played a role in its introduction and expansion into the rainforests of West Central Africa early in the Holocene period (7,000–2,500 BCE). By the late Holocene it had become a common element in the subsistence economy in both West and West Central Africa. According to the archaeobotanist A.W. Sowunmi, it is likely that the human use of fire in rainforest clearings prevented the regrowth of forest trees in the openings and thus brought about an anthropogenically enhanced expansion of the natural oil palm stands. The oil palm, from which edible oils (both palm kernel oil and palm oil) can be extracted and that can be tapped for toddy to make wine, is one of the most economically useful plants in West and West Central Africa.[28] This interpretation of the archaeobotanical evidence for the expansion of the oil palm holds that it is a proxy for the increased human presence in and exploitation of the rainforest biome.[29]

The question of the cultivation origins of the white and yellow Guinea yams, distinguished by their high caloric yields, has attracted the attention of researchers since the 1960s. During the 1960s and 1970s the preeminent scholar of the West African yams, D.G. Coursey, advanced an evolutionary model of yam use that reached far back in time. He held that hunters and gatherers had exploited wild yams even before 60,000 BP, and that in the period 45,000 to 15,000 BP the Late Stone Age peoples had begun to develop ritual concepts and practices to protect the yam plants. According to Coursey, by 9,000 BCE these peoples had begun to develop a "protoculture" based on the replanting of selected wild plants.

In Coursey's model, a "diffusionist" impulse remained important. In his view, by 3,000 to 2,000 BCE Neolithic grain cultivators, influenced by the agriculturalists of southwestern Eurasia, had moved south from the Middle Niger River valley, interacted with the "protoculturalists," and created yam cultivation. For Coursey, this yam culture began to spread deeper into the forest with the advent of iron working, around 500 BCE.

[28] J.G. Vaughan and C.A. Geissler, *The New Oxford Book of Food Plants* (Oxford: Oxford University Press, 1999), 24–25.

[29] M. Adebisi Sowunmi, "The Significance of the Oil Palm (*Elaeis guineensis* Jacq.) in the Late Holocene Environments of West and West Central Africa: A Further Consideration," *Vegetation History and Archaeobotany*, vol. 8 (1999), 199–210. These conclusions are tentative, and Sowunmi calls for palynological studies of terrestrial cores and more extensive archaeological study to confirm or refute them.

For an interpretation that the expansion of the oil palm was owing to climate change, see Jean Maley, with the collaboration of Alex Chepstow-Lusty, "*Elaeis guineensis* Jacq. (Oil Palm) Fluctuations in Central Africa during the Late Holocene: Climate or Human Driving Forces for This Pioneering Species," *Vegetation History and Archaeobotany*, vol. 10 (2001), 117–120.

The forest ecologies favored cultivation of the yam over grain crops, and yam growers could produce more calories and thus achieve numerical superiority over grain farmers and create complex culture systems.[30]

The concept of protocultivation has been revised since the time of Coursey's pioneering work. Recent scholarship argues for early African yam practices that were highly productive but were not a stepping-stone on the path to cultivation. Edmond Dounias has termed this *paracultivation* to distinguish it from the evolutionistically weighted term *protocultivation*. In essence, paracultivation consists of the voluntary reburial of the wild yam head after tuber harvesting. The plant is thereby maintained in its original environment.[31] These practices apparently advanced the "ennoblement" of the guinea yams – that is, the genetic selection of the better yams to harvest and propagate that resulted in harvestable tubers that were far superior for comestible purposes to those produced by wild plants.

Linguists have also developed historical evidence of early yam cultivation. In the 1980s, the linguist Christopher Ehret judged that the words for *cultivation* and *yam* in Proto-Niger-Congo date back to at least 8,000 BCE. Recently, Ehret has synthesized a wealth of archaeological evidence and located the invention of "West African planting agriculture" by at least 8,000 BCE – thousands of years before the arrival of Neolithic seeds and agricultural techniques from the Fertile Crescent or before the emergence of the complex societies that arose in the middle valley of the Niger.[32] These new understandings of early Holocene exploitation of

[30] D.G. Coursey, *Yams: An Account of the Nature, Origins, Cultivation, and Utilisation of the Useful Members of the Dioscoreaceae* (London: Longmans, 1967); D.G. Coursey, "The Origins and Domestication of Yams in Africa," in ed. J.R. Harlan, J.M.J. de Wet, and A.B.L. Stemler, *Origins of African Plant Domestication* (The Hague: Mouton, 1975), 383–408.

[31] Edmond Dounias, "The Management of Wild Yam Tubers by the Baka Pygmies in Southern Cameroon," *African Study Monographs*, suppl. 26 (March 2001), 135–156. Dounias defines the term *paracultivation* as "a combination of technical patterns and social rules which structure the exploitation of wild plants. This term characterizes a particular process of wild plant harvesting which aims at encouraging plant reproduction, so that the plant can be repeatedly exploited. Furthermore, the plant is voluntarily kept within its original environment, in order to better respond to the seasonal mobility of forest dwellers. The maintenance of plants in the forest is the key difference between paracultivation and protocultivation" (137).

[32] Christopher Ehret, "Historical/Linguistic Evidence for Early African Food Production," in ed. J.D. Clark and S.A. Brandt, *From Hunters to Farmers* (Berkeley: University of California Press, 1984), 26–39; Ehret, *The Civilizations of Africa*, 82–83.
    The Middle Niger Valley is an important agricultural region in which some dryland crops (notably pennisetum) and the wet crop, "red rice" (*Orzya glabberima*), were

the rainforest edges and rainforest openings for yam paracultivation and then yam cultivation delink further the African historical experience from the diffusionist model that stressed the adoption of the "Neolithic agricultural revolution" by hunters and gatherers in tropical Africa.

AN IMMUNOLOGICAL GRADIENT IN
TROPICAL AFRICA

Yam paracultivation and then yam cultivation took place in cleared woodlands near the rainforests or in rainforest openings. These microenvironments were created through the use of fire and the stone ax and, beginning in the first millennium BCE, the iron ax. There were direct epidemiological implications. The fire-cleared openings in woodland and rainforest were the ideal environments for the *Anopheles gambiae* and *Anopheles funestus* mosquitoes to breed in. (These mosquitoes do not breed in swamps or full rainforests.) The cultivation of yams entailed lengthier residence and work in sites conducive to anopheline mosquito breeding, and thus encounters with falciparum malaria would have intensified with the shift from paracultivation to cultivation. It seems likely that at this time the increasing pressure of falciparum infections, with many first attacks fatal and others debilitating, began to select for a genetic mutation to mitigate the damage.[33]

New disease dynamics became established within the early tropical woodland and rainforest settlements. When yam paracultivators became yam cultivators and lived nearby their plantings, this created an environment of continual malarial infection, with paradoxical consequences.

---

domesticated. For an excellent overview, see Roderick McIntosh, *The Peoples of the Middle Niger* (Malden, MA: Blackwell Publishing, 1998).

[33] Although it is not possible to specify exactly when the sickle cell mutation first developed or became common, specialists are generally agreed that the falciparum malaria parasites developed from within the tropical African woodland and rainforest environments and later spread into other biomes. The earliest human physical evidence of sickle cell anemia comes from the mummified remains of Egyptians from the fourth millennium BCE (A. Marin, N. Cerutti, and E. Rabino Massa, "Use of the Amplification Refractory Mutation System (ARMS) in the Study of HBS in Predynastic Egyptian Remains," *Bollettino della Società Italiana di Biologia Sperimentale*, vol. 75, nos. 5–6 [1999], 27–30). This evidence suggests that falciparum may have spread from the upper Nile region to the lower Nile region. The issue of whether or not the sickle cell mutation arose separately in the lower Nile valley remains an open question. Today, the incidence of sickle cell along the entire length of the Nile is very low (0.0–2.5%) (Stuart Edelstein, *The Sickled Cell: From Myths to Molecules* [Cambridge, MA: Harvard University Press, 1986], 148, fig. 7.3).

Individuals who survive the initial bouts of falciparum malaria and live in environments of endemic infection, with high parasite loads, develop immunities that greatly reduce suffering from the disease. In this respect, after the initial onslaught of falciparum malaria, the survivors are much safer if they continue to live in a settlement of continuous stable infection. When individuals leave, for periods of even less than one year, their immunities deteriorate.

The yam-based diet may have played a role in the human biological response to malaria pressures and may have shifted some of the falciparum burden. Some scholars have proposed that the "yam complex" is a classic example of coevolution between plants and people – in which people selected plant variants that offered some protection from the damage of falciparum malaria. Yams release chemicals that inhibit both the growth of the falciparum parasite and the sickling of the hemoglobin molecule. The contemporary West African prohibition against eating new yams during the peak season of mosquito infestation and thus the worst period of the malarial season may allow yam-growing communities to have the better of two adaptations. It may achieve a modest reduction in the intensity of falciparum infection, preserving the defenses of those who are heterozygous for sickle cell during the worst malarial season and improving the condition for homozygous sickle cell individuals during the rest of the year. To some researchers this has suggested a profound and ancient cultural adaptation to malarial pressure.[34]

The world of the early yam-growing tropical African village was thus, in epidemiological terms, a different disease world from the rainforest that surrounded it. When hunters and gatherers made even brief contact with villages of stable falciparum infection – where the villagers appeared to be in good health – they experienced sharply elevated mortality and morbidity rates and were at ongoing risk for death and debilitation at successive contacts. Thus, the establishment of permanent settlements in tropical Africa created an "immunological gradient" that shifted steeply from villagers to hunters and gatherers in the rainforests and woodlands around them.

TROPICAL VEGECULTURAL FRONTIERS

From the woodlands of West Africa, pioneers extended the practice of vegeculture, which was centered on yam cultivation, deep into the rainforests. There were two major frontiers of this multiregional, vegecultural

---

[34] Edelstein, *The Sickled Cell*, 60–63.

expansion. One was within West Africa. The West African speakers of languages of the "West Atlantic" grouping of the Niger-Congo language family moved south from the savanna and woodlands into the rainforest belt above the Gulf of Guinea. These rainforests were not entirely unfamiliar to them, and indeed the autochthonous peoples spoke languages from the same language family.[35] From the point of view of historical linguistics, these movements have attracted relatively little scholarly attention.

A second frontier of expansion was initiated from the border of what is today Nigeria and Cameroon. From this region, "Bantu-speakers" spread across tropical Africa to the south and east, into west-central and eastern Africa. They encountered hunters and gatherers who were Batwa-speakers, and, over a period of a few thousand years, in two great migrations (5,000–4,000 BCE and 1,500–500 BCE), the Bantu-speakers spread their languages over the vast expanse of equatorial Africa and much of eastern Africa. Because of the relatively recent periods in which these migrations took place and the phenomenal extension of the Bantu-language zone, the Bantu-speakers' phases of expansion have attracted the attention of scholars from a variety of disciplines.[36]

Recently, Kairn Klieman has brilliantly reconceptualized the relationship between Bantu-speaking villagers and Batwa-speaking peoples ("Pygmies"). She argues from cultural and linguistic evidence that the relationship between Bantu-speaking immigrants and Batwa-speaking hunting-and-gathering autochthons began with the first Bantu migration (5,000–4,000 BCE). It profoundly changed with the introduction of the banana/plantain complex and iron working during the second Bantu expansion, in the Late Stone to Metal Age (1,500–500 BCE).[37]

Probably during the end of the second millennium BCE or the first half of the first millennium BCE, the plantain/banana complex spread west from

---

[35] See, e.g., M.E. Kropp Dakubu, "The Peopling of Southern Ghana: A Linguistic Viewpoint," in ed. Christopher Ehret and Merrick Posnansky, *The Archaeological and Linguistic Reconstruction of African History* (Berkeley: University of California Press, 1982), 245–255; and M.E. Kropp Dakubu, "Linguistics and History in West Africa," in ed. Emmanuel Akyeampong, *Major Themes in West Africa's History* (London: James Currey, 2005), 52–72.

[36] On the expansion of yam farming in early West Africa, see Bassey W. Andah, "Identifying Early Farming Traditions of West Africa," in ed. Thurston Shaw et al., *The Archaeology of Africa: Food, Metals and Towns* (London: Routledge, 1995), 240–254. The expansion of rice farming into the western regions of the West African rainforests is thought to have taken place in the first millennium CE.

[37] Kairn Klieman, *"The Pygmies Were Our Compass": Bantu and Batwa in the History of West Central Africa, Early Times to c. 1900 C.E.* (Portsmouth, NH: Heinemann, 2003).

eastern Africa into the central equatorial rainforests.[38] There it likely became the staple food.[39] The plantain/banana complex, along with the yam cultivation and some use of seed agriculture, provided a robust basis for village settlement. In the same ways that the yam and oil palm played important roles in the opening of the rainforests during the late Holocene, tropical Africans in later millennia widely adopted the plantain/banana complex and incorporated it into the heart of their rainforest village economies.

Over the course of these Bantu migrations, and particularly following the adoption of the banana/plantain complex, rainforest villagers were able to establish larger permanent settlements in the rainforests. These settlements became centers of falciparum infection.[40] This disease process must have been one of the major factors that led to the replacement of non-Bantu-speaking peoples with Bantu-speaking peoples over vast areas of the continent in a very slow process that unfolded over many centuries.[41] Falciparum malaria would have dramatically reduced the numbers of all peoples who visited the village zones of stable malaria, much as it dramatically killed European visitors millennia later, during the years of the Atlantic slave trade, the era of the "white man's grave."

Historians have hitherto sought explanations for the expansion of the Bantu-language speakers in other material processes, such as the adoption of yam cultivation (which yields large numbers of calories and would

[38] E. De Langhe, R. Swennen, and D. Vuylsteke, "Plantain in the Early Bantu World," *Azania*, vols. 29–30 (1996), 318–323; Christophe Mindzie Mbida, "Evidence for Banana Cultivation and Animal Husbandry during the First Millennium BC in the Forest of Southern Cameroon," *Journal of Archaeological Science*, vol. 27 (2000), 151–162; Christophe Mindzie Mbida, "First Archaeological Evidence of Banana Cultivation in Central Africa during the Third Millennium before Present," *Vegetation History and Archaeobotany*, vol. 10 (2001), 1–6.

[39] De Langhe, Swennen, and Vuylsteke, "Plantain," 158, citing Jan Vansina, *Paths in the Rainforests* (Madison: University of Wisconsin Press, 1999).

[40] As Klieman notes: "Bantu populations grew in number, settled into larger more sedentary villages, and began to produce larger quantities and more diverse styles of ceramics. Iron tools and banana cultivation also allowed Bantu villagers to move into forested regions away from the original riverine routes of settlement. This phenomenon resulted in the formation of numerous new speech communities, especially during the Late Stone to Metal Age (1,500–500 BCE). As was the case in other parts of Africa, the introduction of iron engendered a greater centralization of local economies and an increase in economic specialization." *"The Pygmies Were Our Compass,"* 123–124.

[41] Jan Vansina, "New Linguistic Evidence and the 'Bantu Expansion,'" *Journal of African History*, vol. 36, no. 2 (1995), 173–195; Christopher Ehret, "Bantu Expansions: Re-Envisioning A Central Problem of Early African History," *International Journal of African Historical Studies*, vol. 34, no. 1 (2001), 5–41; Roland Oliver et al., "Comments on Christopher Ehret, 'Bantu-History: Re-Envisioning the Evidence of Language'," *International Journal of African Historical Studies*, vol. 34, no. 1 (2001), 43–87.

have contributed to population growth) and the adoption of new iron technologies. The pairing of yams and iron, however, has been criticized on the basis that iron tools are not necessary for yam cultivation. (Wooden digging sticks are admirably suited to the work.) Others have held that in the Bantu migrations the principal use of iron was for weaponry, strengthening the ability of the Bantu-speakers to dominate in war.[42] There is, however, no archaeological or linguistic evidence of such warfare.

A more plausible interpretation emerges if we consider the processes of rainforest exploitation and the dynamics of falciparum infection. The expansion of the zone of Bantu-language speakers appears to be based on the demographic advantages of high-yielding yam and plantain/banana cultivation, in conjunction with a tropical falciparum malarial "immunological gradient." In this light, the processes of the Bantu expansions are direct analogues to the expansions of the disease-experienced peoples of early village Eurasia.[43]

The contemporary distribution of sickle cell mutations in West and Central Africa bears eloquent witness to the end results of these early processes. Today, sickle cell mutations occur in two major independent groups identified on the basis of the location on the gene of the hemoglobin mutation. The major groups are known as 7.6 kb fragment and 13 kb fragment. The first is found in Central Africa in the Zaire basin. The second is found in the Niger delta region. A third independent origin of sickle cell mutation, which is less severe in its consequences for homozygous individuals, is centered in Sierra Leone (Map 1.2).[44]

This map displays the spatial distribution of the three independent mutations of the sickle cell mutations. As Stuart Edelstein, one of the leading authorities on sickle cell, has argued, both the 13 kb and 7.6 kb fragments offer against falciparum malaria the same protection for those who are heterozygous for the mutations and the same costs for those

---

[42] Jared Diamond has recently repopularized this notion of a Bantu military-industrial complex (*Guns, Germs, and Steel: The Fates of Human Societies* [New York: W.W. Norton, 1997], 394–396).

[43] William H. McNeill, *Plagues and Peoples* (Garden City, NY: Anchor Press, 1976), 69–131.

[44] This third mutation was first identified in Senegal. Individuals with the Senegalese pattern of sickle cell anemia produce higher levels of hemoglobin F, and this anemia may therefore be less severe. See Edelstein, *The Sickled Cell*, 148–149.

   Experts are not agreed on whether or not sickle cell hemoglobin mutations have a common ancestor. For the argument for a Middle Eastern origin of hemoglobin S and the diffusion of a single mutant, see F.B. Livingstone, "Who Gave Whom Hemoglobin S: The Use of Restriction Site Haplotype Variation for the Interpretation of the Evolution of the βs-Globin Gene," *American Journal of Human Biology*, vol. 1 (1989), 289–302.

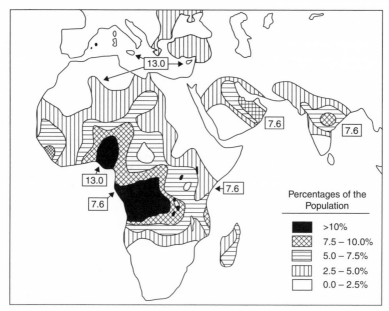

MAP I.2. Distribution of Hemoglobin S (Sickle Cell Gene S)
Source: Adapted from Stuart J. Edelstein, *The Sickled Cell: From Myths to Molecules*
(Cambridge, MA: Harvard University Press, 1986), 149.

who are homozygous. The mutations could not have arisen prior to the
Bantu expansions: otherwise, the 7.6 kb mutation, to establish itself so
prominently, would have had to confer a decisive advantage over the 13 kb
mutation, which it does not. Edelstein estimated that these mutations
arose independently in recent millennia, probably during the first millennium BCE and/or the first millennium CE.[45] This estimate would be
roughly coincident with or follow the full adoption of the plantain/banana
complex. Thus, sickle cell, even if now widely distributed, appears to have
emerged only in the final centuries of, or even in the aftermath of, the
second Bantu expansion.

MALARIA AND TRYPANOSOMIASIS

Malaria has been a heavy disease burden in tropical Africa for many
millennia. In part, this is because the principal malarial mosquitoes,
A. gambiae and *A. funestus*, became highly specialized in feeding on

---

[45] Edelstein, *The Sickled Cell*, 55–56, 147–148. In the 1980s, it was thought that the two Bantu
expansions had taken place in the second and first millennia BCE, respectively.

human beings. This specialization meant that the mosquitoes were able to transmit the malaria parasites with greater efficiency, and thus greater deadliness, because the mosquitoes took few of their blood meals from other animals. When they did bite other animals and inject malaria parasites into them, the parasites died. This specialization in feeding on human blood came about, in part, because when cultivators opened up clearings in the rainforests, the rainforest fauna retreated a safe distance away from the human predators. Thus, in the rainforest clearings, human beings were just about the only meals to be found.

This mosquito specialization – sometimes calculated at an 80 to 100 percent preference for human blood over animal blood – was also the indirect consequence of the tsetse fly (*Glossina morsitans*) infestation in much of tropical Africa. The tsetse fly is the host and vector for the parasites that cause trypanosomiasis, or sleeping sickness. Sleeping sickness was a major disease problem for African communities; the disease caused great human suffering and death across vast stretches of tropical Africa. It weakened the afflicted sufferers, and it intensified the severity of malarial infections, much as human immunodeficiency virus (HIV) intensifies malaria today.

The even greater significance of the great tsetse fly zone for the African malarial burden, however, emerged from the fact that the sleeping sickness parasites proved fatal to all species of livestock that humans were able to domesticate elsewhere across the expanses of Afro-Eurasia. Thus, most tropical Africans lived without regular access to domesticated animal products, including milk and butter. They did not have domesticated pack animals; human beings head-loaded their belongings. In most of tropical Africa, there were no pastoralists and thus no grand divergences in the ways of life of nomadic and sedentary peoples, one of the great organizing principles of life in much of Eurasia.

The barrier of trypanosomiasis, however, was not absolute in tropical Africa. From the mid-fourth millennium BCE, Africans introduced cattle and seed agriculture from the Nilotic Sudan into the plains and highlands of eastern Africa.[46] These early adopters created new systems of agro-pastoralism in the region of what is today Ethiopia and southern Sudan. Eventually, the agropastoralists cleared out a corridor to the east of the tropical rainforests and maintained the corridor with periodic burnings. This destroyed the tsetse habitat as well as encouraged the growth of nutritious new grasses for the herds. Some groups broke away to specialize

---

[46] Ehret, *Civilizations of Africa*, 119–121.

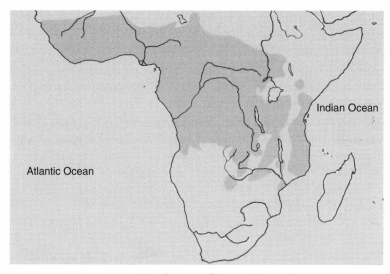

MAP 1.3. Distribution of Tsetse Fly in Africa
Source: Adapted from Roland Oliver, *The African Experience* (New York: Westview Press, 1991), 139.

in keeping cattle and developed distinctive traditions of eastern African pastoralism that included sheep and goats. Over time, pastoralists gradually extended the tsetse-free corridor all the way to the southern tip of Africa by the early centuries of the first millennium CE. In this zone of pastoralism, malarial pressure was relatively light, owing to the mobility of the herders and the ready availability of alternative cattle blood meals for the mosquitoes.

Outside of the cattle corridor, however, tsetse fly infestation created an epidemiological barrier that made it extremely difficult for tropical Africans to incorporate the common domesticated animals such as the cow, horse, sheep, goat, pig, and donkey into their farming economies. In other world regions, these domesticated animals provided alternative blood meals for the malarial mosquitoes, and when this happened, the intensity of transmission sometimes decreased in a process known as zooprophylaxis. This "natural" constraint on malarial infection was absent in most of tropical Africa (Map 1.3).

THE DESICCATION OF THE SAHARA

During the early stages of agropastoralism in eastern Africa, and in the course of the first Bantu expansion in the rainforests, the vast expanse of the Saharan grasslands rapidly began to dry out. The natural biophysical process had probably been ongoing for several millennia, but in the mid-third millennium BCE, the pasturelands that had supported cattle herding turned into a largely arid, rocky, sand-swept expanse. This climate change drove some cattle herders north into the Mediterranean littoral and others southward toward tropical Africa.

The desiccation of the great desert forged an even greater degree of epidemiological distinctiveness for tropical Africa. The Sahara became a buffer zone, where malarial infections were rare because populations were light. From the third millennium BCE until the introduction of the camel in the first millennium BCE, the disease environments to the north and to the south of the Sahara increasingly diverged.

The malarial environments of tropical Africa continued to develop over time. Along the southern shore of the Sahara, in the Niger Bend region, where tsetse fly infestation was light, new styles of life that blended cattle, sheep, and goat pastoralism and sedentary agriculture were forged that proved particularly adaptable to the climatic fluctuations that shaped the region's long-term history.[47] Clustered centers began to form at least by the first millennium BCE, and with the growth of the centers, tropical Africans in the western reaches of the continent became part of the broad range of more densely peopled settlements in which new forms of political power and new possibilities for ecological adaptation would evolve.

Along the banks of the Niger and its swampy tributaries, cultivators began to domesticate the distinctive "red rice" (*Oryza glaberrima*) of West Africa. It thereafter diffused into the coastal lowlands, tidal swamps, and rain-fed uplands.[48] These rice fields, like those in southern China and across the southern rim of Eurasia generally, became important foci for malarial infection. The West African mosquitoes adapted themselves to the new settings. As was often the case, our human quest for food security and our requirement for fresh water propelled us toward greater malarial infection. This distinctive malarial environment of tropical Africa developed separately from and alongside of the Human-Plant-Parasite (H-P-P) complex that stressed the cultivation of yams. The rice cultivators and the millet and sorghum farmers in the

---

[47] Roderick J. McIntosh, *Ancient Middle Niger: Urbanism and the Self-Organizing Landscape* (New York: Cambridge University Press, 2005).

[48] Judith A. Carney, *Black Rice: The African Origins of Rice Cultivation in the Americas* (Cambridge, MA: Harvard University Press, 2001), 34–49.

Niger Bend region lived without the protection that the yam-based diet afforded.

* * *

Malaria was a significant burden in early tropical Africa. The genetic mutation to vivax malaria known as Duffy negativity probably first emerged in communities that practiced seasonal settlement along tropical African riverbanks, long before the Neolithic agricultural revolution. The genetic mutation to falciparum malaria known as sickle cell hemoglobin was a later development. The transition from yam paracultivation to yam cultivation led to the creation of village zones of falciparum infection that exacted high mortality and morbidity costs from hunters and gatherers who could not acquire the limited immunities that came with village life. This immunological gradient played a critical role in the expansion of Bantu-speaking peoples in tropical Africa.

2

Into Eurasia

Between one hundred thousand and fifty thousand years ago, in a replay of the out-migrations of *Homo erectus* that took place one or two million years ago, small numbers of modern humans (*Homo sapiens*) again forsook the continent of Africa for the wilds of Eurasia. Over immense periods of time marked by major transformations in climate and vegetation, including a long, unusually wet interglacial period from circa 57,000 to 25,000 BP, and a dry glacial period that followed from circa 25,000 to 12,000 BP, their progress was likely slow. Their survival strategies of gathering, fishing, and hunting kept them close to exploitable resources, hugging the rivers and coastlines. They built up their numbers slowly. A growing and moveable frontier of our species explored unknown terrains. Over time, small groups here and there broke away to make their own choices about territories and resources. These early human voyagers would become the ancestors of the first modern Eurasians. They brought with them the tool kits and cultural knowledge of their ancestors in tropical Africa, and they brought with them, initially at least, a range of tropical parasites.

Almost all of the parasites died out. As the migrants left the wet tropics, they left behind the tropical insects that carried disease and the tropical animals that served as reservoirs of disease that could afflict humans. They escaped from yellow fever, sleeping sickness, river blindness, elephantiasis, and a host of other maladies. However, they could not flee easily from the malarial infections. They carried these infections in their bloodstreams, and in a spate of intense misfortune, as the migrants rambled through the wilds of Afro-Eurasia, they encountered the never-ending hum of *Anopheles* mosquito species that could play host to malaria parasites.

Over an immensely long period of time, the malarial infections were likely sporadic. Human population densities were low, and populations were mobile. As the habitat of modern humanity expanded in Eurasia, malaria eventually established new roots far outside the African continent. Its fruits for human history were quite different from those in tropical Africa but just as bitter.

In the course of the great expansions throughout Afro-Eurasia, malaria flourished in resource-rich lowlands where groups camped temporarily or even settled on a seasonal basis. The earliest history of modern human malaria in Eurasia, perforce, shares some common elements with that in tropical Africa. Eventually the pressures from malarial infections began to select for protective mutations, and genetic accommodations to vivax and falciparum malaria emerged in some Eurasian populations. These accommodations to malarial pressure, however, never approximated the levels that were found in tropical Africa. This was not because the infections, when contracted, were less severe. In Eurasia, vivax infections made people just as sick, and falciparum infections could be just as deadly as in tropical Africa. However, the levels of endemic infection in Eurasia were typically lower than in Africa. Eurasian malaria was less stable and thus prone to epidemic outbreaks. In part, this was because the Eurasian mosquitoes were less efficient at transmitting the malaria parasites and had lower preferences for human blood meals over animal blood meals.

Life was easiest in humid tropical and subtropical lands. For this reason, the earliest migrants – for perhaps several tens of thousands of years – preferred to explore the southern Eurasian zones, where year-round warmth and plentiful water ensured enough to eat and drink. Some early groups in Southeast Asia discovered the bonanza of yams that, like the yams of tropical Africa, were highly nutritious and rich in calories. As in tropical Africa, it is difficult to date the beginnings of yam harvesting in the Southeast Asian tropics, but it was probably long before the beginnings of seed agriculture. There were likely similar patterns and processes of paracultivation and seasonal settlement there that provided the baseline conditions for infection. In tropical Eurasia, as in tropical Africa, malaria established itself as the oldest of the human infectious diseases. Its effects were large.

MOSQUITOES AND EARLY HUMAN PATTERNS OF LIVING

The early histories of malarial infections are interwoven with one of the most fundamental activities of human life – the quest for potable water. From earliest human times until the development of aqueducts and piping, human beings camped, ranged, hunted, practiced paracultivation, and foraged near water sources. Human beings need to drink about one gallon of water per day in tropical environments, and, for this reason, humans conducted most of their lives within a single day's journey of fresh water. Gourds and hide water containers could sustain hunters and gatherers during daily expeditions, but the sheer weight of water (some eight pounds per gallon) meant that it was impractical to carry sizeable volumes.

Human beings' core economic activities thus were loosely wedded to mosquito habitats. In the same way that the *A. gambiae* and *A. funestus* bred in holes opened up in the rainforest canopies in tropical Africa, some of the principal malarial mosquitoes of tropical Eurasia also specialized in rainforest clearings. Others bred in coastal lowlands that tempted human communities with their rich bounties of shellfish and finned fish. Other mosquitoes bred in the full-canopy rainforests – a variation that did not occur in tropical Africa. Perhaps this is the reason that very deep in time, two or three million years ago, when our earliest hominid ancestors explored the forest wilds of Southeast Asia, vivax malaria was able to jump species – from forest-dwelling primates to hominids.

Throughout deep time, human beings have found mosquitoes a great annoyance, particularly when trying to rest. Today, throughout much of the developed world, it is easy to lose track of this commonplace reality of the past. We have significantly reduced the level of mosquito annoyance by screening windows and doors, spraying local mosquito habitats, and sleeping under nets. Our early ancestors undoubtedly repelled insects by applying animal grease and plant extracts to their bodies. But the most effective defense against nocturnal mosquito bites was probably a smoky fire.

The human need for fire has generally been interpreted as fundamental to our evolution. It may have led to a very substantial increase in meat consumption, a development that some theorists have linked to the increase in human brain size.[1] It is certain that fire could keep large animals at bay and permitted our ancestors to render some plants digestible. Domesticated fire also spread other immediate social benefits. Its smoke drove away mosquitoes and other annoying flying insects. The effect could be enhanced by slowing the dissipation of smoke, by kindling a fire just within the mouth of a lean-to or other rough shelter, a cave, or overhanging ledge. By cutting down on the night whining of mosquitoes,

[1] Vaclav Smil, "Eating Meat: Evolution, Patterns, and Consequences," *Population and Development Review*, vol. 28, no. 4 (2002), 604–605.

these environments provided more than simple shelter from the elements and predators. Smoking fire became an integral element of communal social life.

HUMAN MOBILITY AND MALARIAL INFECTIONS

Because early human groups could be highly mobile, vivax infections had a dominant comparative advantage over falciparum infections. Vivax parasites could reside in the liver for lengthy periods of time and then reemerge, to reignite a malarial infection. Human beings were migrating reservoirs of disease, and as such we should be considered the great disseminators of the infection, rather than the much-maligned anopheline mosquitoes.

New accommodations began when the early Eurasians began to explore the cooler climates. The vivax parasite developed an ability to "winter over" inside its human host. This meant that the range of vivax malaria could be extended, fitfully, into zones with a cold season. The chain of infections was not necessarily broken if and when the mosquito populations died from cold. The large variations in the incubation periods of the various "strains" of vivax that have been studied seem to be the result of such adaptions to severe winter.[2] During the following warm season, the parasite circulating in the human blood could then infect the next generations of vector mosquitoes to repeat the cycle. In Eurasia this meant that vivax infections could be expanded into the northernmost climes during the summer months and recur the following season. On this basis, it seems likely that vivax infections, even if highly discontinuous, extended across the full range of Eurasia, even during the era before the agrarian revolution.

The long history of Eurasian falciparum infections proceeded along a different path. In early tropical Africa, falciparum infections had been highly sporadic. The falciparum chains were much more difficult to sustain than those of vivax. The chains kept breaking, in part because the falciparum infections were far more deadly. The parasites perished with the human host. The infections of those individuals who survived bouts with falciparum malaria were short-lived. The survivors' immune systems

---

[2] The "Madagascar" strain has 1.6% of infections with extended incubation periods; the "McCoy" strain from the southern United States had only 1.1%; the "Dutch" strain had 38%. Richard E.L. Paul, Mawlouth Diallo, and Paul T. Brey, "Mosquitoes and Transmission of Malarial Parasites – Not Just Vectors," *Malaria Journal*, vol. 3, no. 38 (2004), 2.

generally cleared the parasites after the initial series of attacks. In principle, the transmission of falciparum in the warm, humid tropics was greatly enhanced by the fact that falciparum could be transmitted on a year-round basis. The levels of infection in Eurasia seem to have been far lower than those in tropical Africa during the long epochs before the agricultural revolutions in the river basins. The multiple factors of mobility, low population density, short-lived infections, and, later, the domestication of animals that allowed for zooprophylaxis combined to minimize transmission.

The timing of the exodus of falciparum from tropical Africa and its spread into tropical and subtropical Eurasia cannot be established with any certainty.[3] Falciparum probably accompanied many of the emigrant groups that left the African hearth. Falciparum transmission, however, was difficult to sustain among the small numbers of emigrants, and the initial infections must have flickered on and off.

By contrast, the ability of vivax to relapse and produce new infections gave it a comparative survival advantage. Following the infection of human communities with a new strain of simian vivax, malarial infections eventually began to increase, particularly in tropical Asia. There, as in tropical Africa, the most likely venues for infection were the seasonal settlements, along the banks of rivers, near mangrove mudflats, or in coastal regions rich in shellfish. All were breeding grounds for one or another of the many Asian anopheline species that could host the parasites.[4] Throughout the Asian tropics, human beings were also moving into new ecological niches, and from a hearth in Southeast Asia, migrants then moved northward into eastern Asia.[5]

---

[3] On the possible influence of climate change on temperature ranges during the last pleniglacial, see J. de Zulueta, "Changes in the Geographical Distribution of Malaria throughout History," *Parassitologia*, vol. 29 (1987), 193–205.

[4] For Southeast Asia, see I.M. Puri, "Anophelines of the Oriental Region," in ed. Mark Boyd, *Malariology; A Comprehensive Survey of All Aspects of this Group of Disease from a Global Standpoint* (Philadelphia: Saunders, 1949), 483–505.

[5] Specialists dispute the degree to which the contemporary populations of East Asia are descended from migrants from Southeast Asia. All agree that migrants from Southeast Asia made a major contribution to the population of East Asia. Some hold that migrations through Central Asia also played a significant role. See B. Su et al., "Y-Chromosome Evidence for a Northward Migration of Modern Humans into Eastern Asia during the Last Ice Age," *American Journal of Human Genetics*, vol. 65, no. 6 (1999), 1718–1724 and Tatiana Karafet et al., "Paternal Population History of East Asia: Sources, Patterns, and Microevolutionary Processes," *American Journal of Human Genetics*, vol. 69 (2001), 614–628.

Vivax infections initially more intensively parasitized human groups with fishing, hunting, and gathering technologies who settled seasonally to take full advantage of nature's resources. Over time, the practices of gathering and para-experimentation with horticulture at the forest edges came to include the use of fire to expand or renew the habitats at the edge of the rainforests or to open up gaps in the rainforests. This, in turn, created new contexts for seasonal settlement.

These practices, however, did *not* multiply the possibilities for malarial infection. The relationship between deforestation and malaria in tropical Eurasia was different than in tropical Africa, and in some ways it was more complex. By way of broad generalization, because of the different behaviors of the Asian mosquitoes, human beings were more likely to contract malaria *within* the tropical forests rather than in the aftermath of tropical deforestation. Whereas in tropical Africa, deforestation typically increased the transmission of malaria, in tropical Asia it decreased the risk.[6]

It is not possible on the basis of current evidence to establish the general timing of our ancestors' para-experimentation with yams (*Dioscorea alata* and *Dioscorea esculanta*) and taro (*Colocasia esculenta* [true taro] and *Alocasia macrorrhuza* [giant or false taro]) in tropical Asia.[7] Because the early human experiences in tropical Eurasia shared other broad similarities with those of tropical Africa, it seems possible that at some early point our ancestors began to harvest the tastiest nutrient-rich and calorie-rich tubers and also began a process of genetic selection comparable to that in tropical Africa.

In this respect, it probably makes more sense to conceive broadly of a long period of paracultivation – of many thousands of years or even tens of thousands of years – before the experiments with seed agriculture and settled tropical horticulture that we call the "agricultural revolution" came to fruition. Human beings colonized the vast landmass of New Guinea, Australia, and Tasmania known as Sahul at least 40,000 years ago, when sea levels were as much as ninety meters below their current levels. And biomolecular evidence suggests that in the distant past, in what is today New Guinea and islands farther east in Melanesia, human

---

[6] C.A. Guerra, R.W. Snow, and S.I. Hay, "A Global Assessment of Closed Forests, Deforestation, and Malaria Risk," *Annals of Tropical Medicine and Parasitology*, vol. 100, no. 3 (2006), 189–204.

[7] See Patricia J. O'Brien, "Sweet Potatoes and Yams," and Nancy J. Pollack, "Taro," in ed. Kenneth F. Kiple and Kriemheld Coneè Ornelas, *The Cambridge World History of Food*, vol. 1 (New York: Cambridge University Press, 2000), 207–218 and 218–230, respectively.

beings domesticated various species of bananas, plantains, breadfruit, sugarcanes, taros, and yams.[8] The plants are propagated by suckers, cuttings, or shoots – rather than by seed – and our ancestors prepared the terrain by using fire to burn off the vegetative cover. The tasty grasses, which grew back after the fire, attracted animals, and this, in turn, improved the prospects for hunting. These practices apparently preceded by many millennia the origins of agriculture in highland New Guinea.[9]

As early humanity accomplished the domestication of food crops, our ancestors entered more deeply into the grip of a terrible vise. Many of the practices that allowed human groups to exploit more effectively their tropical environments also improved their chances of maintaining a chain of malarial infection. One strategy to lessen the burden of malarial infection was to move to higher ground. By simply moving far up into the forested highlands, it was generally possible to climb above the range of the local varieties of anopheline mosquitoes. The tradeoffs varied from one microregion to another, depending on the local microecologies and species of anopheline mosquitoes. However, higher altitudes meant cooler temperatures and less radiant energy, and, often, gatherers and hunters had to spend more of their time securing enough to eat.

Our understandings of the earliest patterns and processes in the distribution of human malaria across Eurasia in the distant past can only be approximate. What we can know with greater certainty is that these infections were locally discontinuous and regionally continuous. Vivax infections apparently maintained an overall unbroken chain of infection that stretched back more than a million years, punctuated with jumps in the increasing malarial burden. Falciparum, introduced from tropical Africa in the emigrations of *Homo sapiens*, was more difficult to maintain in chains of infection and became anchored in tropical Eurasia only in the aftermaths of these colonizations. In tropical Eurasia, both falciparum and vivax probably emerged as truly chronic infections with expanding cultural and economic consequences only when human beings began to

---

[8] V. Lebot, "Biomolecular Evidence for Plant Domestication in Sahul," *Genetic Resources and Crop Evolution*, vol. 46, no. 6 (1999), 619–628. On the initial colonization of Sahul, see J.F. O'Connell and J. Allen, "Dating the Colonization of Sahul (Pleistocene Australia–New Guinea): A Review of Recent Research," *Journal of Archaeological Science*, vol. 31 (2004), 835–853.

[9] T.P. Denham et al., "Origins of Agriculture at Kuk Swamp in the Highlands of New Guinea," *Science*, vol. 301, no. 5630 (July 11, 2003), 189–193; Tim Denham, Simon Haberle, and Carol Lentfer, "New Evidence and Revised Interpretations of Early Agriculture in Highland New Guinea," *Antiquity*, vol. 78, no. 4 (2004), 839–857.

settle in the earliest subtropical and tropical river basins – along the banks of the Nile, the Tigris-Euphrates, the Indus, and the Yellow rivers – and founded the first great seed-based societies.

NEW PATTERNS IN INFECTION: PERMANENT SETTLEMENT

Why did "agricultural revolutions" take place? Why did our long millennia of experimentation with gathering calories from diverse ecosystems take such a radical turn? What directed our choices to settle near the floodplain soils of the major river systems in southern Eurasia and northern Africa? A generation or so ago, the explanation seemed straightforward. The widely accepted ideas that once held the day still have a façade of plausibility: that there were more calories to be won more easily from agriculture than from hunting and gathering, and that there was more food security. These ideas, however, have run afoul of evidence from studies of contemporary hunters and gatherers that show that it requires less work to glean calories from the wild than from agriculture, and that in the wild, because the sources of food are so varied, there is less food vulnerability during bad seasons and destructive weather.

Why, then, did some human groups decide to take up agriculture and establish permanent settlements? Some scholars have suggested that slow but relentless population growth forced the move, and that population pressure on regional resources drove human beings into agriculture, where they could work longer hours and with less efficiency but still get enough calories to keep more bodies fed.[10] Recent research has called into question the bases for the conceptual categories of "hunters and gatherers" and "agriculturalists" and highlighted the extensive evidence for "low-level food production" that occupied the "middle ground" between hunting and gathering and agriculture.[11] It seems improbable that there can be a single, overarching explanation for the complex of choices that drove the initial processes of sedentarization along the various Afro-Eurasian river basins.

Whatever the first considerations, coercion later came to play a major role. The evolution of social inequality – that is, the creation of social

[10] Mark Nathan Cohen, *The Food Crisis in Prehistory* (New Haven: Yale University Press, 1979).
[11] Bruce D. Smith, "Low-Level Food Production," *Journal of Archaeological Research*, vol. 9, no. 1 (2001), 1–43.

classes and the subjugation of women and most men – went hand in hand with the growth of more complex and densely settled populations. This social and political metastasis was matched by a new epidemiological order.

In the stinking settlements along the banks of the tropical and subtropical Afro-Eurasian river systems, the density of settlement allowed for the evolution of more stable infections. Some of these infections were familiar and had plagued humanity since earliest times. The physical conditions of settlement life were rife with intestinal parasites that were transmitted by fecal-oral contamination. Settlers also suffered from soil-transmitted helminthic infections – such as whipworm (*Trichuris trichiura*) and roundworm (*Ascaris lumbricoides*) – that had been more limited in the earlier epochs when human groups broke camp regularly to move away from their own wastes.

The domestication of animals, however, launched the most wide-ranging transformations in the new epidemiological order. The close familiarity of humans with their animals was critically important in this long-evolving process. Some domesticated animals did not require intimate management and apparently did not make much contribution to human disease. This appears to be true of donkeys, yaks, and water buffalo. But other animals did require close tending, and the results were dire. From chickens came the chickenpox, from horses the common cold, from pigs and ducks influenza, and from cattle came tuberculosis, measles, and smallpox. The new diseases, known as zoonoses, flooded over ancient boundary lines between humans and other animals. The increase in settled population density and the domestication of animals together constituted an epidemiological juggernaut that ruptured the old ecological balances. A welter of microparasites that had long cohabited with the biological systems of animals leaped across species boundaries onto and into human bodies and achieved more or less permanent infections in the early Eurasian and northern African farming communities.[12]

With the creation of permanent settlement, suffering from disease could be more or less continuous and multilayered. Other infections soared because the population density had crept up to a critical level, high enough to support "crowd diseases." For the malaria parasites, the densely settled populations presented a new horizon of opportunity. The

---

[12] William H. McNeill, *Plagues and Peoples* (Garden City, NY: Anchor Press, 1976); Jared Diamond, *Guns, Germs, and Steel: The Fates of Human Societies* (New York: W.W. Norton, 1997).

parasites multiplied in the larger populations and began to achieve the status of endemic diseases.

NEW PATTERNS OF INFECTION: NOMADIC PASTORALISM

Our understandings of the history of animal domestication – like the history of plant domestication – have become more nuanced. Until recently, keeping livestock was considered by most scholars a simple adjunct to an agricultural economy, one that reduced the labor of hunting for meat and hauling animal products back to the settlements. The archaeological evidence from southwest Asia suggested that at some very early point in the domestication of animals, the economic logic of keeping livestock began to demand more pastureland than was close at hand. The keepers of livestock began to separate from the agricultural communities. They ultimately forged an entirely new human lifestyle known as pastoral nomadism that met fundamental human needs for food and shelter in an entirely new way.

The evidence from Africa north of the rainforests suggests a different historical evolution. Pastoralism in Africa seems to have developed *before* settled village farming, as part of an integrated system that incorporated limited hunting and fishing with gathering. Although with profoundly different trajectories, human communities in southwest Eurasia and northern Africa brought the wild cow, sheep, and goat under their control, and the knowledge of animal husbandry eventually spread throughout the Afro-Eurasian ecumene. In the eastern Sahara, in later millennia, herders eventually integrated their mixed herds that included cattle, sheep, and goats in agricultural and agropastoral systems that spread westward into the grasslands of the Sahara and southward into the humid tropics. This pastoral expansion was undoubtedly influenced by climate change, such as the arid phase that brought about the desiccation of the Sahara, particularly from the middle of the third millennium BCE.[13]

The early patterns of Eurasian pastoral nomadism are similarly hazy. On the grasslands of Eurasia, beginning perhaps as early as the fifth millennium BCE, herders began to specialize in the management of mixed herds of livestock. From archaeological studies, there are more or less definitive indications of lifestyles of pastoral nomadism in the grasslands

---

[13] Diane Gifford-Gonzalez, "Pastoralism and Its Consequences," in ed. Ann Brower Stahl, *African Archaeology* (Malden, MA: Blackwell Publishing, 2005), 187–224.

by the third or second millennia BCE. Experts disagree about the timing and the details, but the very broad outline, at least, is clear.[14]

Thus, over the course of several millennia, human beings pioneered the new lifestyles of pastoral nomadism and spread it into the vast grasslands of central Eurasia and Saharan Africa. These new ways of life allowed for a new type of human presence in regions that were only very lightly populated. Although the pastoral nomads initially branched off from the settled communities, with the intent to trade animal products for those of the farmers, the pastoralists must have rapidly adapted to their changed circumstances, which were rich with possibility. They learned that, if necessary, they could draw their sole sustenance for extended periods from their herds alone. They could live from milk, blood, and meat. For their material needs, they learned to use virtually every part of their animals – bone, tooth, hide, and hair. These adaptations inculcated the virtues of independence and offered some relief from the social inequality of the settlements.

From an epidemiological perspective, the pastoral nomadic lifestyle had other advantages. Pastoralists typically moved their animals across the grasslands in great elliptical arcs over the course of the year, to take advantage of seasonal pastures. This ongoing mobility conveyed some health benefits to humans. The temporary nature of the pastoralists' encampments allowed them to move away from their own wastes and those of their animals, and this reduced the extent of fecal-oral contamination. Other benefits flowed from the close contact that the herders had with their animals. For example, the pastoralists' ongoing contact with cattle exposed them to cowpox and thereby provided immunity to smallpox.

The largest health benefits flowed from the fact that the pastoral nomads' lifestyles freed them from the burden of crowd diseases that plagued the agricultural settlements. The nomadic pastoralists were mobile and widely dispersed, and their camps were small. They were unable to sustain the critical population density necessary for crowd diseases to wreak their havoc. These health benefits, along with a spate of other fundamental economic considerations, including the need for pasture, encouraged the eventual separation of pastoral herders from farmers. This separation eventually conferred on the pastoralists a favorable balance of power vis-à-vis the farming communities. They learned to

[14] Anatoly M. Khazanov, *Nomads and the Outside World*, 2nd ed. (Madison: University of Wisconsin Press, 1994), 85–118.

harness the power of their riding animals (particularly horses and camels) for military advantage and were often able to live free from or to exact economic rents from the sedentary authorities in exchange for protection from violence.

With regard to malaria, pastoral nomadism offered nearly a full escape. Domesticated animals were biologically incapable of hosting the malaria parasites. When an infected mosquito bit a herding animal and injected parasites into its bloodstream, the parasites died. The effect of this zoo-prophylaxis was to reduce the malaria cycle of infection. The infected mosquito still retained malaria parasites in her salivary glands and could infect the next human from which she took a blood meal.[15] But zoopro-phylaxis, in conjunction with the regular movements of herders that took them away from infected mosquitoes, meant that herders lived largely free from malaria. The costs to this otherwise happy situation were that pastoral nomadic peoples lived without acquired immunities to malaria. This left them vulnerable to malaria when they came within the disease orbit of the fetid population clusters along the river systems of southern Eurasia and the Saharan edges.

MALARIA AND RIVER-BASIN CIVILIZATIONS

For the expanding populations of the northern African and Eurasian agricultural experiments, malaria was a witches' brew, with rapid onset and an ability to sicken and kill. Over time, malaria spewed out from the early river-basin civilizations into the small villages and the temporary settlements in the close and distant countrysides. This was undoubtedly a broken and discontinuous process. By the first millennium BCE, however, both vivax and falciparum malaria were well on their way to becoming endemic diseases of the Eurasian tropics and subtropics, and, for vivax, the temperate zones as well. This Eurasian expansion was completed roughly in the same era that the Bantu expansions extended throughout the rain-forests of tropical Africa. By the first millennium BCE, zones of malarial infection extended across the Afro-Eurasian landmass. The falciparum infection zone had its center in tropical Africa, although falciparum had become ensconced throughout tropical Asia and probably as far west as along the shores of the Mediterranean. The vivax infection zone was long and wide, ranging across all of Afro-Eurasia, with the exception of the wet African tropics where it was ousted by the spread of Duffy negativity.

[15] Personal communication from Professor John C. Beier.

Within this vast Afro-Eurasian zone were the extensive grasslands of the Sahara and central Eurasia, both largely clear of malaria and nearly surrounded by zones of infection. A zone of mixed infections (vivax, falciparum, and malariae) in northern Africa and a zone of falciparum in tropical Africa enclosed the Sahara Desert. A zone of vivax infections in northern Eurasia and a zone of mixed infections (vivax, falciparum, and malariae) in southern Eurasia wrapped around the great Central Eurasian grasslands.

There was an additional, significant difference in the disease environments that surrounded these two basins of livestock herding. To the south of the Sahara, largely coincident with the zone of falciparum malaria, was a vast zone of trypanosomiasis infection that checked the extension of livestock herding into tropical Africa.[16] Cattle, sheep, and goat pastoralism (and from the first millennium CE, camel pastoralism) could be practiced only in the savanna, where the infestation of the tsetse fly vector was light. Malaria was also seasonal in these savanna drylands, and this epidemiological frontier of both human and animal disease marked off a broad ethnic and cultural frontier that stretched across much of the southern shore of the Sahara.[17]

In eastern Africa, another early pattern is evident. There, early adopters of cattle, perhaps as early as 2000 BCE, used fire to destroy the tsetse fly habitat and reduce vector infestation, which enabled them to manage a zone in which it was relatively safe to pasture cattle. This was possible because the herders understood the ecology of tsetse fly infestation and repeatedly burned off the low bush cover. This reduced the fly habitat and, at the same time, encouraged the growth of nutritious new grasses for their animals. Fire worked wonders on tsetse habitat, but it had no significant impact on the anopheline malaria vectors. There was no malarial frontier in eastern Africa per se, with the exception of some highland zones, above the habitat of the anopheline vectors, where malarial outbreaks were exceedingly rare.

The herding peoples of the Sahara thus inhabited a largely malaria-free zone, and for much of the year they were beyond the reach of the dangerous disease environments of the Nilotic or Sahelian settlements.[18] But

---

[16] John Ford, *The Role of the Trypansomiases in African Ecology* (Oxford: Clarendon Press, 1971).

[17] James L.A. Webb Jr., *Desert Frontier: Ecological and Economic Change along the Western Sahel, 1600–1850* (Madison: University of Wisconsin Press, 1995), 3–26.

[18] Andrew B. Smith, "Origins and Spread of Pastoralism in Africa," *Annual Review of Anthropology*, vol. 21 (1991), 125–141.

pastoral nomadic peoples everywhere rarely produced all of what they consumed, even with their efforts at irrigated agriculture in the oases, and they were often obliged by necessity to venture into agricultural lands during harvest seasons in the agricultural settlements. At least by the second millennium CE this was a seasonal process that hinged on the exchange of animal products and salt for grain and captives.[19] The introduction of slaves into the Saharan environments raised the risks of malarial outbreaks in the oasis areas, although these risks were mitigated by the fact that the desert mosquitoes took their blood meals mostly from the livestock.

ZONES OF ENDEMIC MALARIA

The development of the falciparum, vivax, and mixed infection zones depended on critical population densities and agricultural styles of life. Because the parasites completed one part of their life cycles within the female mosquito, and the life cycles of the mosquitoes outside of the tropics were sharply constrained by ambient temperatures and seasonality, climate was a major limiting condition. Temperature also played an important role in development of the parasites within the mosquito, for both falciparum and vivax. The development of the falciparum parasites within the vector mosquito occurs in the temperature range between 19 and 35 degrees C. At the warmer temperatures, the parasites complete their cycles more rapidly. Below 19 degrees C the falciparum parasite does not develop. Above 35 degrees C the falciparum parasite reproduces much less efficiently, and the mosquitoes die off at about 40 to 42 degrees C. The vivax parasite has a somewhat extended lower range, down to 15 degrees C.[20] Because of the narrower range of falciparum, and the fact that it does not have a dormant liver stage, falciparum malaria is largely confined to a broad belt in the tropics and subtropics. It is possible to introduce falciparum beyond this belt, but these infections will be episodic and ephemeral.

Even within the zone of mixed infections, where malaria is often unstable, falciparum epidemics proved broadly destructive as endemic

---

[19] Webb, *Desert Frontier*, 27–67.
[20] Experts differ as to the lower temperature at which vivax sporogony ceases – either 15 degrees C or 16 degrees C. See Robert W. Snow and Herbert M. Gilles, "The Epidemiology of Malaria," in ed. David A. Warrell and Herbert M. Gilles, *Essential Malariology*, 4th ed. (London: Arnold Press, 2002), 91–92 [16 degrees C] and George MacDonald, *The Epidemiology and Control of Malaria*, (London: Oxford University Press, 1957), 10–11 [15 degrees C].

infections spread. George MacDonald, the leading malaria epidemiologist in the 1950s, calculated that a single infected individual introduced into a settlement of immunologically naïve people would be capable of infecting more than 1,100 other individuals in the course of a given season.[21] Small wonder, then, that in the first or second millennium BCE, at the beginnings of interregional trade, falciparum malaria – introduced by a merchant, soldier, or child captive – insinuated itself into the early human population clusters and created short-lived havoc. Only slowly, and after repeated infections and intense suffering, with high death rates spiking through the entire age pyramid of the settlement population, did some individuals acquire functional immunities. These centers of infection probably became established by the first millennium BCE and probably were fixed even earlier in the first river-basin societies. From these pro-tourban centers, falciparum malaria was likely extended, fitfully, throughout the southern reaches of Eurasia.

This extension of malaria was driven in part by the developing patterns of economic growth and exchange. The early patterns anticipated those of more recent millennia: the gradual pressures of population growth, even under the conditions of the new crowd diseases, meant that broader swaths of surrounding lands were adapted to agricultural and pastoral use. The early principal technology was fire – to clear brush, to return inorganic nutrients to the soil, to encourage the new growth of grasses. Following the development of furnaces circa 1500 BCE in Anatolia that burned hot enough to make iron, the new technology diffused throughout the societies of Afro-Eurasia.

Along the frontiers of these agricultural sectors in expansion, malarial fevers raged. In the Asian tropics, the fevers were year round. Conditions were poor in the rice zones. Those who produced two crops of irrigated rice annually had high levels of exposure because throughout the rice zones there were anopheline mosquitoes that could breed in the standing irrigation waters. Many rice farmers must have acquired immunities to the local strains of malaria. It is also possible that the integration of domesticated livestock into the farming settlements may have had a significant impact on the rates of malarial infection. One strategy employed by Chinese farmers was to keep animals at the periphery of the village, between the rice fields and human dwellings, which had the effect of providing the mosquitoes with a blood meal near their breeding grounds. This early, unintentional experiment with zooprophylaxis was probably

[21] MacDonald, *The Epidemiology and Control of Malaria*, 17–18.

only partially effective. Everywhere along the southern rim of Eurasia, malaria plagued the lowlands and was checked at higher altitudes.

The patterns of malarial infection that became established in tropical Asia, however, were profoundly different from those in tropical Africa. Rather than the African pattern of heavy endemic falciparum infection, in tropical Asia the patterns of malarial infection were generally more unstable and have remained so to the present day. This may be due, in part, to the fact that the anopheline vectors there had more opportunities to take their blood meals from domesticated animals. At all events, there was considerable regional variation in the stability of malarial pressure. Northern India and Sri Lanka even today remain at the far extreme of the continuum, with extremely unstable epidemic malaria. Throughout the rest of tropical Asia, the malarial infections were moderately unstable. The only parallel in tropical Africa was in highland regions, where malarial infections were also highly unstable. There, the lower temperatures created much lower survival rates for the vectors and, consequently, lower rates of transmission, and thus they allowed for little acquired immunity. When unusual conditions obtained, such as an unusually warm summer, epidemic malaria could break out in the highlands of tropical Africa.[22]

In tropical Asia, the agricultural lowland riverine areas, including those crafted for rice cultivation, were among the most afflicted. However, depending on the regional anopheline mosquitoes' behaviors, local rainfall patterns, and a host of other factors, even in densely populated areas, the local malarial patterns might be either stable or unstable. This was true along the course of every river system in southern Eurasia – in the Punjab and along the Ganges, Brahmaputra, Irawaddy, and Mekong.

These lowland regions were the centers of intense infection, whether they were stable or unstable. They were also the regions with the most complex political and military systems, and for these reasons they were able to extend their zones of political influence fitfully into neighboring regions, incorporating at times, if only briefly, the highland zones. The lowland civilizations multiplied and extended the infections throughout the susceptible zones of Eurasia. In northern India, the malarial zone extended from the Indo-Gangetic plain into the terai – the lowlands that served as a defensive disease bulwark for the highland kingdoms in Nepal. In southeastern Eurasia, it reached throughout the regions known today as northern Burma, Vietnam, and Laos.

---

[22] On the measures of stability, see ibid., 33–43.

The expansionist tendencies of the lowland settlements in southern Eurasia thus facilitated the extension of malaria. In the highlands, the commitment to highland styles of life may have limited the exposure of these communities to the longer-lived and more efficient anopheline vectors that multiplied in the lowlands. This differential vulnerability to malarial infection may have been one of the reasons that shifting cultivation remained a preferred pattern of economic activity for many in southern and southeastern Eurasia, well after the establishment and growth of lowland settlements.[23] The most dramatic near-contemporary example of this differential comes from New Guinea, where highland populations lived at elevations above the ranges of the anopheline vectors, practiced horticulture, and had little regular contact with the malarial lowlands, until the 1930s.[24]

EURASIAN OBSERVATIONS AND CONCEPTIONS OF MALARIA

By the first millennium BCE, observations about malarial fevers began to appear in different Eurasian regions. In northern India, two celebrated medical authors, Caraka and Susruta, conceptualized malaria as similar to a seed sown in the ground: Malaria came to fruition in one day as a quotidian fever, two days as a tertian, and three days as a quartan. Moreover, both authors recognized that individuals frequently contracted malaria in lowland regions and at the feet of mountains – and thereby made the earliest contribution to what we might think of as malarial geography.[25]

Chinese and Greek authors also offered observations about malaria during the course of the first millennium BCE.[26] These observations indicate that Greek and Chinese societies had very different early experiences

---

[23] J.E. Spencer, *Shifting Cultivation in Southeast Asia* (Berkeley: University of California Press, 1966), *passim*. For a comparison with Sri Lanka, see James L.A. Webb Jr., *Tropical Pioneers: Human Agency and Ecological Change in the Highlands of Sri Lanka, 1800–1900* (Athens: Ohio University Press, 2002), 11–13, 38–41.

[24] Bob Connelly and Robin Anderson, *First Contact* (New York: Penguin, 1987).

[25] B.L. Raina, *Introduction to Malaria Problem in India*, 2nd ed. (New Delhi: Commonwealth Publishers, 1991), 1–4, 135–141.

[26] The *Zhou li* (Ritual of the Zhou Dynasty), from the eighth century BCE, mentions what translators have rendered as "malaria" in the context of the seasonality of disease ("malaria and cold diseases in autumn"). See Cai Jingfeng and Zhen Yan, "Medicine in Ancient China," in ed. Helaine Selin, *Medicine across Cultures: History and Practice of Medicine in Non-Western Cultures* (Dordrecht, Holland: Kluwer Academic Publishers, 2003), 51–52.

with malaria. Robert Sallares has recently suggested that malaria became established in Greece as early as the eighth century BCE.[27] At least by the fifth century BCE, malariae, vivax, and falciparum were all present in the zone of mixed infections.[28] The emerging northern Chinese civilization, at the eastern end of Eurasia, was developing in the zone of predominantly vivax infection. In the third century BCE, in this northern region, only malariae and vivax were present. Falciparum malaria was noted in the southern regions that today are the provinces of Kweichow and Yunnan.[29]

Most peoples of eastern Eurasia, like the inhabitants of most regions in Afro-Eurasia, had no idea that malaria was mosquito-borne.[30] The principal anopheline vectors in eastern Eurasia bred in a variety of environments and were interspersed among many nonmalarial mosquitoes. The causes of malarial infection were thought to vary. According to early Chinese medicine, for example, malaria was caused either by ghosts and spirits, climate, weather, specific localities, improper diet, disharmony between yin and yang, an enlarged spleen (an apparent confusion of cause and effect), or by "Mother Malaria."[31]

The early Vedic civilization in southern Eurasia likewise had a complex view of disease causation. The early Ayurvedic system of medicine, developed sometime in the second millennium BCE, focused on the restoration of balance within the body through the treatment of opposite qualities. As in Ayurvedic medicine today, the various forms of fever were

[27] Robert Sallares, *Malaria and Rome: A History of Malaria in Ancient Italy* (Oxford: Oxford University Press, 2002), 20–22; Robert Sallares, Abigail Bouwman, and Cecelia Anderung, "The Spread of Malaria to Southern Europe in Antiquity: New Approaches to Old Problems," *Medical History*, vol. 48, no. 3 (2004), 311–328.

[28] The Hippocratic corpus, written by a number of persons during the late fifth century and early fourth century BCE, described all three fevers with a precision sufficient to convince contemporary medical historians that it was malaria under description.

[29] The Chinese term for falciparum malaria was *changch'i*. It was probably known to the civilized Chinese from the third century BCE, when they first traveled to Kweichow.

According to Y.T. Yao and L.C. Ling, native physicians in Kweichow described the disease as follows: "When a man is attacked by the poisonous gas he feels feverish and headache first and then becomes comatose. He may come out of his coma and recover afterwards, or he may die from the acute symptoms in a few days. But more commonly he will suffer from the chronic symptoms, such as jaundice, swelling of abdomen, emaciation, etc, and die within a year or so. The disease is also believed to run a more acute and deadly course among strangers and travelers than among the natives of the endemic area" (Y.T. Yao and L.C. Ling, "Studies on the So-Called Changch'i. I. Changch'i in Kewichow and Kwangsi Border," *Chinese Medical Journal*, vol. 50 [1936], 729).

[30] One exception is the Bai people of Yunnan. See Mark Elvin, *The Retreat of the Elephants: An Environmental History of China* (New Haven: Yale University Press, 2004), 262.

[31] R. Hoeppli, "Malaria in Chinese Medicine," *Sinologica*, vol. 4, no. 2 (1955), 91–101.

thought to reflect the underlying constitution of the afflicted individual, and disease was diagnosed on the basis of symptoms that the individual's constitution expressed.[32] Medical observers in the early Vedic civilization may have achieved the earliest knowledge of some of the basic "facts" of malaria, linking the disease with mosquitoes, in a collection of the South Asian oral texts known as the Atharva Veda, although both the dating and interpretation of these texts are in dispute.[33]

Across Eurasia, various theories competed to explain the onset of malarial fevers. All of the rubrics of explanation – except that of an enlarged spleen – also existed in early Mediterranean medical thinking.[34] The mode of explanation of any disease, including malaria, as a consequence of biophysical imbalance – whether expressed as yin and yang, humors, or chakras – was widely shared across the early civilizational societies and is probably best interpreted as elements of a common intellectual expression across the culture of settlement in early Eurasia.[35]

[32] Ananda S. Chopra, "Ayurveda," in Selin, *Medicine across Cultures*, 75–83.

[33] The dating of the early Vedic oral texts is problematic but is currently thought to lie sometime from the middle of the second millennium BCE to the middle of the first millennium BCE (Romila Thapar, *Early India: From the Origins to AD 1300* [Berkeley: University of California Press, 2002], 104). These texts appear to include some observations about the mosquito and fever and death, although they are expressed in language that is susceptible to diverse interpretation, and scholars disagree about whether or not the texts refer to malaria.

B.L. Raina finds abundant evidence of malaria in the early texts. "From the numerous references to it and analysis of its characteristics it would appear that malaria was the commonest type of fever. Its association with mosquito may be surmised by the descriptions which give nearly all the characteristics and habits of mosquitoes, especially the needle-like proboscis (kusulu), bloody mouth (lohitasyan) and the habit of visiting the dwellings after sunset (salah parinrtyanti sayam). There is also reference to the odourous or fumigating medications used to destroy them" (Raina, *Introduction to the Malaria Problem in India*, 1–3; see also 135–141).

Professor Ganesh Thite of the Bhandarkar Oriental Research Institute in Pune, India, a specialist on the magico-religious aspects of Indian medicine reads the same evidence differently, finding evidence of "demons," rather than mosquitoes (personal communication from Professor Harry J. Walker).

The ancient Indian physicians Susruta and Caraka, writing in later periods – but impossible to date with certainty – refer to the periodicities of different malaria infections. (For excerpts from the writings of Susruta and Caraka, see Raina, *Introduction to the Malaria Problem*, 138–141.)

I am grateful to my classicist colleague Harry J. Walker and to Professor Thite for sharing their observations about these Sanskrit texts.

[34] R. Hoeppli, "Malaria in Chinese Medicine," *Sinologica*, vol. 4, no. 2 (1955), 91–101.

[35] In southwestern Asia, Greece, India, and China, societies developed distinctive, great traditions of ethical reflection during the first millennium BCE. The philosopher Karl Jaspers introduced one explanation of this macrophenomenon: that the evolution of these great traditions took place within the major settled zones – those of dense

The observations in Chinese texts are additionally interesting because they indicate a range of treatments. Some apparently had no direct chemotherapeutic value: "Take one dog fly. Remove the legs and wings. Roll it in wax so as to form a pellet which is to be taken with cold rice-wine on the day of the attack."[36] Other treatments identified plants with antifever properties. In the period up to the fall of the Northern Sung dynasty in 1126 CE, *ch'ang-shan* (Dichroa roots) were the principal plant therapy, and researchers in the twentieth century established that these roots contain antimalarial alkaloids.[37] The sweet wormwood plant (*Artemisia annua*) known as *qinghao*, which is emerging as the frontline drug artemisinin in the contemporary antimalaria campaigns of the early twenty-first century, also had a place in the Chinese pharmacopoeia.[38] The knowledge of these therapies, however, was limited to medical elite. These therapies played no role in the control of malaria. They undoubtedly brought relief to individual sufferers, but the plant drugs were too little used to have had an impact on the extent of general suffering from malaria. By contrast, in the malarial environments of ancient Greece and Rome, no drugs that were effective against malarial infections were ever discovered.[39] The Greeks and Romans did, however, invest considerable efforts in draining swamps, in an attempt to eliminate the environments that were associated with disease.[40]

After the fall of the Northern Sung, the center of Chinese civilization shifted into what is today central China. There, in the aftermath of the wars and famines that wracked northern China, malaria became a much more widespread and serious problem, particularly for the emigrants

population settlement – in response to the threat of nomadic peoples. Jaspers referred to this period as the age of axial thought. See Karl Jaspers, *The Origin and Goal of History* (New Haven: Yale University Press, 1953).

The suggestion made here is that the concept of biophysical imbalance as an explanation for disease may distinguish the more densely settled societies of the first millennium BCE, along the southern axis of Eurasia, from societies elsewhere in the world.

[36] Jacques Gernet, *Daily Life in China on the Eve of the Mongol Invasion, 1250–1279* (Stanford: Stanford University Press, 1962), 169.

[37] Saburdo Miyasita, "Malaria (*yao*) in Chinese Medicine during the Chin and Yuan Periods," *Acta Asiatica*, vol. 36 (1979), 103.

[38] [Anonymous], "Rediscovering Wormwood: Qinghaosu for Malaria," *The Lancet*, vol. 339 (March 14, 1992), 649.

[39] Sallares, *Malaria and Rome*, 48.

[40] Jean-Nicolas Courvisier, "Eau, Paludisme et Démographie en Grèce Péninsulaire," in ed. René Ginouvès et al., *L'Eau, la Santé et la Maladie dans le Monde Grec* (Athens: Ècole française d'Athènes, 1994), 314–315.

from the upper classes who fled the chaos.[41] In Guizhou, malaria was said to be rife in the southern half of the province, but it almost certainly was vivax rather than falciparum.[42] The Chinese who moved into Yunnan province, however, immigrated to the northernmost reaches of the zone of mixed infections. They were fated to encounters with falciparum.[43] In the south, *ch'ang-shan* (*Dichroa febrifuga*) grew wild throughout the provinces south of the Yangtze River and continued to be used for treatment.[44]

At some point, malaria crossed from mainland Eurasia into Japan. The first accounts of Japanese malaria date back only to the tenth century CE, but it is possible that the introduction of malaria is older. It may be linked to the introduction of rice, dated to circa 400 BCE. At all events, malaria entered into the bloodstreams of the rice farmers in Japan as it had in mainland Eurasia. In Japan, as in China, experimentation with native plants was successful. The *ch'ang-shan* plant did not grow in Japan; but the roots of plants native to Japan such as *kusagi* (*Clerodendron trichotomum* THUMB.) and *kokusagi* (*Orixa japonica* THUMB.) are reported to have been in use as antimalarial medicines from ancient times.[45] Even in China and Japan, these natural cures do not appear to have been in general use, and thus they appear to have had no discernible impact on the epidemiological history of malaria before the twentieth century. There is no evidence to suggest that these natural cures in any way broke the chains of transmission.

In western Eurasia, in particular around the Mediterranean basin, malaria was largely a lowland phenomenon, and there it was the only disease that was transmitted by mosquitoes. (This was quite different from the environments of tropical Africa or southern and southeastern Eurasia, where mosquitoes could transmit a range of other serious diseases.) For this reason, the association of malaria with lowlands (inland swamps, in particular) was deeply anchored in the common experience, and the Romans sought to limit the damage from malaria by draining some inland swamps into rivers. In ancient Italy, although there were no explicit connections made between mosquitoes and malaria, from the learned

---

[41] Gernet, *Daily Life in China*, 147.
[42] Mark Elvin, *The Retreat of the Elephants* (New Haven: Yale University Press, 2004), 262–264.
[43] David A. Bello, "To Go No Where No Han Could Go for Long: Malaria and the Qing Construction of Administrative Space in Frontier Yunnan," *Modern China*, vol. 31, no. 2 (2005), 1–35.
[44] Miyasita, "Malaria (*yao*) in Chinese Medicine," 94, 97.
[45] Ibid., 108–110.

authors we know that some Romans used nets, burned wormwood, and daubed themselves with extracts of wormwood in oil to ward off mosquitoes.[46] Although Mediterranean communities built up local and idiosyncratic knowledge concerning the therapeutic properties of a wide range of natural products including herbs, roots, barks, and fermented and distilled beverages, there were no cures for malarial fevers, only palliatives.

EURASIAN DIETARY INFLUENCES ON MALARIA AND TREATMENTS

Recent research has suggested that dietary patterns and culinary practices may have been able to mitigate the impact of malaria. One line of inquiry indicates that the interactions among vitamins and foods, for example, can have important influences on malarial infections. Vitamins A and E, for example, occur naturally in a range of foods and are antioxidants. It is now known that these vitamins can reduce the effectiveness of antimalarial drugs and thereby contribute to higher parasite loads among infected persons. Conversely, deficiencies of these vitamins may help to protect against infections. This is just part of the spectrum of interactions. Foods high in iron or cooked in iron or copper pots can help mediate the production of free radicals and act as oxidants to suppress the parasite load.

Common tropical spices also release oxidants in the blood, in much the same way that modern antimalarial medicines do. These oxidants promote a toxic environment for the asexual (schizodontal) stage of the malaria parasites. The increased oxidation interrupts the development of the plasmodia within the host red cells and leaves immature parasites that cannot infect other red blood cells.[47] A wide array of spices and plants including clove, nutmeg, cinnamon, basil, and onion have oxidant properties and are common medicines for fever in the southern and southeast Eurasian pharmacopoeias.[48] These spices, plants, and vitamins did not prevent infection. However, in regions of endemic malaria they may have had a hand in reducing the severity of infection.

---

[46] Sallares, *Malaria and Rome*, 47–48.
[47] Nina L. Etkin, "Plants as Antimalarial Drugs: Relation to G6PD Deficiency and Evolutionary Implications," in ed. Lawrence S. Greene and Maria Enrica Danubio, *Adaptation to Malaria: The Interaction of Biology and Culture* (Amsterdam: Gordon and Breach, 1997), 153.
[48] Nina L. Etkin, "The Co-Evolution of People, Plants, and Parasites," *Proceedings of the Nutrition Society*, vol. 62 (2003), 311–317, esp. 314; Etkin, "Plants as Antimalarial Drugs," in Greene and Danubio, *Adaptation to Malaria*, 139–176.

In some Eurasian regions of mixed infections, some major foodstuffs may have mitigated the severity of the falciparum burden, much as did the yams of tropical Africa. The best-known example is that of fava beans (*Vicia fava*). In the western Mediterranean region, the consumption of fava beans was commonplace. This was also a region in which falciparum pressure had selected for an inherited red blood cell disorder known as the G6PD hemoglobin mutation. This mutation also arrests the development of immature falciparum stages, although because it compromises the integrity of the red blood cells, it carries substantial health risks to the bearer. Like the sickle cell mutation, it occurs as a balanced polymorphism. For those who carried the G6PD hemoglobin mutation, the consumption of fava beans could further stress the bearer's hemoglobin and produce a condition known as favism. For the majority population that did not carry the mutation, however, eating fava beans was purely beneficial in that it suppressed the parasite load.[49]

It is likely that our understandings of the significance of the oxidizing spices and plants will improve with further research. At this point, perhaps only a cautious, interim judgment can be advanced: It may not be pure happenstance that peoples who were subject to endemic malaria developed cuisines that conveyed some advantages in lightening the malarial burden.

THE EARLY GLOBALIZATION OF MALARIA

After the establishment of densely settled population centers at numerous sites across Eurasia and North Africa and the rise of more regular trade contact between them from the beginning of the first millennium CE, the web of infectious disease thickened. Some of these trade connections may have involved a simple transfer back and forth of known infections across Eurasia. Others probably involved new patterns of disease. The particulars are lost to the historical record, but there can be little doubt that evolution of a global diaspora of African captives, transferred from the East African coast to Persia, India, and beyond, to China, as well as across the Sahara into the Mediterranean zone, introduced new infections.[50] Because most of

[49] S.H. Katz, "Fava Bean Consumption: A Case for the Evolution of Genes and Culture," in ed. Marvin Harris and Eric B. Ross, *Food and Evolution* (Philadelphia: Temple University Press, 1987), 139–159.

[50] On the volume of slave exports, see Ralph Austen, *African Economic History* (Portsmouth, NH: Heinemann, 1987), app., table A2, 275. For evidence of Africans in China from the fourth century CE, see Graham W. Irwin, *Africans Abroad* (New York: Columbia University Press, 1977), 170–176.

malarial infections were falciparum, it is likely that the trade in African slaves bequeathed a lethal inheritance for the receiving societies.

Another major mixing of infections took place through military conquest and political expansion. This must have been the case with the phenomenal expansion of Islam across northern Africa and much of the southern rim of Eurasia, beginning in the seventh century CE.[51] The new zone of Islamic civilization also encouraged the movement of peoples and brought about an increased mixing of infections, although the levels of malarial infection across the entirety of the Islamic world remained unstable, and societies from Morocco to Indonesia remained subject to epidemic outbreaks.

In the first millennium CE, vivax became more firmly anchored in northern Europe with the (at first) limited adoption in the sixth century CE of the moldboard plow that could be pulled by oxen through heavy soils.[52] This allowed farmers to open up the river-basin soils of northern Europe to agriculture. With agriculture came more settlements, increased river travel, and denser smatterings of peoples organized in webs of relationships, in lands that were climatically less hospitable than those in southern Europe. In northern Europe, as would later be the case in the Americas, malaria followed the plow.

* * *

Human migrants had long been traveling bandwagons of infection. From eastern Africa, they carried malaria into the wider Eurasian world, where a thickening web of interactions between settled peoples gradually created two new discrete zones of malarial infections. In northern Eurasia, the malaria parasites were principally vivax. Following permanent settlement in the river basins of southern Eurasia and northern Africa, a vast zone of mixed infections that included falciparum stretched across the southern expanses of the Eurasian continent to envelop the islands of South and Southeast Asia. The great herding grasslands and deserts of central Eurasia and northern Africa remained largely free of malaria, owing in part to pastoral nomadism.

---

[51] On the general expansion of Muslim commerce and culture, see Patricia Risso, *Merchants and Faith* (Boulder, CO: Westview Press, 1995).

[52] The moldboard plow, with its critically shaped share, cut and turned the soil. The moldboard plow was in use in northern China since at least the third century BCE. Vaclav Smil, *Energy in World History* (Boulder, CO: Westview Press, 1994), 61.

3

Into the Americas

For many millennia after the great extension of malaria from tropical Africa into Eurasia, biological limitations kept the malaria genies bottled up. Early Eurasian voyagers had set out on oceanic missions to explore and colonize the far-flung Pacific islands to the east, and some of these sailors must have carried malaria parasites in their bloodstreams. Throughout the Pacific islands, however, there were no indigenous anopheline mosquitoes and thus no prospect for transmitting malaria. No mosquitoes could have survived the windswept ocean crossing in an open canoe. The malarial infections that the ocean-going migrants carried with them were eventually suppressed by their immune systems. The communities founded in the Pacific islands by the ocean migrants lived free from malaria.

There were also biological constraints on malaria farther to the north. There, the winter temperatures militated against year-round infection. Depending on the species, a few of the fertilized female mosquitoes that harbored malaria parasites might succeed in hibernating indoors, or all the adults died out at the onset of cold weather, and the population overwintered as larvae.[1] In this second case, the new season of infection depended on a relapse of malaria in a sufferer or the arrival of infected migrants who hosted the parasites. For these reasons, the ongoing transmission of malaria within northern Eurasia was fraught with difficulties.

Some of these same northern biological constraints prevented the overland transfer of malaria and other diseases from northern Eurasia to the Americas. During the last glacial maximum circa 19,000 BCE, global

[1] Mike W. Service and Harold Townson, "The Anopheles Vector," in ed. David A. Warrell and Herbert M. Gilles, *Essential Malariology*, 4th ed. (London: Arnold Press, 2002), 69.

ocean levels were about 120 meters below their current levels, and a vast, wide landmass that is today under water connected North America with northeastern Eurasia. Recent microbiological evidence suggests that a small group of Eurasian pioneers crossed the Bering Land Bridge into the Americas at approximately 12,000 BCE, although some scholars have proposed a much earlier arrival.[2] At all events, the arrival of the migrants took place well before the domestication of livestock, and the subsequent thawing out of the glaciers and the submersion of the Bering Land Bridge in about 9000 BCE sealed off the Americas from later waves of migrants who might have crossed from Eurasia with their animals. The Americas thus remained free from the wide array of infectious diseases that were transferred from domesticated animals – the zoonoses – to livestock-keeping human communities in Afro-Eurasia.[3]

The Americas also remained free of malaria. The hunters and foragers who traveled to the Americas were relatively few in number. The migrants departed from northern Eurasia, and some may have been infected with vivax or malariae parasites. But if so, most infections would have died out on their northern journey through Eurasia and across the Bering Land Bridge. Although there were many species of anopheline mosquitoes in the Americas that could host the parasites, early human population densities in the Americas were apparently too low to support any vivax infection that might have reemerged.

Many millennia later, the difficulties of introducing malaria into the Americas remained daunting in the early age of trans-Atlantic voyaging. It is possible that Scandinavian ocean-going vessels might have introduced malaria to Greenland or perhaps even the northeastern expanses of North America during the early contacts that began in the tenth century CE. However, the cold weather and the scant and mobile populations would have ruptured the chains of infection, just as in the northern reaches of Eurasia.[4]

---

[2] Charles C. Mann, *1491: New Revelations of the Americas before Columbus* (New York: Vintage, 2005), 137–173.

[3] Recent research has shown, however, that the populations of the Americas suffered from a variety of illness in the pre-Columbian era. See Richard H. Steckel and Jerome C. Rose, eds., *The Backbone of History: Health and Nutrition in the Western Hemisphere* (New York: Cambridge University Press, 2005).

[4] The Viking sagas and archaeological evidence suggest substantial and well-insulated dwellings in early Norway (personal communication from Professor Richard C. Hoffman, May 2007). It is thus possible that the early Norsemen suffered from malaria; if the vivax parasite were present in Scandinavia in this era, the vector mosquitoes may have found indoor shelter during the winter months and may have been able to circumvent the

By the era of European maritime exploration in the South Atlantic, malaria had taken hold firmly across much of Europe. In southern Europe, vivax and malariae mixed with falciparum, in a witches' brew. Explorers from Spain, Portugal, Italy, and southern France hailed from these zones of mixed infection. But in southern Europe, falciparum was a seasonal infection, and many sufferers cleared the parasites from their systems after surviving a bout of illness. Survivors could be subject to reinfection, but in southern Europe there were no zones of chronically heavy, year-round endemic falciparum infection, as was the case in tropical Africa. Falciparum infections were less prevalent among the European seafarers than vivax or malariae – the run-of-the-mill, common "agues."

The major malaria problem north of the Mediterranean zone stemmed from vivax and, to a lesser degree, malariae parasites. In northwestern Europe, vivax in particular had had considerable success in adapting to the cooler climes. South of Scandinavia, below the 55 degree parallel, the vivax parasite developed an extended incubation period that allowed it to reemerge from the liver after the long winter.[5] Explorers who unfurled their sails in the port harbors of Europe carried vivax parasites with them, and because of the long dormancy of these parasites, vivax infections could break out during a Mid-Atlantic voyage or within the distant landscapes of the New World. This was true of the voluntary immigrants who crossed the Atlantic in search of religious freedoms, profits, and opportunity; the poor who sold themselves into indentured contracts; and the convicts who were banished across the seas.

---

limiting 16 degree C. isotherm below which the vivax parasite could not complete its life cycle.

  In Finland, malaria began to appear at the end of the seventeenth century and grew in importance during the nineteenth century, when workers on large projects became infected and returned to their sending communities. See Lena Huldén, Larry Huldén, and Kari Heliövaara, "Endemic Malaria: An 'Indoor' Disease in Northern Europe. Historical Data Analysed," *Malaria Journal*, vol. 19, no. 4 (2005). This can be found online at http://www.malariajournal.com/content/4/1/19.

[5] These adaptions were complex and varied according to the individual biology of the human host. However, the overall picture is clear enough. People infected with the "Dutch" strain were more than thirty times more likely to have a protracted incubation period than were those infected with the "McCoy" strain, once common in the southern United States. Richard E.L. Paul, Mawlouth Diallo, and Paul T. Brey, "Mosquitoes and Transmission of Malaria Parasites – Not Just Vectors," *Malaria Journal*, vol. 3, no. 1 (2004), 2. This can be found online at http://www.malariajournal.com/content/3/1/39. On the adaptation of vivax, see V.A. Snewin, S. Longacre, and P.H. David. "*Plasmodium Vivax*: Older and Wiser?," *Research in Immunology*, vol. 142 (1991), 631–636.

Falciparum malaria was the great African contribution to the malarial mix in the Americas. From the very beginnings of the dismal Atlantic slave trade, a very high percentage of all West Africans who arrived in the Americas hailed from subregions of intense, continuous endemic infection and carried falciparum parasites in their blood, even though they had achieved functional immunities. These enslaved adults and children also carried the genetic mutation for Duffy negativity that made them unable to contract vivax malaria.

Thus from the late fifteenth century, the initial trickle of explorers, seamen, and adventurers inaugurated a new chapter in the global history of malaria, to be written on the vast Americas. As the transfer of the Afro-Eurasian malarial inheritance to the western hemisphere began, Africans and Europeans extended their patterns of suffering across the Atlantic. To the great misfortune of immigrants and indigenous peoples, throughout the Americas there were anopheline mosquitoes that could host the malaria parasites.[6] The principal constraint to transferring these infections to the New World was a sufficient settled population density. The establishment of malaria in the New World thus fundamentally depended on either of two possibilities: (1) making contact with densely settled indigenous populations, or (2) creating new settlements of European and African free and forced immigrants.

NEW WORLD MALARIAL PATTERNS, 1500–1600

During the sixteenth century, the earliest Iberian activities in the Americas focused on searching out the population concentrations in the Americas, with the hope of discovering great caches of wealth. In the Caribbean, the Spaniards found populous Arawak and Carib settlements. They carried out savage conquests and imposed brutal labor regimes on the conquered, although to the Spaniards' disappointment, they discovered no significant deposits of precious metals on any of the islands.[7] In the process of establishing their dominance on the Caribbean islands, the Spaniards

---

[6] The success of the trans-Atlantic transfer of parasites depended on the anopheline mosquitoes' infectivity. Studies have shown the difficulty that African strains of *P. falciparum* incur in infecting some European mosquitoes. See C.D. Ramsdale and M. Coluzzi, "Studies on the Infectivity of Tropical Strains of *Plasmodium Falciparum* to Some Southern European Vectors of Malaria," *Parassitologia*, vol. 17, nos. 1–3 (1975), 39–48.

[7] The historical demographic evidence does not permit reliable quantification. For a critical exploration of the historiography of the historical demography of the Americas, see David Henige, *Numbers from Nowhere: The American Indian Contact Population Debate* (Norman: University of Oklahoma Press, 1998).

inadvertently introduced a welter of Eurasian diseases that brought about the demographic collapse of the Caribbean peoples within two generations. This collapse was so complete that it threw open the door to the large-scale importation of workers – both Africans and Europeans.[8]

Owing to the limitations of evidence, it is not possible to weigh the contribution of malaria in the population collapse, but it was likely minor. Other infectious diseases such as smallpox and measles were more immediately lethal and probably were responsible for most Carib and Arawak deaths.

In the Central American lowlands surrounding the Caribbean basin, malaria may have become established through the early contacts with explorers even before the arrival of Hernando Cortés in 1519. These contacts, however, were episodic and infrequent, and it is far from certain that malaria made its way to the mainland during these early years.[9] The armies of Cortés most likely extended malaria into the heart of Mexico through the process of conquest, from 1519 to 1521. From Cortés's infected soldiers, malaria eventually spread through both the lowlands and uplands, probably with a higher incidence and greater mortality in the lowlands, in keeping with a global pattern of less efficient transmission at higher altitudes.[10]

The highland anopheline mosquitoes in Central America are capable of transmitting the disease at considerable altitude – up to 2,400 meters or so in the valley of Mexico, and the extended stay of Cortés's army in Tenochtitlan likely provided more than sufficient opportunity to introduce malaria parasites to *A. pseudopunctipennis* and *A. maculipennis* var. *aztecas*, which bred in the lakebeds and extensive swamplands around the Aztec capital city.[11] These vectors were not highly efficient at transmitting

---

[8] The Caribbean was the principal destination for migrants from the British Isles in the period to 1660. Henry A. Gemery, "Emigration from the British Isles to the New World, 1630–1700: Inferences from Colonial Populations," *Research in Economic History*, vol. 5 (1980), 179–231, table A-5.

[9] Nicholás Sanchez-Albornoz suggests that the introduction of malaria may have helped to bring about the depopulation of these regions. He does not, however, produce supporting evidence for this interpretation. See his essay "The Population of Colonial Spanish America," in ed. Leslie Bethell, *The Cambridge History of Latin America, vol. 2, Colonial Latin America* (Cambridge: Cambridge University Press, 1984), 13.

[10] This was the pattern discovered in the 1940s in the state of Veracruz. See Ernest Carroll Faust, "Malaria Incidence in North America," in ed. Mark Boyd, *Malariology* (Philadelphia: Saunders, 1949), 758.

[11] Robert Briggs Watson and Redginal Hewitt, "Topographical and Related Factors in the Epidemiology of Malaria in North America, Central America, and the West Indies," in ed. Forest Ray Moulton, *A Symposium on Human Malaria* (Washington, DC: American

malaria, however, and it seems likely that malaria in Central America was of minor importance during the conquest and probably even during the initial waves of the Eurasian disease epidemics, as in the Caribbean islands.

From Central Mexico, the Spaniards advanced with armies both south and north. By 1524, the southward movement had extended into Guatemala and El Salvador. From there, the Spaniards moved into the Mayan territory of the Yucatan. This was a lengthy process. The Spanish completed their conquest of the Yucatan only in 1547, after the suppression of a large-scale uprising.[12] It is likely that during these decades malaria gained a foothold and then became established throughout Central America and the Yucatan peninsula.[13]

Into northern Mexico, Nuño de Guzman launched a destructive campaign of conquest and carved out the vast kingdom of New Galicia between 1529 and 1536. The Spaniards then sent out two further expeditions: that of Hernando de Soto toward the southeast of North America and that of Francisco Vásquez Coronado to the west of the Mississippi in futile searches for wealth. Their malaria parasites almost certainly died out in the thinly peopled landscapes of the American deserts.

A second wave of mainland conquest started in Panama. The Spaniards moved briefly northward to pillage Nicaragua and then took a Pacific Ocean route south to Peru. From the Peruvian coast, Francisco Pizarro and his fellow conquistadores ascended into the towering Andes Mountains. There, in a political and military coup, Pizarro murdered the Inca, established the murdered ruler's half-brother as Inca, and ruled through him. The installation of a new political regime was accompanied by a new epidemiological order. The malaria parasites that were introduced into western South America were largely confined to the coastal plains and

Association for the Advancement of Science, 1941), 142–143. The same species transmit malaria in the highlands of Guatemala, at elevations of up to 5,000 feet.

[12] Nancy M. Farriss, *Maya Society under Colonial Rule: The Collective Enterprise of Survival* (Princeton: Princeton University Press, 1984), 14.

[13] Ernest Carroll Faust noted of the mid-twentieth-century distribution of parasites: "In the interior of Mexico, in Guatemala, Nicaragua, Costa Rica and Panama, *Plasmodium vivax* preponderates; in Nicaragua it is reported to constitute 79.5 percent of the total infections. In Cuba, extensive surveys indicate that *P. vivax* and *P. falciparum* are about equal. In the littoral areas of Mexico and in Yucatan, in El Salvador, Honduras, Haiti, Republica Dominica and the Less Antilles, *P. falciparum* is much the more common species, or at least is the species most commonly found in blood examinations" (Ernest Carroll Faust, "The Distribution of Malaria in North America, Central America and the West Indies," in Moulton, *A Symposium on Human Malaria*, 16).

foothills of the Andes. Its southward extension was checked by the aridity of the Chilean coastal desert. *A. pseudopunctipennis* could breed in the river valleys that were fed by the snow-capped mountains of the Andes, but it could not breed southward across the long stretches of desert and could only extend its range as far as 20 or 21 degrees south latitude along the Pacific coast, as opposed to 31 degrees south latitude along the Atlantic riverine coasts in northern Argentina. Nowhere in South America did vivax malaria approach its maximum theoretical extension, as estimated by the limiting summer isotherm of 15 degrees C.[14]

At the upper elevations malaria probably continued to fluctuate from year to year, owing to changes in temperature. *A. pseudopunctipennis* is the highest vector of malaria in the world with endemic malaria reported in Bolivia above 2,600 meters. Although highland malaria was common in Peru and Bolivia, it became increasingly rare to the north of Ecuador. There was little malaria in the Colombian highlands, and this inability to transmit malaria extended north to Guatemala, for reasons that are not well understood.[15]

In eastern South America, the historical patterns of malarial infection were different. Following Pedro Álvares Cabral's voyage in 1500, Portuguese and other traders regularly began to make landfall along the lightly peopled Brazilian coast, taking on fresh water and supplies and seeking to stimulate a trade in dyewoods, particularly the brilliant reddish violet hue that could be extracted from the tree known as brazilwood. The early trading encounters intensified into a system of modest exports by the mid-sixteenth century. The small bands of indigenous peoples that the Europeans contacted probably remained largely and perhaps entirely malaria free, because the trading contacts were brief and episodic.[16]

---

[14] L.W. Hackett, "The Malaria of the Andean Region of South America," *Revista del Instituto de Salubridad y Enfermedades Tropicales*, vol. 6, no. 4 (1945), 241–242.

[15] Ibid., 249–250.

[16] The size of the population of Amazonia at first contact with the diseases of Africa and Europe is unknown. William Denevan has estimated its population at 6.8 million and, in an addendum that incorporates the idea of the buffer zone between Amazonian peoples, at 5.1 million (William M. Denevan, "The Aboriginal Population of Amazonia," in ed. William M. Denevan, *The Native Population of the Americas in 1492*, 2nd ed. [Madison: University of Wisconsin Press, 1992], 205–234). This is considerably higher than earlier estimates. See Maria Luiza Marcílio, "The Population of Colonial Brazil," in ed. Leslie Bethell, *Cambridge History of Latin America, vol. 2, Colonial Latin America* (Cambridge: Cambridge University Press, 1984), 39. The political significance of the size of the precontact Amazonian population is explored in Mann, *1491*, 280–311.

A turning point in the epidemiological relationship with indigenous peoples took place in the mid-1530s, when the first Portuguese colonists arrived in Brazil and began to search for laborers, in addition to brazilwood. This developed into a tradition of slave raiding deep into the interior of the continent. This slaving tradition was countered by the efforts of missionaries to protect the indigenous peoples from these depredations by concentrating them in settlements and converting them to permanently settled ways of life.[17]

A pivotal change took place in the middle of the sixteenth century, when Portuguese entrepreneurs introduced sugarcane to the coastal lowlands of Brazil. Indigenous peoples caught up in the Bandeirantes' slave-trading operations were sold to the newly created plantations.[18] The sugar industry demanded laborers, and the indigenous peoples of Brazil who were captured were few in number, relative to the demand, and they did not survive long. They were poorly prepared to weather the mixed malarial infections and other Eurasian and African diseases that battered the plantations.

The sugar plantations, grinding mills, and boiling houses of northeast Brazil were the sites of the earliest intensive use of African labor in industrial agriculture. By the 1550s, Africans began to replace indigenous Brazilians as plantation workers.[19] There, by the end of the sixteenth century, plantations produced soaring profits so high that the plantation technologies and the use of African slave labor became a kind of economic and social template that could be transferred to other lowland regions in the South Atlantic basin. These profits fueled the extraordinary growth of the sugar-and-slave economy in the New World.[20]

The significance of the plantation complex for malarial infections was large. The imported African workers carried the genetic mutation for Duffy negativity and were unable to contract vivax malaria. Most arrived in Brazil with some functional immunity to falciparum malaria, although most carried parasites in their bodies and were highly infectious, even if asymptomatic. They produced a lethal falciparum zone in northeast Brazil that was quite distinct from the highland and lowland pattern of mixed

---

[17] Warren Dean, *With Broadax and Firebrand: The Destruction of the Brazilian Atlantic Forest* (Berkeley: University of California Press, 1995), 59–60.

[18] Richard M. Morse, "Introduction: The Historical Role of the Bandeirantes," in ed. Richard M. Morse, *The Bandeirantes: The Historical Role of the Brazilian Pathfinders* (New York: Knopf, 1964), 3–36.

[19] Dean, *With Broadax and Firebrand*, 83.

[20] Philip D. Curtin, *The Rise and Fall of the Plantation Complex* (New York: Cambridge University Press, 1990), 48–53.

infections that characterized the early Caribbean, Central America, and western South America. By the late sixteenth century, these zones of fever blended across parts of the northern and southern fringes of the Caribbean. Even the "wild coast" of Guyana, so-called because it lay outside of the jurisdiction both of the Spanish possessions on the Orinoco and the Portuguese in Brazil, was fever ridden by the late sixteenth century.[21]

NEW WORLD MALARIAL PATTERNS, 1600–1700

The history of malarial infections along the eastern seaboard of British North America shares some similarities with that of Spanish America, although its evolution took place later, in the course of the seventeenth century. There is no evidence to suggest that early sparse contacts produced malarial infections among the indigenous peoples during the sixteenth century. Neither the handful of Spanish Jesuit missionaries who visited the Chesapeake Bay in the 1570s nor the English colonists who founded the short-lived community at Roanoke in the 1580s succeeded in establishing malaria. In the case of the Spanish Jesuits, although it is possible that some carried malaria parasites – because Spain was awash in infections – their contacts with the indigenous peoples were extremely limited. The Roanoke settlers were recruited from the county of Devon, outside of the malarial zone in England. They probably arrived in the New World malaria free.

Malaria seems to have first gained a foothold in the ecological systems of the middle seaboard of North America at the Jamestown settlement, founded in 1607. Many of the original colonists at Jamestown were originally from Kent, Essex, Somerset, and greater London, all of which were hotbeds of English malaria, and thus were accustomed to the "ague," as the fits of malaria were known. Other colonists apparently were not. After Governor De La Warr arrived in Jamestown in 1610, he "was welcommed by a hote and violent Ague."[22] Other seventeenth-century observers also noted that Virginians were subject to "agues."[23] From the feverish colonial settlement, malaria was probably extended, at least episodically, to the local Native American communities.

---

[21] David Watts, *The West Indies: Patterns of Development, Culture, and Environmental Change since 1492* (New York: Cambridge University Press, 1987), 136.

[22] Thomas West De La Warr, *The Relation of the Right Honourable the Lord De-La-Warre, Lord Governour and Captaine Generall of the Colonie, Planted in Virginea* (London: W. Hall for W. Welbie, 1611), n.p.

[23] Jon Kukla, "Kentish Agues and American Distempers: The Transmission of Malaria from England to Virginia in the Seventeenth Century," *Southern Studies*, vol. 25 (1986), 135–147.

Historians of early America have closely examined the evidence for these early North American malarial infections. To the north of Jamestown, in the Chesapeake region, malaria became endemic during the seventeenth century and was a part of the gruesome "seasoning" that newcomers had to undergo. Even immigrants from the malarial estuarine regions of eastern and southern England had to submit to these malarial trials, because they encountered new variants of vivax and malariae to which they had no immunities.[24]

The historical evidence also suggests a shift toward more virulent malarial infections by the second half of the seventeenth century that included falciparum.[25] The first tropical Africans began to reach the North American seaboard colonies as early as 1619, but only from the 1660s did substantial numbers of tropical African unfree laborers arrive, and Virginia began to evolve toward a slave society.[26] South Carolina apparently went through a similar transition to a more virulent malarial environment in the 1680s.[27] There, too, with the arrival of African slaves, the falciparum parasites more fully entered the mix. The establishment of denser settlements allowed infections to increase in the late seventeenth century and early eighteenth century when malaria emerged as the most important killer in the North American colonies.[28]

By the end of the seventeenth century, the three great zones of Afro-Eurasian malaria had been transferred to North America. The New England region lay squarely in the vivax-predominant zone.[29] Malarial outbreaks occurred first in Massachusetts in 1634, and then in 1647, 1650,

[24] For a discussion of the changing strains of infection within England, see Mary J. Dobson, *Contours of Death and Disease in Early Modern England* (Cambridge: Cambridge University Press, 1997), 356–357.

[25] Darrett B. Rutman and Anita H. Rutman, "Of Agues and Fevers: Malaria in the Early Chesapeake," *William and Mary Quarterly*, vol. 33, no. 1 (1976), 42–43.

[26] Anthony Parent, *Foul Means: The Formation of a Slave Society in Virginia, 1660–1740* (Chapel Hill: University of North Carolina Press, 2003).

[27] Peter H. Wood, *Black Majority: Negroes in Colonial South Carolina from 1670 through the Stono Rebellion* (New York: Knopf, 1974), 87–91.

[28] John Duffy, *Epidemics in Colonial America* (Port Washington, NY: Kennicat Press, 1972), 213–214.

[29] This pattern held into the mid-twentieth century. As Ernest Carroll Faust noted, "In North America P. falciparum and P. malariae are not normally indigenous north of the Ohio River Valley in the region east of the Mississippi River, while their distribution west of the Mississippi probably extends northward only into southern Missouri and to the northern boundary of Oklahoma" (Faust, "The Distribution of Malaria in North America, Central America and the West Indies," 8).

and 1668.[30] Vivax only fitfully was extended farther north into northern New England and Canada.[31] It remained episodic, severely constrained by the cooler temperatures.

The zone of mixed infections that reached across the upper-Mid-Atlantic colonies marked the most northward extension of the zone of mixed malaria that included falciparum. Along the British North American seaboard, in this zone of mixed infections, there were two significant gradients of intensity. One ran from the coast into the interior. The most intensely infectious environments were in the tidewater zone, and infections became fewer and less intense as one moved westward.[32] The other gradient stretched from the south to north. Falciparum became less prevalent as one moved north from Virginia into Maryland, Pennsylvania, and New Jersey.

In the rice-growing areas of South Carolina, to the south of Virginia, falciparum became the dominant infection, owing to the arrival of substantial numbers of parasitized tropical Africans who came to constitute a black majority population. This zone extended south from South Carolina down to the Caribbean islands.

The shift toward greater virulence in South Carolina and Virginia was part of a major transformation of the Caribbean malarial environment that took place in the mid-seventeenth century. Before the mid-seventeenth century, indentured servants from the British Isles made up the principal flow of workers to the British Caribbean and British North America. After the establishment of yellow fever and malaria in the American tropics, the nonimmune European laborers suffered greatly increased mortality and morbidity. The upshot was that tropical African laborers gained a reputation for living longer and remaining healthier than European workers. This brought about a transition in labor use that substituted enslaved African workers for indentured Europeans.[33]

---

[30] M.J. Quinn, "Malaria in New England," *Boston Medical and Surgical Journal*, vol. 193 (1926), 244–247.

[31] In New England, malaria declined in incidence in the late eighteenth and early nineteenth centuries (see Oliver Wendell Holmes, "Dissertation on Intermittent Fever in New England," *Boylston Prize Dissertations* [Boston: C.C. Little and J. Brown, 1838]). Interestingly, Holmes's correspondent who reported on malaria in the state of Maine was a professor of classics at Waterville College. This institution was later renamed Colby College and is the employer of the present author.

[32] Mary J. Dobson, "Mortality Gradients and Disease Exchanges: Comparisons from Old England and Colonial America," *Social History of Medicine*, vol. 2 (1989), 272.

[33] Philip R.P. Coelho and Robert A. McGuire, "African and European Bound Labor in the British New World: The Biological Consequences of Economic Choices," *Journal of Economic History*, vol. 57, no. 1 (1997), 83–115.
     Some scholars have asserted that there was a similar cost to African American workers

The volume of the Atlantic slave trade to the islands increased dramatically when other Europeans adopted the sugar plantation template, and French, British, Dutch, and Danish capitalists purchased tens of thousands of enslaved Africans annually and put them to hard labor growing tropical produce – first and foremost, sugar, but also coffee, tobacco, indigo, and an array of minor crops. On the plantations in the South Atlantic basin, the influx of African slaves with vivax resistance meant that falciparum parasites out-competed vivax in areas where Africans outnumbered Europeans. This, in turn, intensified the danger for nonimmunes, who were Europeans. The arrival of large numbers of African workers thus hastened the demise of the earlier system that had depended mostly on white indentured workers. Europeans were susceptible to both vivax and falciparum; tropical Africans were completely refractory to vivax and most had functional immunities to falciparum. This translated into a powerful epidemiological differential that underwrote the dependence of the plantation system on the importation of African slaves.

The establishment of a predominantly falciparum zone in the Caribbean also required anopheline mosquitoes that could transmit the parasites. The principal vector, A. *albimanus*, was limited to low altitudes and coastal regions, but its habitat was extensive and spread across most of the Greater Antilles of the central and western Caribbean. In the Lesser Antilles of the eastern Caribbean and in Trinidad, the main vector was A. *aquasalis* whose habitat was restricted to coastal regions.[34] For this reason, the islands of the Lesser Antilles were deemed healthier than

in the United States who lived in northern climes, where the crude death rate for blacks was higher than the crude death rates for whites – the obverse of the malarial gradient. The most likely disease candidate responsible for this differential would seem to be tuberculosis. Although recent research has confirmed a greater susceptibility of blacks than whites to tuberculosis infection, no higher percentage of blacks than whites who are exposed to infection progress to clinical symptoms of the disease. This suggests that other variables – including income level, material conditions of housing, and diet (all of which are not quantifiable in the historical records and which contribute to tububerculosis becoming symptomatic) – may have played determinative roles. For a race-specific interpretation, see Christian Warren, "Northern Chills, Southern Fevers: Race Specific Mortality in American Cities, 1730–1900," *Journal of Southern History*, vol. 63, no. 1 (1997), 23–56.

Studies of aboriginal Canadian populations have suggested that some populations carry an inherited predisposition to the progression of clinical tuberculosis. See Laurent Abel and Jean-Laurent Casanova, "Genetic Predisposition to Clinical Tuberculosis: Bridging the Gap between Simple and Complex Inheritance," *American Journal of Human Genetics*, vol. 67, no. 2 (2000), 274–277.

[34] Philip D. Curtin, "Malarial Immunities in Nineteenth-Century West Africa and the Caribbean," *Parassitologia*, vol. 36 (1994), 70.

elsewhere in the Caribbean basin. Within the Lesser Antilles, Antigua and St. Vincent apparently enjoyed lower rates of malarial infection. To the north of the Lesser Antilles, the Bahamas apparently did as well.[35] This was likely owing to the limited swampy mosquito habitat on these islands. Another distinction, valid throughout the Caribbean, drew on the differences between the highlands and lowlands. As ever, the highlands were generally considered to be healthier.[36] Neither *A. albimanus* nor *A. aquasalis* had a particularly strong preference for human blood, and thus the intensity of malarial infection throughout the population was lower than in tropical Africa.

The major anomaly in the Caribbean basin was Barbados. The island did not have anopheline mosquitoes, and thus malaria transmission was nil. Any infected Europeans or tropical Africans who arrived on the island with malaria were unable to infect others. For this reason, Barbados – although subject to yellow fever epidemics and a host of other tropical diseases like the rest of the Caribbean – gained a reputation as a salubrious colony. In the period to 1675, it attracted more British immigrants than any other New World colony. Barbados even established itself as a sanatorium for malaria sufferers.[37]

---

[35] August Hirsch, *Handbook of Geographical and Historical Pathology*, vol. 1 (London: New Sydenham Society, 1883), 220.

[36] In the first half of the nineteenth century, preventive medicine, built on a foundation of empirical observation, won a notable victory when the British opened a barracks in the Blue Mountains above Kingston, Jamaica in 1841 (Curtin, "Malarial Immunities," 75).

In the Usambara mountains in Tanzania, researchers discovered that the intensity of exposure to falciparum malaria parasites and infection was negatively correlated with a 100-meter increase in elevation between 300 and 1,700 meters. See René Bødker et al., "Relationship between the Intensity of Exposure to Malaria Parasites and Infection in the Usambara Mountains, Tanzania," *American Journal of Tropical Medicine and Hygiene*, vol. 74, no. 5 (2006), 716–723.

[37] This reputation continued at least into the late nineteenth century (Hirsch, *Handbook of Geographical and Historical Pathology*, 220). A medical visitor's report from 1867 states that "Yellow fever seldom occurs in the island, and intermittent very rarely" (J.B.S. Jackson, "Diseases of the Island of Barbadoes," *Boston Medical and Surgical Journal*, vol. 76, no. 22 [July 4, 1867], 447).

Apparently, it was only in the twentieth century that the vector *A. albimanus* was introduced, by steamship, to the island. In 1927, an epidemic of more than one thousand cases of falciparum racked the island. See Mark F. Boyd, "Historical Sketch of the Prevalence of Malaria in North America," *American Journal of Tropical Medicine*, vol. 21 (1941), 228; Rubert W. Boyce, *Health Progress and Administration in the West Indies* (New York: J. Murray, 1910), 144–146.

Richard S. Dunn, on the basis of fragmentary surviving documentation, has judged that English life expectancies in the English West Indies in the seventeenth century

The broad picture thus is that falciparum infections became most intense in the South Atlantic, in regions where tropical Africans became numerically significant. The New World came to mirror the tropical and subtropical distribution of malaria in the Old World. This was owed in part to warmer temperatures and in larger part to the fact that tropical African workers were settled to work rice, coffee, tobacco, and sugar plantations in the South Atlantic basin.[38] Beyond the plantation complex lay the patterns of forced resettlement of indigenous peoples, by dint of missionary zeal or the conquistadores' ruthless demands for the control of Amerindian labor. These settlements also produced nodes of infectious disease, of which malaria was one.

The biological constraints to the transfer of malaria from Europe and from Africa to the New World thus were remarkably few. The trans-Atlantic transfer of malaria was accomplished early in the Columbian Exchange. This chapter in the history of malaria stands in stark contrast to the difficulties – the near impossibility – of transferring strains of falciparum malaria from tropical Africa to Europe.[39] Southern Europeans took tropical African captives in considerable numbers to Portugal in the fifteenth and sixteenth centuries but never succeeded inadvertently in introducing the tropical African falciparum strains to the Mediterranean region.

MALARIAL CONSEQUENCES OF THE TRANSFORMATION OF NEW WORLD ECOLOGIES

Europeans, Africans, and Native Americans were agents of continuous ecological change in the Americas. The broad themes in the globe-altering exchange of plants and animals – as well as diseases – have become known as the Columbian Exchange since the publication of Alfred W. Crosby's book with this title in 1972.[40] More recent scholarship has highlighted the significance of Africans and Native Americans, supplementing and broadening the literature that initially stressed the impact of European agency.[41]

(including on Barbados) were significantly shorter than in England (Richard S. Dunn, *Sugar and Slaves* [Chapel Hill: University of North Carolina Press, 1972], 301).

[38] Curtin, *The Rise and Fall of the Plantation Complex*.

[39] C.D. Ramsdale and M. Coluzzi, "Studies on the Infectivity of Tropical Strains of *Plasmodium Falciparum* to Some Southern European Vectors of Malaria," *Parassitologia*, vol. 17, nos. 1–3 (1975), 39–48.

[40] Alfred W. Crosby, *The Columbian Exchange: The Biological and Cultural Consequences of 1492* (Westport, CT: Greenwood Publishing, 1972).

[41] For an example of African ecological agency, see Judith A. Carney, *Black Rice: The African Origins of Rice Cultivation in the Americas* (Cambridge, MA: Harvard

The transfer of Old World domesticated livestock animals – in particular the cow, horse, goat, and sheep – reworked the ecologies of the New World. The sheep and the goat likely made their principal contributions by compacting soil and selectively grazing, thereby broadly influencing the regional composition of plant mosaics. The horse served initially as a war animal and signified European military dominance. However, as early as the end of the sixteenth century, beginning in northern Mexico, the horse also became a working animal to herd cattle. Over the course of the late seventeenth century through the eighteenth century, some Native American groups on the Great Plains of North America adopted the horse and created their own culture of pastoral nomadism. The cow made three major contributions: as a herded animal, it allowed subsistence-oriented cattle keepers to launch processes of exploration into the Brazilian interior; as a draft animal, it made possible the working of the sugar mills, through the hauling of fuel wood and harvested cane and the turning of the giant sugar presses, and it facilitated the movement of goods to market; and as a commercialized meat animal, it provided protein for workers in mines (as well as leather and tallow, as fuel for underground torches) and on plantations.

The introduction of Old World animals also helped to shape three very broad patterns of land-use change in the Americas, and these in turn had decisive influences on the epidemiology of New World malaria. The first was the Spanish pattern found throughout mainland Central America. It was based on the fact that the Spaniards, while exploiting the precious metal deposits in Mexico and Peru, took the agricultural reorganization of the Central American peoples under their authority. The conquistadores received large land grants known as *encomiendas* that included rights to the labor of the peoples on their land. Old World animals were integrated into the *encomiendas*, following on the collapse of Native American populations. A new economic order emerged in Central America, after the failure to find exploitable gold and silver deposits and after a brief effort to force Native Americans into villages for purposes of conversion to Christianity or to enslave them to grow cacao. The net result was to regroup Native Americans into denser

University Press, 2001); on African influence more generally, see John Thornton, *Africa and Africans in the Making of the Atlantic World* (New York: Cambridge University Press, 1998). On Native American agency and precontact historical processes, see Mann, *1491*.

settlements for agricultural labor that rendered the inhabitants more vulnerable to crowd diseases.[42]

A similar pattern, with variations, appeared in the Andes and in Mexico. In both regions, the Spaniards found exploitable silver deposits, and laborers were brought in and concentrated in mining camps. The most famous of these settlements, Potosí (in what is today Bolivia) grew to a population of roughly 150,000 by 1600. Elsewhere, the general model was that of the *encomienda*, a concentration of Native Americans and a new order of agriculture, shaped by the use of draft animals. The predominant malarial infections were vivax and malariae, but their intensities undoubtedly varied greatly over time and space. In the highlands of the Andes as on the plains of central Mexico, there were highland anopheline mosquitoes, but the incidence of malaria – judging by twentieth-century evidence – was probably low, compared to the malarial zone of the coastal plains of Central America, the northern and southern reaches of the Pacific coast of South America, and the Amazon basin.[43]

A second pattern of land-use change in the Americas can be traced back to the agricultural fields of tropical Africa. The slave ships that transported the Africans in chains also carried foodstuffs from Africa to keep the captives fed in transit across the Atlantic. These foodstuffs made their way into the garden fields that were spotted around the slave settlements, near the sugar fields and the placer mines.[44] Present in these gardens were the Guinea yams, part of the great H-P-P complex that had emerged over millennia of tropical African experience. In the South Atlantic basin, however, yams never made up the principal foodstuff, and tropical Africans in bondage never reconstituted the new yam festivals or the prohibitions on eating new yams that had been a feature of some West African cultures. Whatever the effect of yams on the falciparum parasites in West Africa, it was muted in the South Atlantic basin.[45]

---

[42] Murdo J. MacLeod, *Spanish Central America: A Socioeconomic History, 1520–1720* (Berkeley: University of California Press, 1973).

[43] Hackett, "The Malaria of the Andean Regions," 240.

[44] Watts, *The West Indies*, 115, 162. Watts states on p. 115 that yams from Africa were introduced into the Spanish settlements in the early sixteenth century and on p. 162 that "African yams (probably *Dioscorea alata* and *D. bulbifera*)" were introduced into the early Northwest European plantations shortly after 1630.

[45] A similar biological relationship seems to have developed following the introduction of cassava (*Manihot esculenta*) from Brazil to Africa during the era of the Atlantic slave trade, although the African adoption of cassava has been too recent for a truly coevolutionary relationship to develop. Cassava also releases chemicals that appear to have had a similar double effect. These mutual symbioses are probably a simple fortuity, reinforced by the

A third pattern of land-use change was rooted in the sugar plantations in both the French and British Caribbean, which held surprisingly often to the same basic pattern. They were ideally sited with ample pastureland around the cane fields to provide forage for the draft animals on whose power the mills and plantations turned. The draft animals, as well as goats and sheep, were penned. This provided an alternate blood meal for the mosquitoes, and thus probably reduced the pressures on the anopheline mosquitoes to specialize in human blood.[46] This was far from the "mixed

more obvious and appreciable high caloric yields from cassava cultivation.

As Fatimah Jackson notes: "It is highly probable that important sequential changes have occurred in the quality and quantity of H-P-P relationships during the last 150,000 years of human evolution. . . . [T]hese changes reflect changes in human identification and use of particular plants, modifications in plant biology associated with the domestication process, changing patterns of human contact with plant secondary compounds (allelochemicals), alterations in human residential patterns influencing contact with various human parasites, transformations in various parasites to accommodate changes in human behavior and physiochemistry, and the effects of reciprocal changes in all of the above." Fatimah Jackson, "Ecological Modeling of Human-Plant-Parasite Coevolutionary Triads: Theoretical Perspectives on the Interrelationships of Human HbßS, G6PD, *Manihot esculenta, Vicia faba,* and *Plasmodium falciparum,*" in ed. Lawrence S. Greene and Maria Enrica Danubio, *Adaptation to Malaria: The Interaction of Biology and Culture* (Amsterdam: Gordon and Breach, 1997), 180; Stuart J. Edelstein, *The Sickled Cell: From Myths to Molecules* (Cambridge, MA: Harvard University Press, 1986), 61–64; W.H. Durham, "Testing the Malaria Hypothesis in West Africa," in ed. J.E. Bowman, *Distribution and Evolution of Hemoglobin and Globin Loci* (New York: Elsevier, 1983), 45–76.

[46] The zooprophylactic impacts are larger when the mosquito preference for human blood is moderate or low. The reasons are as follows: for malaria to be transmitted, a mosquito must take two successive blood meals from different human beings. The first allows the mosquito to take up the malaria parasites (gametocytes) with her human blood meal; the second allows the mosquito to inject the malaria parasites (sporozoites) into a human being. If one pens livestock, and provides a large stock of potential blood meals for the mosquitoes, it is possible to cause malaria transmission among humans to drop considerably. As in all malariological matters, there are many other important variables, including the density of anopheline mosquitoes, the constraints of the larval habitat, and the distance of the animal pens from human dwellings. (For a recent modeling effort that reformulates some of the classic epidemiology of George MacDonald, *The Epidemiology and Control of Malaria* [London: Oxford University Press, 1957], see Allan Saul, "Zooprophylaxis or Zoopotentiation: The Outcome of Introducing Animals on Vector Transmission Is Highly Dependent on the Mosquito Mortality While Searching," *Malaria Journal,* vol. 2 [2003]; this can be found online at http://www.malariajournal.com/content/2/1/32).

It is possible that an increase in anopheline density as a result of blood meals from domesticated livestock could produce an increase in malaria infections. This "zoopotentiation" has been documented in a few areas where livestock are kept within a human compound, in which people sleep outside (see Menno Bouma and Mark Rowland, "Failure of Passive Zooprophylaxis: Cattle Ownership in Pakistan Is Associated with a Higher Prevalence of Malaria," *Transactions of the Royal Society*

farming" model that integrated livestock with agriculture that was credited centuries later with reducing the malarial burden in Europe, but its effect was likely similar.[47] The lower rates of transmission meant that peoples of African and mixed African and European descent in the Caribbean ("West Indians") never acquired the fully functional immunities that Africans did in the holoendemic regions of tropical Africa. Immunities acquired in Africa could protect one, however, in the Caribbean malarial environment.[48]

The Caribbean Basin developed into a lethal environment for non-immunes. This was true for military expeditions as well as for efforts at settlement. The epidemiological consequences were severe. In 1655, the English took the island of Jamaica from the Spaniards with seven thousand men and later added eight hundred reinforcements, but by January of 1656, more than five thousand had died from malaria and dysentery.[49] The disease environment remained deadly into the nineteenth century. From 1794 to 1795, the British invaded the French colony of Saint Domingue to suppress an uprising by African slaves and people of mixed race that threatened the slave system throughout the South Atlantic. The British force lost an estimated one hundred thousand troops to yellow fever and malaria.[50] In 1801, the rebels declared the independent state of Haiti, and the following year, the French tried to reimpose their control over the island of plantations. A similar epidemiological disaster befell the troops of Napoleon. Some sixty thousand troops were reduced to seven thousand by malaria and other tropical diseases.[51] The epidemiological disasters suffered by the Europeans helped to solidify the insurgents' new structures of authority.

---

of *Tropical Medicine and Hygiene*, vol. 89 [1995], 351–353). To my knowledge, there is no historical evidence of this pattern in the Americas.

[47] Watts, *West Indies*, 387–390; L.W. Hackett, *Malaria in Europe: An Ecological Study* (London: Oxford University Press, 1937).

[48] Curtin, "Malarial Immunities," 79–80.

[49] S.A.G. Taylor, *The Western Design: An Account of Cromwell's Expedition to the Caribbean*, 2nd ed. (London: Solstice Productions, 1969), 16–17. Cited by John F. Richards, *The Unending Frontier: An Environmental History of the Modern World* (Berkeley: University of California Press, 2003), 442.

[50] Watts, *West Indies*, 255–256. Interestingly, in Saint Domingue, the causes of mortality were surprisingly localized. As commonly known at the time, yellow fever occurred only in the towns and malaria was found near the swamps (David Geggus, "Yellow Fever in the 1790s: The British Army in Occupied Saint Domingue," *Medical History*, vol. 23 [1979], 56).

[51] Tim Matthewson, "Napoleon's Haitian Guerilla War," *Military History*, vol. 18, no. 6 (2002), 30–36.

The importation of millions of African slaves thus extended the epidemiological zone of tropical Africa across the South Atlantic Ocean into the Americas.[52] Falciparum malaria was only one of the diseases from which West Africans suffered the indignities of insult and eventually built up immunities. The mid-seventeenth-century introduction of the *Aedes aegypti* mosquito-borne viral infection of yellow fever also underscored the huge epidemiological differential between Europeans and tropical Africans in the South Atlantic. Most tropical Africans brought to the Americas had been exposed in childhood to a mild form of yellow fever in Africa and had achieved life-long immunity. Europeans, by contrast, were immunologically naïve.

It is possible that peoples of African descent born in the Americas may have inherited some resistance to yellow fever.[53] If so, some difference in susceptibility to yellow fever between peoples of European and African descent may have persisted – even absent the importation of new immunes. In any case, the large-scale importation of enslaved Africans with yellow fever immunities over the course of the seventeenth, eighteenth, and much of the nineteenth century maintained this differential. The presence of a large number of Africa-born immunes reduced the possibility of endemic transmission of yellow fever on the slave plantations. The result was that yellow fever struck principally as an epidemic disease and seems to have targeted principally Europeans. It may have been as large a killer – or larger – of Europeans as malaria. It is impossible to sort out the relative weights of these two diseases, because their symptoms were often similar, and the diseases were often confused with one another. The upshot was that as early as the late seventeenth century the double barrier of yellow fever and falciparum malaria closed the door to a large-scale presence of European laborers in the Caribbean islands.

[52] The malariologist Marshall Barber estimated that the proportions of falciparum, malariae, and vivax infections in Haiti in the first half of the twentieth century were about the same as in West Africa (Marshall A. Barber, *A Malariologist in Many Lands* [Lawrence: University of Kansas Press, 1946], 30–31).

[53] Donald B. Cooper and Kenneth F. Kiple, "Yellow Fever," in ed. Kenneth F. Kiple, *The Cambridge World History of Human Disease* (New York: Cambridge University Press, 1993), 1101–1102. This issue has been hotly contested. See Sheldon Watts, "Yellow Fever Immunities in West Africa and the Americas in the Age of Slavery and Beyond: A Reappraisal," *Journal of Social History*, vol. 34, no. 4 (2001), 955–967; Kenneth F. Kiple, "Response to Sheldon Watts," *Journal of Social History*, vol. 34, no. 4 (2001), 969–974; Sheldon Watts, "Reply to Kenneth Kiple," *Journal of Social History*, vol. 34, no. 4 (2001), 975–976.

A similar long-standing barrier had guarded the interior of tropical Africa. The danger of falciparum malaria along the African coasts fore-closed the effective exploration of the interior of tropical Africa and the possibility of European-dominated plantations in tropical Africa during the long centuries of the Atlantic slave trade.[54] As recent scholarship has shown, the coastal balance of power in Africa between Europeans and Africans during the course of the Atlantic slave trade was decisively in favor of the Africans.[55] It was extremely difficult even to maintain European trading communities along the coast.[56]

The epidemiological disaster that lay in wait for European merchant seamen who were delayed in taking on their cargoes along the African waterways and in the African ports-of-call established the rhythms of the slave trade along the African coasts. One of the ironies of the Atlantic slave trade was that African workers were hired on as crew – because of their immunological resistance. Africans from the Caribbean and Africans and African Americans from North America also served on the ethnically mixed ships, some as slave workers and some as free men.[57]

NEW WORLD MALARIAL FRONTIERS, 1700–1800

Major frontiers of malaria developed over the course of the eighteenth century that pushed malarial infections deep into both the South American and North American continents. In Brazil, owing to the rise of competing Caribbean plantations run by British and French rivals, the fortunes of the Portuguese sugar plantation complex went into a period of decline in the mid-seventeenth century. This downturn was soon followed, however, by the discovery of surface deposits of gold in the late seventeenth century and then diamonds in the early eighteenth century. These deposits were in the distant hinterlands of the littoral towns of São Vicente and São Paulo, located several hundred kilometers in the interior of the continent.

---

[54] Philip D. Curtin, "Epidemiology and the Slave Trade," *Political Science Quarterly*, vol. 83 (1968), 190–216.

[55] John K. Thornton in his book *Africa and Africans in the Making of the Atlantic World* (New York: Cambridge University Press, 1998) has presented convincing evidence that the older interpretations that stressed European agency in wresting African workers from the continent need to be fundamentally revised.

[56] George E. Brooks, *Eurafricans in Western Africa* (Athens: Ohio University Press, 2003).

[57] On African and African American crew and the multicultural world of the slave ships, see Emma Christopher, *Slave Ship Sailors and Their Captive Cargoes* (New York: Cambridge University Press, 2006), 51–90.

These discoveries set off a massive scramble for wealth. Portuguese immigrants flooded into Brazil. Some moved into the interior on their own, as wildcat prospectors. Most Portuguese immigrants, however, purchased African slave workers, who were beginning to be brought across the South Atlantic from central Africa in large numbers. These population movements launched the Brazilian "mining century" of the 1700s, a process of internal colonization through which Portuguese immigrants and their African workers trekked into the interior province, later known as the General Mines (Minas Gerais), and set up mining camps, where they panned for gold and diamonds. More than one million tropical Africans flowed with their masters into the heart of the continent.[58]

New farms were established to feed the miners. A cattle industry expanded westward, to provide meat, leather, and beasts of burden. The migrants adopted slash-and-burn agriculture with profligacy, and in short order the Atlantic forest of Brazil succumbed to the ax.[59] There were significant consequences for the malarial environment. No indigenous anopheline mosquitoes bred in the full-canopy forest, but the great deforestation created new habitat for what would become the major anopheline vector, *Anopheles darlingi*.[60] Malaria spread rapidly into the newly cleared regions. At the mining camps and frontier towns, the sedentary populations were ideally sited to transmit the disease. The frontier of mining and farming became one of fever and death.

These massive population movements and temporary settlements introduced vivax and falciparum infections and other Afro-Eurasian diseases to the heartlands of Atlantic Brazil. The region became a hothouse of disease, a multiplier of malaria. European and tropical African immigrant populations trekked into the Brazilian rainforests to mine and, after the initial surface deposits were exhausted, moved on to new locations to create new camps. The miners and slaves depended on livestock farmers who supplied these temporary pioneer settlements with food and tools. These cattle drivers and mule drivers circulated new infections among the constellations of camps.

---

[58] Richards, *The Unending Frontier*, 377–411.
[59] Dean, *With Broadax and Firebrand*.
[60] Only 10 of 54 *Anopheles* species described in Brazil have been reported to be naturally infected with malaria parasites, and 9 of these 10 are zoophilic and/or exophilic and thus appear to be of limited epidemiological significance. See C.A. Guerra, R.W. Snow, and S.I. Hay, "A Global Assessment of Closed Forests, Deforestation, and Malaria Risk," *Annals of Tropical Medicine and Parasitology*, vol. 100, no. 3 (2006), 191.

Other settlers broke away from the mining and plantation systems. Africans fled in considerable number into the interior and set up their own communities known as *quilombos*. These militarized communities also created zones of endemic malarial infection. Thus did the populations of Portuguese, tropical Africans, and their progenies of mixed race accomplish the "occupation" of the interior of Brazil and extend the zone of malarial infection.[61]

These eighteenth-century Brazilian epidemiological processes were very different from those to the south in Argentina, where there were no anopheline vectors capable of transmitting malaria, no lands suitable for sugar production, and no influx of enslaved Africans. The banks of the Río de la Plata marked the southernmost extent of the distribution of *A. darlingi* and thus the southernmost extent of the malarial zone of eastern South America.[62]

The second major eighteenth-century malarial frontier in the Americas was in North America. The frontier moved west with pioneers from the tidewater settlements in British North America. Malaria had become well ensconced along the Atlantic coast from the early seventeenth century, a full century after the infection of the Caribbean basin. In the colonies of Virginia, Maryland, and Pennsylvania during the eighteenth century, white landowners imported indentured Europeans and enslaved Africans as farm laborers. For the European immigrants who arrived principally from the British Isles and northwestern Europe, the Mid-Atlantic colonies of the North American eastern seaboard were far less epidemiologically dangerous than South Carolina or Georgia or elsewhere in the British South Atlantic. The era of white indentured servitude ground to a halt in the decade before the British North American colonies revolted against the rule of Great Britain (1776–1787).[63] This transformation in labor took place approximately a century later than in the Caribbean basin.

---

[61] For a fine overview of Brazilian Atlantic history, see Dean, *With Broadax and Firebrand*.

[62] The range of the principal anopheline vector for the Andes, *A. pseudopunctipennis*, extended into northern Argentina, but the cold winter and the succession of seasons (a dry winter and heavy rains during the summer) were unfavorable to the mosquito. Had this not been the case, L.W. Hackett judged that malaria would have been so intense as to have prevented the development of the rich Tucuman irrigation area (Hackett, "The Malaria of the Andean Regions," 240).

[63] Many of the "indentured servants" sent to the British North American colonies were criminals deported from the United Kingdom. Following the success of the British North American colonial revolt, the criminals were sent to Australia. For an overview, see Robert Hughes, *The Fatal Shore: The Epic of Australia's Founding* (New York: Knopf, 1987).

By the late eighteenth century, an ecological line that divided the zone of mixed infections was drawn through the Mid-Atlantic United States, roughly at the Maryland-Pennsylvania border. In the southern half lay the subregions of slave economies. In the northern half the economies were dominated by freeholders of European descent, where the cooler climate and poorer soils helped to foreclose the possibility of the use of bonded labor on a large scale as on the tropical and subtropical plantations.

Malaria also helped to undergird the ideology of slavery throughout the South Atlantic zone of mixed infections. Africans were largely immune to vivax infections, and thus it was possible for epidemics of vivax malaria to erupt among the white populations and for Africans to be untouched. This "racial" difference, in conjunction with the immunity to yellow fever that most first-generation African immigrants had acquired in Africa, helped to underwrite the nineteenth-century medical thinking that blacks were biologically and "racially" different from whites. According to white North American nineteenth-century thinkers, blacks could withstand the rigors of the southern climate better than whites and could be put to harder labor.[64]

During the late eighteenth century, the malarial zones of vivax and mixed infections in the Mid-Atlantic States were extended by migration and the westward extension of the agricultural frontier to the Mississippi River. In the first half of the nineteenth century, these zones pushed westward, beyond the Mississippi. By the mid-nineteenth century, the division between malarial zones also demarcated a line between the legality and illegality of slave labor, and an economic divide between the production of subtropical agricultural goods such as tobacco and cotton using slave labor and the mixed livestock and food grain econ-omies of the "free" whites. This division also contributed to a political cleavage between the South and the North, on either side of which states aligned to fight for and against the right of political secession in the U.S. Civil War (1861–1865).

The westward movement of the Euro-American pioneers in the United States, like the frontier expansion in Brazil, produced a high incidence of malaria. In Brazil, the destruction of the Atlantic forest in the eighteenth

---

[64] White perceptions of differential racial vulnerability were based on a multitude of factors, including the location of black housing that caused greater exposure, immunities to malaria, the white propensity to evacuate during the malarial season, and white immigration. See Kenneth F. Kiple and Virginia Himmelsteib King, *Another Dimension to the Black Diaspora: Diet, Disease, and Racism* (New York: Cambridge University Press, 1981), 50–58.

century had created habitat for *A. darlingi.*[65] A similar process was responsible for the nineteenth-century expansion of malaria in the United States. It, too, was owed to the conversion of forest to agricultural land.

In North America, the only important malaria vector across the trans-Appalachian west into the Great Plains was *A. quadrimaculatus.* It bred in streams and small depressions in the soil, some so small that they were the result of cattle hooves trodding wet soil. However, unlike the malarial frontier in tropical Africa that experienced intensified malarial infections over time, which provoked immunological and genetic responses, the malarial frontier in the United States was ephemeral. It lasted a generation or so, sickening and killing the pioneers, causing the westward movement to slow to a crawl. It was the principal and characteristic disease of the North American agricultural frontier. In the zone of mixed infections, there was enough falciparum to exact a heavy toll in mortality. It was the number one killer in Illinois, for example, until the 1850s.[66]

The intense malaria of the first generation of pioneers rolled forward across the Midwest. In the wake of the westward movement, malarial infections receded fitfully. This was true in the prairie grasslands as well as in the regions stripped of their forests. In Kansas, for example, the earliest pioneers moved into an ecological zone that had been shaped by Native American management practices. Euro-Americans came to claim the buffalo ranges, where the buffalo wallows served as a breeding ground for anopheles mosquitoes.[67] When the pioneers contributed the malaria parasites, a malarial firestorm erupted. As the plow turned the prairie soils, rainwater percolated into the soils, the habitat for mosquito breeding shrunk, and the increase in farm livestock helped to deflect the anopheles mosquitoes from their human blood source. Here, too, the malarial burden lasted only a few generations.

In the deep U.S. South, the malarial frontier likewise rolled westward, with the opening up of the Mississippi delta lands for cotton planting in the early nineteenth century. This subtropical forest biome shared the

---

[65] The Brazilian expansion of malarial mosquito habitat continues into the present. It entered a new phase in the second half of the twentieth century, as Brazilians seeking land launched pioneer migrations to convert the interior Amazonian rainforests to ranchland.

[66] M.A. Urban, "An Uninhabited Waste: Transforming the Grand Prairie in Nineteenth Century Illinois, USA," *Journal of Historical Geography*, vol. 31 (2005), 653.

[67] Barber, *A Malariologist in Many Lands*, 12, citing Dr. A.E. Hertzler who had a malarial practice in Kansas.

same mosquito vector, *A. quadrimaculatus*, with the U.S. Midwest. However, this southern part of the agricultural frontier differed in some important ways. That many of the richest bottom lands were along the floodplains of the Mississippi River and its meandering rivulets (or "bayous") meant that there were a nearly infinite number of mosquito breeding sites that could not be drained by routine agronomic practices. The shorter winters meant longer seasons of malaria transmission. The result was that malaria developed into an endemic disease of the newly opened southern states.

Throughout much of the U.S. South, malaria was stable.[68] The southern populations – those of European, African, Native American, or mixed-race descent – all bore in different ways the malarial burden of mixed infections. Those born in regions of stable infection submitted to malarial trials in childhood. Their communities suffered the losses of childhood mortality and adult debility. Some African Americans carried the sickle cell gene that afforded some protection against falciparum. Most African Americans remained unable to contract vivax malaria. Over time, however, some lost this protection. One of the many human costs that were borne by the African American communities during slavery was that interracial sex between master and slave resulted in a loss of Duffy negativity, and a larger percentage of the U.S. black population eventually became susceptible to vivax infection.[69]

The U.S. South retained a distinctive epidemiological profile into the twentieth century. For whites born outside of the zone of mixed infections, it was still necessary to pass through the "seasoning" process in the South. This was well appreciated by contemporary observers. As a mid-nineteenth-century physician observed of the South Carolinian plantations: "those who have resided for some time in a malarial district are less liable to it, and its severity less with them, than those who have

---

[68] Anthony Kiszewski et al., "A Global Index Representing the Stability of Malaria Transmission," *American Journal of Tropical Medicine and Hygiene*, vol. 70, no. 5 (2004), 491, fig. 2.

[69] The historical evidence, although certainly problematic, suggests that during the U.S. Civil War, blacks were subject to intermittent (presumably vivax) malaria (see Smart, "Paroxysmal Fevers," 77). In the late twentieth century, 70% of African Americans were estimated to carry the mutation for Duffy negativity (Peter F. Beales and Herbert M. Gilles, "Rationale and Technique of Malaria Control," in ed. David A. Warrell and Herbert M. Gilles, *Essential Malariology*, 4th ed. [New York: Arnold Press, 2002], 125; Dobson, *Contours*, 329); an estimated 97% of West and West Central Africans carry the Duffy mutation.

recently arrived from a healthy region of country."[70] For northern whites, the U.S. South had a well-deserved reputation as a dangerous disease environment.

* * *

Over the course of the early centuries of European and African immigration to the Americas, the three great Afro-Eurasian zones of malaria were extended to the New World. The levels of endemic infection in the Americas were not as high as those in tropical Africa. Most tropical Africans carried the gene for Duffy negativity that protected them against vivax, and some carried the sickle cell mutation that afforded some protection against falciparum. Europeans did not. This epidemiological differential helped to shape the peopling of the Americas. Its logic underwrote the importation of Africans to the plantations of the South Atlantic system and the tragedy of African enslavement and racial discrimination in the Americas.

[70] Thompson McGown, *A Practical Treatise on the Most Common Diseases of the South* (Philadelphia: Grigg, Elliot, 1849), 27–28.

4

Bitter Medicines

Early European immigrants looked on the Americas as a vast botanical storehouse of useful natural products – particularly dyestuffs, stimulants, and medicines. Early Portuguese explorers in South America traded for wood from a rainforest tree (*Caesalpinia echinata*) that, when boiled, yielded a prized reddish-purple dye very similar to that from the heartwood of a closely related Asian tree (*Caesalpinia sappan*) known in Europe through long-distance trade. The South American tree became known as brazilwood and lent its name to the Portuguese colony. The Spaniards followed with their own "discovery." In the course of their military expeditions into Mexico, the Spaniards learned the source of the brilliant red that decorated the Aztec garments. In the postconquest centuries, the Spaniards encouraged the indigenous farmers to produce large quantities of the insects (*Dactylopius coccus*) that fed from the prickly pear cactus and then crushed the insects to yield a dye known as cochineal that, like brazilwood, dazzled the European visual palate.

Europeans also hit a bonanza in their search for stimulants. Indigenous peoples in parts of North America, South America, and the Caribbean smoked tobacco. Europeans, Africans, and Asians soon enthusiastically took up the smoking habit and launched tobacco on an extraordinary, global career. Over time hundreds of millions of people on all continents became addicted. Other powerful and addictive stimulants remained for centuries within the orbit of their original New World societies. Amazonian and Andean peoples chewed coca leaves to produce mild euphoria and greater power of endurance. In the mid-nineteenth century European chemists learned to isolate cocaine, the active alkaloid in the coca leaf, and a significant international trade in the drug developed in the late nineteenth century.[1]

---

[1] David T. Courtwright, *Forces of Habit* (Cambridge, MA: Harvard University Press, 2001), see 14–19 on tobacco; see 46–52 on coca.

In their search for medicines, however, the Europeans had their greatest successes. Tree barks were an important source of indigenous medicines throughout the Americas, and some barks were in common use over large regions. In North America, the Caribbean, and the Amazon, for example, before 1492 the ill had drunk tinctures from the bark of the dogwood tree (*Cornus florida*) as a painkiller and sleep-aid. After the introduction of malaria into the Americas, sufferers employed dogwood bark as a remedy. It apparently dulled the pain from malarial symptoms, although it was ineffective against the parasites. Over a wide stretch of the Americas, it became a culturally accepted palliative malarial treatment, and in North America, dogwood bark remained in wide use in the U.S. South throughout the Civil War.[2]

Other bark and root tinctures were used to treat an array of maladies. In North America, for example, poplar tree bark and sarsaparilla tree root were employed to fight fever, and they contained active chemical compounds similar to those in aspirin.[3] In the Caribbean, the heartwood of the *Guaiacum officinale*, known as the "wood of life," was an all but universal treatment for illness.[4] These barks, roots, and heartwood entered into the regional pharmacopoeias of early European New World empires and had broad applications, although later studies have concluded that, like dogwood bark, they were ineffective against the malaria parasites.[5]

---

[2] Michael A. Flannery, *Civil War Pharmacy* (New York: Pharmaceuticals Products Press, 2004), 226–227. It remained part of the herbal *materia medica* into the twentieth century. See Finley Ellingwood, *The American Materia Medica, Therapeutics, and Pharmacognosy* (Chicago: Ellingwoods Therapeutist, 1919), 272–273.

[3] Aspirin, first produced in 1897, is acetylsalicylic acid. It is a synthetic analog of the naturally occuring salisylic acid that is found in the poplar, willow, and myrtle trees; salicylic acid, like aspirin, has antiinflammatory and antibacterial properties.

[4] David Watts, *The West Indies: Patterns of Development, Culture, and Environmental Change since 1492* (New York: Cambridge University Press, 1987), 134. The flower of this tree is one of the national symbols of Jamaica.

[5] Daniel Drake noted in 1850 that "Many of our native bitters have been more or less extensively used to arrest the paroxysms of intermittent fever. The favorites are, or have been, the bark of the Cornus Florida, or dogwood; Liriodendron tulipifera, or yellow poplar; Prunus Virginiana, or wild cherry tree, and the herbs Eupatorium perefoliatum, or thoroughwart, and Sabbatia angularis (formerly Chironia ang.) or American centaury. As it was an old professional opinion that the superior efficacy of the cinchona bark, over other bitters, arose from the union of an astringent principle, it has been customary to combine, with the bark of the trees just mentioned, a quantity of oak or some other astringent bark, and to render the whole stimulating with wine or whisky; frequently, indeed, to administer them in the form of tincture" (Daniel Drake, *A Systematic Treatise, Historical, Etiological, and Practical, of the Principal Diseases of the Interior Valley of North America* [Cincinnati: W.B. Smith and Co, 1850], 749–750).

The Spaniards made the most important medical "discovery" in the Americas during the turbulent sixteenth century. In the aftermath of their conquest of the Incan Empire, the Spaniards "discovered" the bark of one of the tropical trees that grew on the eastern slopes of the Andes. Its astonishing property was that it could bring a quick end to cyclic malarial fevers. Hard evidence about the "discovery" is scant, and legends have blossomed. The most popular romantic legend had the Countess of Chinchon, the wife of the Spanish Viceroy in Peru, stricken with a tertian fever that was cured by powdered cinchona bark. Following her cure, she dispensed the bark to the suffering citizens of Lima. Alas, painstaking historical research in the 1940s revealed that there was no basis for the legend.[6]

The reality was undoubtedly more prosaic. In the epidemiological disaster caused by the introduction of African and Eurasian diseases, sick and dying peoples throughout the Americas sought remedies from their indigenous pharmacopeia in the hope that the known medicinally active plants could counter the strange and horrifying new diseases. It thus is likely that the Incans, knowledgeable about the fever-reducing properties of cinchona bark, sought relief from fevers and thereby discovered the "cure." The stroke of great good fortune was that cinchona bark killed the malaria parasites, in addition to reducing fever.[7]

Cinchona bark *was* something of a miracle. It contained four natural alkaloids – quinine, cinchonine, cinchonidine, and quinidine – all of which killed the malaria parasites during their blood stages. Treatment must have been something of a hit-or-miss affair. Some cinchona trees were potent, others not. There was a large number of subspecies of cinchona tree, and the alkaloids occurred in different quantities in the different subspecies. The proportions also varied a great deal among individual trees within the same subspecies, and the amount of total alkaloids in a given quantity of bark varied from one tree to the next. But irrespective of the alkaloid mix, the powdered cinchona bark worked against all of the

[6] A.W. Haggis, "Fundamental Errors in the Early History of Cinchona," *Bulletin of the History of Medicine*, vol. 10, no. 3 (1941), 568–587.

[7] An analogous process took place in Brazil: sufferers sought remedies for malaria from the local pharmacopoeia. Of the noncinchona plant species used for malaria treatment, researchers testing the antimalarial activity of the ethanol crude extracts of these plant species in mice infected with *Plasmodium berghei* found that only one, *Remijia ferruginea*, showed antimalarial activity, reducing parasitaemia and mortality at the highest dose tested (V.F. Andrade-Neto et al., "Antimalarial Activity of *Cinchona*-like Plants Used to Treat Fever and Malaria in Brazil," *Journal of Ethnopharmacology*, vol. 87 [2003], 253–256).

malaria parasites, and if sufferers found that the dose was inadequate, they could ingest more bark as necessary.

The results were astonishing. In the case of vivax, malariae, or falciparum infections, the cinchona alkaloids produced a "cure." The sufferer could be retrieved from the nightmare of fevers and, except in the case of vivax, be spared the recurrences – at least until reinfection.[8] The bark, however, was intensely bitter in taste and difficult to ingest. It tended to produce nausea, and if the powder was vomited out, the alkaloids could not work their magic. If the sufferer was suffering from malaria and could keep the powder down, the relief could be full, profound, and nearly immediate.

THE EARLY THERAPEUTIC USE OF CINCHONA

The discovery of the medicinal powers of cinchona, however, did not gain immediate traction. In sixteenth-century Spanish America, there were many disease-causing pathogens scourging wide swaths of the Andes Mountains and surrounding lowlands – and against most of these diseases, cinchona bark was ineffectual. Many who suffered from malaria were additionally afflicted with diseases other than malaria, and any relief won from cinchona bark in these circumstances would have been buried under the symptoms of other afflictions.

Early documentary sources that seem to describe the cinchona tree suggest that cinchona bark may have been known and appreciated by Spaniards in the late sixteenth century. It was not until the early 1640s, however, under the aegis of the Order of the Society of Jesus, that the "Jesuit's powder" gained a therapeutic foothold in Rome, and only then did knowledge of the medicine diffuse more widely through Jesuit networks.[9] Throughout most of the seventeenth century, owing to the grand array of possibilities for confusion among the barks, the frequent inaccuracy of diagnoses, the skepticism on the part of Protestants that any fundamental boon could pass to them through the hands of the Jesuits, and the intellectual dissonance with humoral theory created by the use of a

---

[8] The ovale parasite also had a dormant liver stage like the vivax parasite and could produce a relapse. The ovale parasite seems to have remained in West Africa.

[9] For an analysis of the early documentation concerning cinchona, see Fernando I. Ortiz Crespo, "Fragoso, Monardes and Pre-Chinchonian Knowledge of Cinchona," *Archives of Natural History*, vol. 22, no. 2 (1995), 169–181. See also Saul Jarcho, *Quinine's Predecessor: Francesco Torti and the Early History of Cinchona* (Baltimore: Johns Hopkins University Press, 1993).

"hot and dry" powder to treat a malarial fever, when a "cool and moist" remedy should have been appropriate, there were widely disparate assessments of "the bark."

At length, however, the reported (and very real) successes of cinchona therapy overcame doctrinal resistance. By the 1650s the bitter bark made its way to England, where the elite of London experimented with its use.[10] This was to be a familiar pattern throughout the seventeenth and eighteenth centuries: the medicine proved to be a miracle, but its use was extremely restricted, to those who could afford it. In England, most malaria sufferers were peasants who lived near the salty southeastern marshlands. They were poor, and they got little benefit from the glorious introduction of the Jesuit's Bark to England. They tried to alleviate their sufferings with herbal cures, alcohol, charms, opium, and a variety of concoctions.[11]

During the second half of the seventeenth century, cinchona therapy spread into the elite circles of France, Germany, Switzerland, and Russia. The English physician Robert Talbor treated hundreds of members of European royalty for malaria in the 1670s, and he kept secret that the key ingredient of his cure was cinchona bark. The Jesuits, too, deployed the miracle of cinchona widely. They treated the Qing Emperor for malaria with success in 1693.[12] The finer details of the spread of cinchona therapy have not yet been teased out of the masses of commercial and missionary evidence, but it is clear that at least by the late seventeenth century the knowledge about cinchona bark was becoming a part of nonelite European culture in the wider Atlantic world. In 1681, for example, the English buccaneer surgeon, Lionel Wafer acquired several bundles of

---

[10] Jarcho, *Quinine's Predecessor*, 44–58.

[11] Mary J. Dobson, *Contours of Death and Disease in Early Modern England* (Cambridge: Cambridge University Press, 1997), 316–317.

[12] J.W.W. Stephens, "Pâtes Médicinales and Quinquina: The Treatment of K'ang Hsi, Emperor of China (1662–1723)," *The Journal of Tropical Medicine and Hygiene*, vol. 40, no. 16 (August 16, 1937), 187–188.

Interestingly, Chinese knowledge of *qinghao*, the traditional blue-green herb of the wormwood plant known in the fourth century CE, was rediscovered during the Chinese Cultural Revolution of the mid-twentieth century. It was mentioned in Li Shizhen's *Ben Cao Gang Mu* (1596) as an effective counter to the chills and fever of malaria (see Daniel L. Klayman, "Qinghaosu Artemisisin: An Antimalarial Drug from China," *Science*, new series, vol. 228, no. 4703 [May 13, 1985], 1049). One may doubt, however, how widely it was employed. Paul U. Unschuld's *Medicine in China: A History of Pharmaceutics* (Berkeley: University of California Press, 1986) makes no mention of the drug. On its "rediscovery," see Elisabeth Hsu, "Reflections on the 'Discovery' of the Antimalarial Qinghao," *British Journal of Clinical Pharmacology*, vol. 61, no. 6 (2006), 666–670.

cinchona bark in what is today northern Chile and went on to put it to good use in Virginia and elsewhere.[13]

The reputation and demand for cinchona continued to grow. At least by the early eighteenth century, ships' surgeons and apothecaries of the East India Company began to treat fevers with cinchona bark. In the second half of the eighteenth century, new sources of supply opened up in the Andes. More bark flowed into international markets, and militaries in the North Atlantic began to use the bark to stay healthy enough to fight their enemies. During the American War for Independence (1776–1783), both colonial insurrectionists and British troops swallowed the "Peruvian bark" to rid themselves of malarial fevers.

Even toward the end of the eighteenth century, medical appreciations of the virtues of cinchona bark were clouded. Physicians normally began their therapeutic interventions with bleeding and purging and administered the bark thereafter. Some patients' responses to the bark were thereby mitigated by the rigors of the depletions. Moreover, the response of the feverish to cinchona bark was quite variable, in part because of the confounding, similar symptoms of malarial and nonmalarial fevers. As the physician Robert Jackson noted,

During the late American war, even in the southern and more unhealthy provinces of that extensive country, Peruvian bark, properly administered, seldom failed of cutting short the course of the disease; the same effect was not obtained with certainty, from the same means in the remitting fever of Jamaica; but the exhibition of bark, notwithstanding was even there, generally attended with benefit: in the island of St. Domingo on the contrary, its benefits were very uncertain, as the circumstances, which ensure its success, were not perhaps in general sufficiently regarded: the solution of arsenic was infinitely more effectual; and nothing occurred to furnish suspicion that the use of arsenic was unsafe.[14]

Adding to the confusion was the fact that some professionals disagreed about the superiority of cinchona barks over other barks thought to possess febrifugal attributes.[15] These misunderstandings were fueled by the difficulties of identifying the genuine article.[16] A flood of "bad bark"

---

[13] Lionel Wafer, *A New Voyage and Description of the "Isthmus of America"* (London: Printed for James Knapton, 1699), 98–99.

[14] Robert Jackson, *An Outline of the History and Cure of Fever* (Edinburgh: Printed for Mundell, 1798), 276.

[15] Richard Kentish, *Experiments and Observations on a New Species of Bark* (London: J. Jackson, 1784).

[16] E.g., trees in the Bahamas were thought incorrectly to be cinchona. See Henry Pitman, *A Relation of the Great Sufferings and Strange Adventures of Henry Pitman, Chyrurgion to the late Duke of Monmouth* (London: Andrew Sowle, 1689), 29.

hit the British market in late 1779 or early 1780; one estimate held that spurious bark led true bark by a ratio of 4:1.[17] Moreover, drug grinders commonly adulterated the barks with sugar, lime sulphate, starch, or other alkaloids or acids. Chemical detection of this fraud was, by and large, beyond the means of the sufferers or the attending physicians, and for this reason it was usually possible to buy cinchona powder less expensively by weight than cinchona bark.[18] In the late eighteenth century, the British East India Company launched a search for substitutes in both the East and West Indies, and for a short while the bark of a newly catalogued species of mahogany seemed promising.[19]

THE SUPPLY OF CINCHONA BARK
FROM THE ANDES

The cinchona trees grew in remote Andean regions that were accessible only with considerable difficulty. Local Amerindians found the trees, stripped off the barks, loaded bundles of bark onto mules, and then caravanned them out of the Andes. Much of the bark flowed to ports controlled by the Spaniards. However, a substantial quantity flowed east as contraband via the Amazon basin river tributaries and then downstream to Portuguese and Dutch merchants.

The Spanish Crown made early efforts to impose a royal monopoly on cinchona bark exports from the New World but without broad success. During the reign of Charles III (1759–1788), cinchona imports skyrocketed, and from 1768, when the Grand Pharmacist of the Ministry of the Marine and American Indies began to order fixed annual amounts and took efforts to prevent fraud, the Crown achieved greater control over supply and delivery.[20] Cinchona bark in excess of the quantity ordered by the

---

[17] George Baker, "Observations on the Late Intermittent Fevers; To Which Is Added a Short History of the Peruvian Bark," *Medical Transactions* (1785), 154.

[18] Dennis G. Carlson, *African Fever: A Study of British Science, Technology, and Politics in West Africa, 1787–1864* (Canton, MA: Science History Publications, 1984), 47.

[19] "A botanical description of a new species of Swietenia (mahogany), with experiments and observations on the bark thereof, in order to determine and compare its powers with those of Peruvian Bark, for which it is proposed as a substitute. Addressed to the Honourable Court of Directors of the United East-India Company, by their most obedient, humble servant Wm. Roxburgh (1793)," cited by D. J. Mabberley, "William Roxburgh's 'Botanical Description of a New Species of Swietenia (Mahogany)' and Other Overlooked Binomials in 36 Vascular Plant Families," *Taxon*, vol. 31, no. 1 (1982), 65.

[20] In 1768, royal instructions were sent to the Indies requiring the bark to be wrapped in cloth, put into cases, affixed with wax and sealed, and then wrapped in leather and marked with the Crown seal. The bark cases carried two forms of notation: one that

Spanish Crown went into the broader European and North American markets.[21]

The early supply of cinchona bark had probably originated along the eastern Andean slopes in Ecuador. Beginning in the late 1770s, the demand for cinchona bark rose sharply. A new source of supply began to be cut from the eastern Andean slopes of Colombia, farther to the north. The volume of Colombian exports grew tenfold in little more than a decade, from less than fifty tons in the early 1780s to more than five hundred tons by 1794.[22]

With the regional shift in supply, a different mix of cinchona barks began to reach the market. The earlier supply had been grey in color; some

corresponded to the expedition and the other to the number of cases. Cases were shipped from Cartagena, Montevideo, and particularly from El Callao.

The Spanish Crown had the cinchona bark graded into four categories. The best was reserved for gifts for foreign courts; the second best was reserved for the Spanish royal family; the third for alms; and the fourth was destroyed. Most of the bark was graded in the third category, and the Crown gave significant quantities to hospitals and to religious orders. A few pharmacists made applications to make special formulations such as medicinal wines that were introduced into England, France, and elsewhere (Carmen Frances et al., "Le quinquina: son commerce et son emploi en Espagne au cours de l'histoire," in *Acts of the International Congress for the History of Pharmacy* [Padova, Italy: Accademia italiana di storia della farmacia, 1989], 52–53).

[21] In prerevolutionary France, cinchona imports were doled out through a system of privileges granted by the king. The Hôpital de Lyons, e.g., dispensed cinchona through a regional network. As a late-eighteenth-century observer noted: "The Hospital of Lyons had an exclusive privilege from the Kings of France, exempting it from paying duties on any article imported for its use: this enabled the administrators to keep the most complete pharmaceutical collection in Europe: it was the Hall which supplied not only all the apothecaries shops in Lyons, but those also in all the surrounding towns; for the druggists and apothecaries found it much cheaper and less troublesome to deal with the administrators, that to import their drugs, and prepare them themselves. The profits which accrued to the house from this branch of trade alone, amounted to an hundred pounds sterling a week, exclusive of all kinds of remedies furnished to the patients, the number of whom exceeded very often twenty thousand yearly. The stores, particularly of simples, were immense; that of choice Bark was very considerable, its prime cost amounted nearly to a thousand pounds; of course, had the Yellow Bark been found by experience and observation to surpass it, the loss sustained by the Hotel Dieu might have been very considerable" (Letter of Michael O'Ryan to Dr. John Relph, dated London, July 11, 1794, reproduced in John Relph, *An Inquiry into the Medical Efficacy of a New Species of Peruvian Bark* [London: J. Phillips, 1794], 162–163).

[22] For a recent overview, see Carlos Gilberto Zárate Botía, *Extracción de Quina: La Configuración del Espacio Andino-Amazónico de Fines des Siglo XIX* (Bogotá: Universidad Nacional de Colombia, Sede Leticia, Instituto Amazónico de Investigaciones, 2001). On the eighteenth century, see Alba Moya, *Auge y Crisis de la Cascarilla en la Audencia de Quito, Siglo XVIII* (Quito, Ecuador: Facultad Latinoamericana de Ciencias Sociales, Sede Ecuador, 1994).

of the new supply had a reddish caste. Without a rigorous standard of comparison, and with great variation between individual trees of the same subspecies, apothecaries freely asserted the superiority of one type or batch of bark over another, and there were vogues for different colored cinchona barks in the late eighteenth century.[23] In the early 1790s, bark prices in Great Britain ranged widely from eighteen pence to nine shillings per pound.[24]

The sources of supply were also unstable. In part this was owing to the destructive harvesting practices that killed the trees and forced the bark strippers into ever more remote regions. The Andean slopes were also troubled by the tumultuous colonial wars for independence from Spain (1810–1826). In the 1820s, cinchona bark from Bolivia began to reach the markets, and in the aftermath of political disengagement from Spain, a struggle over the cinchona trade became a key part of the political brawl for control of the Bolivian state.[25] The administration of Santa Cruz (1829–1839) attempted unsuccessfully to restrict cinchona exports in order to establish a national quinine industry. When this administration was swept from power, Bolivia became the largest exporter of bark until 1853,

---

[23] William Saunders defended the new "red bark" that arrived in Europe in 1779 and 1780. He noted: "The introduction of the Red Bark into this country was the effect of chance. In the year 1779, a Spanish Ship from Lima, bound to Cadiz, was taken by the Hussar frigate, and carried into Lisbon; her cargo consisted chiefly of this Bark, some part of which was immediately imported into this country, and a considerable quantity was bought at a very low price at Ostend, by some of our London Druggists. The Boxes in which it was brought to Europe were of the same kind as those in which the common Peruvian Bark was contained, and all sold by the general title of Quinquina. The Druggists in whose hands the Red Bark at first was, found it difficult to dispose of it, its appearance was so unlike that of common Bark; at last they offered it by way of trial to such Apothecaries as reside in counties where agues are frequent; the success attending its use soon convinced them of its superior efficacy. It was early introduced into the hospitals, and its greater powers became universally acknowledged. It has continued ever since in general use in the Hospitals of St. Bartholomew, St. Thomas, Guy, and the London" (William Saunders, *Observations on the Superior Efficacy of the Red Peruvian Bark in the Cure of Agues and Other Fevers* [London: Robert Hodge, for William Green, 1782], 18–19).

[24] John Relph, *An Inquiry into the Medical Efficacy of a New Species of Peruvian Bark* (London: J. Phillips, 1794), 4–5.

[25] The Bolivian Santa Cruz administration (1829–1839) tried to restrict bark exports, in an effort to promote quinine manufacturing and to stimulate internal industry.

In the late 1830s, one of the principal bark traders supplying the U.S. market was David Keener. Some of his correspondence with the firm of Rosengarten and Denis can be found in the archives of the Historical Society of Pennsylvania (hereafter, HSP).

In 1838, Santa Cruz attempted to impose a five-year prohibition on the cutting of bark [HSP, Rosengarten and Denis, box 9, August 1838 folder. Keener to Rosengarten, dated Baltimore, August 4, 1838].

when Colombia regained its premier role.[26] The demand for cinchona bark from South America continued to grow, and it appears that Colombia exported the large majority of the bark from South America that arrived on the international markets until the 1880s.[27]

The cinchona bark export trade had a powerful economic influence in the Andes. During the expansion of the trade in the late eighteenth century, the frontier between the Amazon and the Andes developed into a region of export-oriented economic activity. Mission stations became centers for the cinchona trade. New towns grew up and new transportation routes were carved into the forests. When the efforts to refine the bark and create quinine industries in the postrevolutionary South American states came to naught, the bark was shipped from South American ports directly to markets in the United States, Great Britain, and continental Europe. The upshot was that the remote interior regions of the Andes were more connected to the emerging global economy than the more densely populated "core" regions of the Andean states.

The highland cinchona regions, however, remained thinly populated. The bark strippers operated without oversight, and their crude techniques killed the cinchona trees, in a classic example of the overexploitation of a highland "commons." This was not lost on contemporary observers. Even by the 1830s, some traders had grown concerned about the prospects for cinchona bark exports,[28] and in the 1850s, the Dutch and the British sent botanists on expeditions to bring back cinchona seedlings or seeds in order to found imperial cinchona plantations elsewhere in the tropics.[29]

---

[26] See Carlos Pérez, "Quinine and Caudillos: Manuel Isidoro Belzu and the Cinchona Bark Trade in Bolivia, 1848–1855" (PhD diss., University of California, Los Angeles, 1998).

[27] For an overview of cinchona production in the Colombian Andes, see C. Dominguez and A. Gómez, *La Economica Extractiva en la Amazonia Colombiana, 1850–1930* (Colombia: TROPENBOS; Araracuara: Corporación Colombiana para la Amazonia, 1990), 19–76.

Colombia saw a dramatic increase in its exports from 1850 until the collapse of the world market price in 1883/1884. During these years, Colombia's exports filled the gap created by the collapse of Bolivian exports, owing to political crisis. (Dominguez and Gómez, *La Economica Extractiva*, 38.)

[28] In an 1838 letter to Rosengarten, Keener notes the scarcity of bark from "the great destruction of Trees" [HSP, Rosengarten and Denis, box 9, August 1838 folder. Keener to Rosengarten, dated Baltimore, August 10, 1838].

[29] Mark Honigsbaum, *The Fever Trail: In Search of the Cure for Malaria* (New York: Farrar, Straus, and Giroux, 2001), 63–157.

QUININE AND THE RISE OF THE EARLY
PHARMACEUTICAL COMPANIES

In 1820 in Paris, the conceptual basis of malaria therapy was radically altered at the laboratory bench. At the École de Pharmacie in Paris, Pierre-Joseph Pelletier and his student Joseph Bienaimé Caventou isolated two of the medically active cinchona alkaloids – quinine and cinchonine – by boiling the bark in alcohol and dilute sulfuric acid.[30] This laboratory success allowed for further experimentation with the purified alkaloids, and this in turn confirmed that there were "active principles" at work in plant and animal substances that could be released through chemical manipulation. This understanding was central to the emergence of modern alkaloidal chemistry. The astonishing laboratory results were duplicated the same year in the Netherlands.[31]

Pelletier called for studies to determine the medical efficacy of quinine and cinchonine. Two French physicians took up the call. Working independently, and without modern understandings of the concept of a randomized trial, they administered quinine to a total of nineteen patients and cinchonine to one. The cinchonine-treated patient had been suffering from a difficult, chronic fever, and the treating physician found that large doses were required to suppress the illness. This patient recovered, as did the large majority of those to whom quinine had been given.[32] The larger number of cases treated with quinine, combined with the fact that the cinchonine-treated patient had a chronic illness, lent to quinine the reputation as the superior medicine.[33]

[30] The other two major cinchona alkaloids were quinidine and cinchonidine. Quinidine was isolated in 1833 and cinchonidine in 1847. See George King, *Manual of Cinchona Cultivation in India* (Calcutta: Office of the Superintendent of Government Printing, 1876), 4. Cited by José Antonio Ocampo, *Colombia y la Economia Mundial 1830–1910* (Mexico City: Siglo Veintiuno Editores, 1984), 255n2.

[31] Jan Peter Verhave, "The Use of Quinine for Treatment and Control of Malaria in The Netherlands," *Tropical and Geographical Medicine*, vol. 47, no. 6 (1995), 252.

[32] Pinel, Thénard, and Hallé, "Rapport fait à l'Académie des Sciences par MM. Pinel, Thénard et Hallé, Sur un Mémoire de M. Chomel, intitulé: Observations sur l'emploi des sulfates de quinine et de cinchonine dans les fièvres intermittentes," *Journal de pharmacie et des sciences accessories*, vol. 7 (1821), 226–231.

[33] In the years following the isolation of quinine, the wastage of the cinchona alkaloids was understood to be a major problem. In Rome, in 1830, Pietro Peretti made a mélange of the cinchona alkaloids (an "antifever powder") that was tested by the colleges of medicine in Rome and Bologne and approved by the Cardinal Camerlengo, after which its use became general in Rome (League of Nations, O.H./Malaria/95, Geneva, November 14, 1927. Commission du Paludisme, Fascicule II [D'après les actes de la société pour l'étude

The techniques for isolating the cinchona alkaloids spread rapidly in the North Atlantic world. In France, the physiologist François Magendie published detailed instructions on how to isolate quinine, and his *Formulary for the Preparation and Mode of Employing Several New Remedies* was widely disseminated in translation and in the original French.[34]

In the early to mid-1820s, quinine production began in the United Kingdom, France, Germany, the Netherlands, and the United States of America.[35] A fledgling attempt was also made to produce quinine in Peru in the 1820s.[36] At first, quinine was a simple addition to the offerings of the local "manufacturing chemists." At least in the early decades of the

du paludisme], "Quinetum. Histoire, découverte et emploi du quinetum dans les traitement du paludisme en Italie," 2–3).

Cinchonine, cinchonidine, and quinidine were tested repeatedly in clinical trials during the nineteenth century. All tests confirmed the specific efficacy of the alkaloids in the treatment of malaria. Some tests indicated that these alkaloids were equally efficacious in the same doses as quinine; other tests indicated that larger quantities were necessary to achieve the same efficacy.

[34] François Magendie, *Formulary for the Preparation and Mode of Employing Several New Remedies*, translated from the French of the 3rd ed. of Magendie's "Formulaire" by Robley Dunglison (Philadelphia: J. Webster, 1824).

Magendie had earlier used cinchona bark and was familiar with its drawbacks. He advocated the use of quinine soon after its isolation by Pelletier and Caventou. See François Magendie, "Fièvre intermittente pernicieuse, guérie par une faible dose de sulfate de quinine," *Journal de physiologie expérimentale et pathologique*, vol. 1 (1821), 393–395.

[35] On early quinine manufacture in the United Kingdom, see David Lloyd Howard, "The History and Development of the British Fine Chemical Industry," *Pharmaceutical Journal and Pharmacist* (August 7, 1926), 8–9; London Metropolitan Archives, Acc1037/854a, letter from D.L. Howard to Dr. W. Sieger, dated October 9, 1937. Joseph Jewell established the commercial manufacture of quinine in Great Britain in 1823.

Also in 1823, quinine was first produced in the United States, in Philadelphia, the city that would become the cradle of the national chemical industry. (For the earliest document on quinine production in the United States, see John Farr, "On Extract of Quinia," *Journal of the Philadelphia College of Pharmacy*, vol. 1, no. 2 [1826], 43–45.) The Amsterdam pharmaceutical firm, D'Ailly and Nieuwehuis (later, D'Ailly and Sons), produced quinine from 1825 to 1830.

Details on the business history of Rosengarten and Sons, which began as Seitler and Zeitler in 1822, can be found in [n.a.], *A Century or Longer in Business* (Philadelphia: Insurance Company of North America, 1922).

[36] Abel Victorino Brandin, a former surgeon in Napoleon's armies, traveled to Buenos Aires in 1823, quinine sulphate in hand, with the intention of establishing a quinine factory. He visited Chile, Peru, and Ecuador, and ultimately found a collaborator in the Peruvian pharmacist D. Augustine Cruzate, who was the first to produce quinine sulphate in Peru. The industry eventually failed (Carlos Enrique Paz Soldán, "La Vida Aventura de Abel Victorino Brandin, el Introductor del Sulfato de Quinina en la América Meridional," *Anales de la Sociedad Peruana de Historia de la Medicina*, vol. 2 [1940], 10–29).

quinine industry, the largest quantities were manufactured in France. Pelletier had started a company, whose product set the standard for purity in the wider North Atlantic market. French quinine production in the late 1830s was estimated to be in excess of 120,000 ounces of quinine per year.[37]

The early success of quinine underwrote a major shift in the subspecies of cinchona bark making its way to North Atlantic markets. Around 1824, "yellow" bark (*C. calisaya* and *C. officinalis*) probably from Andean Bolivia – with a higher proportion of quinine than the other barks – won a growing percentage of the market, challenging the "grey" bark (*Cinchona micrantha* and *C. nitida*) and "red" bark (*C. succirubra*).[38] At least by the end of the 1830s, the yellow bark was in high ascendancy.[39]

The market for quinine proved highly profitable, and, over the course of the 1830s and 1840s, the more successful firms either consolidated with their competitors or drove them out of business, and a pattern of oligopoly

---

[37] The French manufacturers enjoyed a comparative cost advantage because of the inexpensiveness in France of alcohol, the solvent used to isolate the alkaloid (William Dawson Hooker, *Inaugural Dissertation upon the Cinchonas, Their Uses, History, and Effects* [Glasgow: Khull, 1839], 23–24).

A similar estimate of 120,000 ounces as the annual French quinine sulphate production was made in 1851 (Lloyd Bullock, "On Amorphous Quinine," in ed. Edward Latham Ormerod, *On the Pathology and Treatment of Valvular Disease of the Heart and Its Secondary Affections: Being the Gulstonian Lectures Delivered at the Royal College of Physicians in February 1851* [London: Wilson and Ogilvy, 1851], 2).

[38] Sir D. Prain, "The Botanical Aspect of the Quinine Question," League of Nations Malaria Commission, C.H./Malaria/16 (I), 4, 9; Félix-Célestin Silvy, *Dissertation sur l'emploi du sulfate de quinine dans le traitement des fièvres intermittentes*. Thèse pour le doctorat en médecine, Faculté de médecine de Paris (1828), 8.

The yellow bark was not unknown. It had been introduced to Great Britain in 1792 or 1793; it is believed to have been known in Spain earlier, perhaps as early as 1786 (Walter Vaughan, *The Evidence of the Superior Efficacy of the Cinchona Flava, or Yellow Peruvian Bark* [London: Printed for T. Cox, Borough, 1795]; Letter of Michael O'Ryan to Dr. John Relph, dated London, July 11, 1794, reproduced in John Relph, *An Inquiry Into the Medical Efficacy of a New Species of Peruvian Bark* [London: J. Phillips, 1794], 162–163).

[39] As W.D. Hooker noted in 1839: "The comparative efficacy of the different species of barks, has been much disputed; the diversity of opinion being perhaps mainly attributable to the uncertain state in which they are found in the shops. At its first introduction, the *Red bark* was represented as far superior to the pale and yellow barks, and was esteemed accordingly; but the great preference given to it, led to so general an adulteration, that it lost much of its reputation. It was a common practice, also, to offer the bark for sale after having extracted the active properties, by making tinctures, infusions, &c. [etc.] from it. The *grey* or *pale Bark* next came into notice and use, and perhaps similar causes depreciated its value in like manner; so that now the Yellow bark has superseded all the others; and so long as Quinine alone is employed in the cure of intermittent fever, it must hold its place in popular favour" (Hooker, *Inaugural Dissertation*, 25–26).

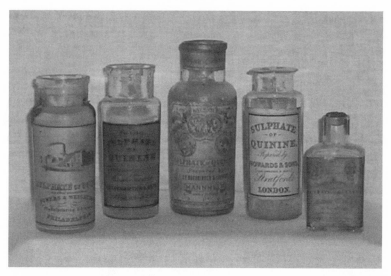

FIGURE 4.1. Nineteenth-Century Quinine Manufacturers' Bottles
Source: Personal collection of the author.

emerged. By the mid-1830s, the establishment of Howard and Kent (later, Howards and Sons) emerged as the largest manufacturer of quinine in Great Britain.[40] In the United States, by the 1840s, two competing manufacturing chemical companies emerged as the major quinine-producing firms: Rosengarten and Denis (later, Rosengarten and Sons) and Farr, Powers and Weightman (later, Powers and Weightman). These firms supplied the chemical wholesalers and retail pharmacies.[41] By the 1850s, four French manufacturers produced quinine, including the firm of Pelletier, Delondre, and Levaillant (Figure 4.1).

[40] The firm manufactured 6,000 ounces in 1836, 43,000 ounces by 1847, and more than 100,000 ounces in 1848. According to an internal history of the company, quinine provided "an enormous proportion of the total gross profit." Bernard F. Howard, "Howards 1847 to 1947: A Treatise Compiled by Bernard F. Howard in 1956," Redbridge Borough Archives, Ilford, 3; [n.a.], *Howards 1797–1947*, printed privately for Howards and Sons Ltd. (Plaistow, UK: Howards and Sons, 1947).
[41] In late 1843, these two firms entered into a contractual agreement to share the market for quinine sulphate. The agreement was to last "as long as it may be found to operate to our mutual advantage." It is not known how long this agreement remained in effect (Merck Archives, Merck and Co., Inc., Whitehouse Station, New Jersey, R6–2.4.4 PWR, contractual agreement, dated Philadelphia, December 27, 1843, and signed by Rosengarten and Denis and Farr, Powers and Weightman).

THE USE OF QUININE TO 1860

From the mid-1820s onward, the demand for the intensely bitter antimalarial drug grew rapidly. In Western Europe and the United States, owing to the long and generally positive experience with cinchona bark, quinine insinuated itself easily into the *materia medica*. Some early adopters embraced the use of quinine within a year or so of its first manufacture in Philadelphia.[42] Initially, quinine was quite expensive, and physicians were not agreed as to the size or timing of the appropriate doses. The oral method of ingesting the drug became nearly universal, after a period of experimentation with other methods such as applying quinine powder to skin that had been rubbed raw.[43] Over the decades of the 1830s and 1840s, the use of quinine in the North Atlantic world came largely to replace the use of the bark. As the chemical manufacturers ramped up production, they experienced economies of scale, and the price for quinine dropped.[44]

Quinine use slowly began to filter into the expatriate European communities in the tropical colonies. British India at first appeared to be a promising market.[45] This proved chimerical, however, because the high price of quinine kept it out of the hands of the vast suffering native populations of India (as had earlier been the case with cinchona bark). The resident Europeans, who could afford the medicine, were relatively few. Moreover, some were under the sway of a "scientific" prejudice, promulgated by Dr. James Johnson. In 1813 Johnson had published an

[42] Thompson McGown noted in 1849: "I believe it was about the year 1824 or '5, when a very fatal form of fever prevailed about Huntsville, Ala. The usual mode of treatment was of so little avail, that Dr. Thomas Fearn was induced to try large doses of quinine, which proved successful; and it appears that he is the first who used large doses of this article, a practice which has since become very popular in the southern and western States, amongst the most enlightened and successful practitioners" (*A Practical Treatise on the Most Common Diseases of the South* [Philadelphia: Grigg, Elliot, 1849], 15).

See also H. Perrine, "Fever Treated with Large Doses of Sulphate of Quinine in Adams County near Natchez, Miss.," *Philadelphia Journal of Medical and Physical Science*, vol. 13 (1826), 36–41, cited by Dale C. Smith, "Quinine and Fever: The Development of the Effective Dosage," *Journal of the History of Medicine and Allied Sciences*, vol. 31 (1976), 356–357.

[43] This method was inspired by a mercury treatment for yellow fever (Silvy, "Dissertation," 12–13).

[44] See note 69.

[45] In 1827, Pelletier and a British manufacturer sent quinine to Calcutta, flooded the market, and drove its price to ruinous levels. Local brokers bought up the surplus in hopes of limiting the damage (London Metropolitan Archives, Acc 1034/853/2, James Low to Dr. Alexander Low, Island of Jersey, dated June 2, 1828, Calcutta).

influential book on tropical diseases in which he violently condemned the use of cinchona. For the next twenty years or so, physicians at the European General Hospital at Calcutta followed Dr. Johnson's lead, and malaria patients were violently purged with mercury compounds, bled, and administered alcoholic stimulants. This prejudice against cinchona and its alkaloids was reversed only in 1835, when cinchona was reinstituted as a malaria treatment at the hospital. Immediately, the patient death rate from malaria dropped by more than 90 percent.[46]

A similar breakthrough took place in Algeria in the early 1830s. The French military physician François Maillot began to treat malaria-stricken soldiers with quinine and conclusively demonstrated the value of the drug. In Algeria, quinine treatment for French soldiers became the norm, and later authorities acknowledged the importance of Maillot's reform in the success of French colonization.[47]

Along the West African coast below the Sahara, at least by the 1840s, resident Europeans had begun to self-medicate with quinine. As the chief medical officer for the British Navy along the West African coast, Alexander Bryson, noted in 1847: "So general has the use of quinine now become, that there is hardly any part of Western Africa, where there are resident Europeans, in whose houses it is not to be found; it is in fact considered to be one of the necessities of life, where life is of all things the most uncertain."[48] Bryson's *Report on the Climate and Principal Diseases of the African Station* shifted the policy of the British military. From 1848 onward, larger doses of cinchona-infused wine bitters were issued, standard doses were specified, and the decision to use cinchona products was no longer left up to the individual commander or captain.[49]

---

[46] James Johnson, *The Influence of Tropical Climates, More Especially the Climate of India, on the Constitutions of Europeans* (London: J.J. Stockdale, 1813); [Anon.], "The Romance of Cinchona," *Indian Medical Gazette*, April 1931, 213.

Dr. Royle, author of the *Materia Medica*, first recommended the introduction of the cinchona plant into India in 1835 (No. 16. "Report by Dr. Royle on the Introduction into India of the Quinine-yielding Cinchonas, and of the Means Which Have Hitherto Been Adopted for the Purpose," *Parliamentary Papers*, House of Commons, 1863, vol. 45, paper 118, 1–272; "Cinchona Plant in India: Correspondence, 1852–1863").

[47] Philip Curtin, *Death by Migration: Europe's Encounter with the Tropical World in the Nineteenth Century* (New York: Cambridge University Press, 1989), 64.

[48] Alexander Bryson, *Report on the Climate and Principal Diseases of the African Station* (London: W. Clowes, 1847), 244.

[49] Dennis G. Carlson, *African Fever: A Study of British Science, Technology, and Politics in West Africa, 1787–1864* (Canton, MA: Science History Publications, 1984), 45–53; Curtin, *Death by Migration*, 64–65.

The largest demand for quinine was in North America. As we have seen, the westward movement of Euro-American settlers across the Appalachian Mountains distributed malarial infections from the Gulf of Mexico north to the Great Lakes. The demand for quinine spread from the eastern seaboard states to the frontiers of settlement. There, its use was first sponsored by physicians, who experimented with dosages and timing. By the mid-nineteenth century, quinine was often administered with opium, the Asian palliative for malaria, and as Daniel Drake noted in his classic medical treatise on the diseases of the North American interior, medical analogies between opium and quinine helped to determine the timing of drug administration.[50]

John Sappington, an entrepreneurial Missouri physician, spearheaded the use of quinine on the Santa Fe Trail, set up a small factory where his slaves produced antifever pills, and popularized the use of his product by sending out agents on horseback through the wider region, although he kept secret his use of quinine as the medically active ingredient.[51] In 1838, 1839, and 1841, Sappington ordered and distributed roughly the same quantity of quinine as several of the larger brokerage houses in Philadelphia or New York combined.[52]

In the European tropical colonies, administrators, missionaries, and merchants took up the use of quinine. In the falciparum zone in western Africa, quinine undoubtedly played a significant role in reducing European mortality, although as Philip Curtin has documented in his study of European military mortality in the tropical world, the largest decreases in mortality over the course of the nineteenth century should be attributed to the use of screens to keep insects out of sleeping quarters, water filtration systems, and improve sanitation, rather than to biomedicine. (Curtin, *Death by Migration*, passim.)

[50] Daniel Drake, *A Systematic Treatise, Historical, Etiological, and Practical, of the Principal Diseases of the Interior Valley of North America* (Cincinnati: W.B. Smith and Co., 1850), 748–749.

[51] Thomas Findley, "Sappington's Anti-Fever Pills and the Westward Migration," *Transactions of the American Clinical and Climatological Association*, vol. 79 (1968), 34–44; Thomas B. Hall Jr. and Thomas B. Hall III, *Dr. John Sappington of Saline County, Missouri 1776–1856* (Arrow Rock, MO: The Friends of Arrow Rock, 1975), 24.

[52] In May 1838, Sappington placed an order with Farr, Powers and Weightman for six hundred pounds of quinine sulphate (9,600 ounces), an unprecedently large order, to be delivered by September first of that year. The firm was producing quinine sulphate "faster than last year" at the rate of 100 ounces per day, and thus this order claimed nearly the entirety of their productive capacity over the summer of 1838. In 1839, Sappington placed an order with Rosengarten and Denis for 1,000 ounces, for 100 ounces in early March 1841, and for a second 100 ounces in late April 1841 (Merck Archives, R6–2.4.1. Thomas H. Powers to William Weightman, Philadelphia, May 30, 1838; R6–2.4.1. John Sappington to G.D. Rosengarten, Jonesboro Saline County Missouri, April 1, 1839; PWR. HSP, Rosengarten and Denis, box 12. John Sappington and Sons to Messrs. Rosengarten and Denis, Arrow Rock, MO, April 29, 1841).

In the U.S. Army, field surgeons also experimented with quinine, and as early as the Second Seminole War (1835–1842) quinine was administered with good results – it kept the troops functioning in the field.[53] The use of quinine, however, was blended with elements from the indigenous pharmacopoeia. William H. Van Buren noted how, in 1840, as an assistant surgeon on duty at Fort King in Florida, he had mixed a few ounces of quinine, dogwood bark (*Cornus florida*), wild-cherry bark (*Prunus virginiana*), and the dried peel of a dozen native oranges to each barrel of whisky with good effect:

> From one to two ounces of this preparation was given to every man at the post, morning and evening, with the effect, in a very short time, of rendering the relapses of fever less frequent and milder in their character, lengthening the interval between the attacks, and in many instances preventing their occurrence entirely during its use.[54]

Quinine, however, was not incorporated into the standard practice of U.S. military medicine for another twenty years. The alkaloid did not play a role during the Mexican-American War, for example, even though the U.S. troops were battered by malarial infections during the autumn of 1846.[55] The U.S. Sanitary Commission finally recommended quinine as a preventive medicine for the military in 1861 because of its curative powers against "malarial or miasmatic disease," although quinine was considered to have a much broader effective field of therapeutic action.[56] It was

---

[53] Smith, "Quinine and Fever," 361–363.

[54] William H. Van Buren, "Quinine as a Prophylactic Against Malarious Diseases," in ed. William A. Hammond, MD, *Military, Medical and Surgical Essays Prepared for the United States Sanitary Commission* (Philadelphia: J.B. Lippincott and Co., 1864), 93. This essay was first issued as the U.S. Sanitary Commission, Report No. 31, *Report of a Committee Appointed by Resolution of the Sanitary Commission to Prepare a Paper on the Use of Quinine as a Prophylactic Against Malarious Diseases* (New York: Wm. C. Bryant and Co., 1861).

[55] Louis C. Duncan, "A Medical History of General Zachary Taylor's Army of Occupation in Texas and Mexico, 1845–1847," *Military Surgeon*, vol. 48 (1921), 96.
Duncan's account is based on a series of memoirs by Surgeon John B. Peters, who accompanied Taylor's expedition to Mexico. There is no mention of quinine in Duncan's account.
Also in 1846, R.S. Holmes, a U.S. Army physician based in Florida, communicated his positive experience in treating malaria there with large doses of quinine. See his "Remarks on the Use of Quinine in Florida, and on Malaria and Its influence in that State; Being the Substance of a Report Made to the Surgeon-General U.S. Army," *American Journal of the Medical Sciences*, no. 24 (October 1846), 297–309.

[56] U.S. Sanitary Commission, Document No. 17, "Rules for Preserving the Health of the Soldier," para. 25. Issued July 13, 1861. The U.S. military lagged behind British naval practice. From the middle of the eighteenth century, British sailors on tropical duty in

regarded rather "like a nutritious food" that permanently conferred increased strength and the power to resist disease.[57] In this view, quinine was a tonic that would stimulate the body to a more robust condition. This was in direct conflict with the idea that fever was a kind of bodily excitement, and for this reason many physicians refused to administer quinine *during* an attack of fever.[58]

During the first decades of quinine manufacture (1820–1860), the disease-specific alkaloid brought relief for Europeans stationed in the tropics or living in Western Europe or the United States who, through dint of economic circumstance, had access to it. Those lucky ones made up a small percentage of sufferers in the broad trans–North Atlantic region, and an even smaller percentage of sufferers around the globe. By mid-century, the successful use of quinine in the tropics had convinced some imperial governments that the time had come to experiment with the production of cinchona bark in their own colonies.

CINCHONA: FROM THE ANDES TO ASIA

From the 1830s onward, some Western merchants and observers became convinced that the stocks of Andean cinchona trees were dwindling. Botanists and seed prospectors traveled into the Andes and tried to smuggle out cinchona seeds and seedlings to start plantations elsewhere in the tropics and subtropics. There were many false steps, and the difficulties of establishing the hard-to-grow rainforest cinchona tree outside of its original habitat were far greater than anticipated. From the late 1840s, cinchona plantations failed in Algeria, Réunion, Mauritius, Jamaica, California, and elsewhere.

The prize of successful cinchona production loomed large, however, and the quest continued. In time, cinchona production eventually became the largest project of nineteenth-century imperial botany. The British in

West Africa (and thus at risk of infection from falciparum malaria) had been issued wine bitters (wine soaked in cinchona bark). In 1847, on the suggestion of Dr. Alexander Bryson, the British navy adopted the use of quinine.

Some private firms in the American tropics, however, did embrace the use of quinine to reduce morbidity and mortality among their workers. In 1855, e.g., the Panama Railroad Company issued orders to provide wine bitters to the crews operating between Aspinwall and New York and thereby reduced the incidence of morbidity from close to 100% down to well below 10%. Quinine was also used by the administrators and employees of the company in Panama (Letter from David Hoadley to William H. Van Buren, cited in Van Buren, "Quinine as a Prophylactic," 97–98).

[57] Van Buren, "Quinine as a Prophylactic," 94.
[58] Smith, "Quinine and Fever," 364.

South Asia launched the first successful initiatives. They established a government plantation in the Nilgiri Hills of southern India in the early 1860s. Later in the decade, in the island colony of Ceylon off the southeastern coast of India, British planters set up private cinchona plantations in the highlands using stock from the government botanical gardens. At the time there was little understanding that the alkaloidal composition of the cinchona barks varied considerably by subspecies. To their great misfortune, the British later discovered that the trees that they had propagated and planted in British India and Ceylon were low in quinine, compared to the other alkaloids – cinchonine, cinchonidine, and quinidine. By the time this awkward fact became well appreciated, the die was cast. The British planters in Ceylon had 128 million cinchona trees and plants in the ground by 1883, when problems of subsoil drainage encouraged them to cut down their cinchona trees to salvage what they could, flooding the markets with bark.[59] The government plantation in southern India soldiered on, ultimately opting to produce a variable mixture of cinchona alkaloids instead of quinine. Later, the British government in India opened up new plantations in northern India and in Burma that were committed to follow the same path. These plantations rarely exported alkaloids outside of British India, and they never produced alkaloids in quantities that met more than a tiny percentage of the local needs.[60]

---

[59] James L.A. Webb Jr., *Tropical Pioneers: Human Agency and Ecological Change in the Highlands of Sri Lanka, 1800–1900* (Athens: Ohio University Press, 2002), 108–128.

The flood of these barks into the market sparked new interest in the "other" cinchona alkaloids. Powers and Weightman, in particular, sought to improve the reputation of these antimalarial alkaloids and to develop the U.S. market (Merck Archives, R6-24.4. PWR, dossier 15: Cinchonidia. Powers and Weightman, *On Sulphate of Cinchonidia and Other Cheap Alkaloids of Cinchona Barks* (Philadelphia [n.d. (c. 1875)]). The British in India likewise moved to endorse the use of the other alkaloids for the treatment of Indian troops, because it promised to reduce the government expenditure on quinine. As the Officiating Secretary to the Government of India noted: "After review of the papers the Government of India are of opinion that, so far as dispensaries and hospitals for Native troops are concerned, the indent on the Home Government for sulphate of quinine may be reduced to one-half, the other half being made up on cinchonidine and quinetum" (Arthur Howell, Esq., Offg. Secretary to the Government of India, to the Surgeon-General, Indian Medical Department – No. 19, dated Fort William, January 18, 1877. *Collection of Papers Showing the Recent Results of the Trial of Cinchona Febrifuge, Quinetum Alkaloids, and Sulphate of Quinetum* [Calcutta, 1878], 5. See also *Further Collection of Papers Showing the Recent Results of the Trial of Cinchona Febrifuge, Quinetum Alkaloids, and Sulphate of Quinetum* [Calcutta, 1881]). Both documents available in the British Library, India Office Records, V/27/623/11.

[60] J.M. Cowan, "Cinchona in the Empire," *Empire Forestry Journal*, vol. 8, no. 1 (1929), 46–48.

On the island of Java, the Dutch colonial government also undertook a major effort in tropical Asia to produce quinine. It would turn out to be vastly more successful than that of the British, although this was far from evident in the early years. The Dutch had tried to introduce cinchona to the Dutch East Indies as early as 1852, but the plants had failed. Better results had come in the 1860s, when the Dutch colonial government felicitously acquired the seeds of a species particularly rich in quinine, after the British had failed to express interest.[61] But even then the Dutch struggled to create a profitable industry. Dutch scientists developed a program of alkaloid testing of individual trees, destroying all but the highest-yielding specimens, and grafting the high-yielding sapling stalks on to the root stock from other cinchona species. They began to produce groves of super trees with many times more quinine than occurred in the natural environment.[62] By the late 1870s, the Dutch were ready to permit private planters to grow the improved cinchona. The timing could not have been worse.

Private Dutch planters on Java began to take up cinchona cultivation in the same heady years of optimism as had British planters in Ceylon, and in the mid-1880s, when the glut of bark from the highlands of Ceylon hit the market, some of the Java planters with their superior tree stocks were driven to desperation and closed down their plantations.[63] The reverberations were felt as far away as the Andes. Several years after the downturn, the prospect of a revived cinchona trade from the Andes caused planters in Peru and Bolivia to take up cinchona cultivation. In the 1880s this was a considerable challenge, owing to the greatly diminished stocks of cinchona trees in the Andes. Some Andean planters imported their seeds and plants from India, rather than go through the tedious and uncertain work of collecting plants in the mountain forests.[64]

THE MARKET FOR CINCHONA ALKALOIDS

The Asian and South American cinchona plantations shipped their barks to wholesale markets in Europe and the United States where quinine manufacturers bid to meet their requirements. By the early 1880s, there were

---

[61] Gabriele Gramiccia, *The Life of Charles Ledger (1808–1905): Alpacas and Quinine* (Basingstoke, UK: Macmillan, 1988).

[62] Norman Taylor, *Cinchona in Java: The Story of Quinine* (New York: Greenberg, 1945), 45–79.

[63] Webb, *Tropical Pioneers*, 126, table 5.3.

[64] H.H. Rusby, "The Cultivation of Cinchona in Bolivia," *Pharmaceutical Record* (October 1, 1887), 305.

fifteen privately owned quinine factories in the world, all situated around the North Atlantic. There were two firms in the United States, two in the United Kingdom, four in France (all in Paris), two in Italy, four in Germany, and one in the Netherlands. Altogether they produced somewhere between fifteen and twenty-five metric tons of quinine per year.[65]

The market structure of the quinine manufacturers in the United States, however, was in the midst of change. In 1879, the U.S. Congress abolished duties on quinine imported into the United States, left in place the high taxes on alcohol that was used as a manufacturing solvent, and thereby opened wide the door to inexpensive European competition.[66] The two grand old firms of Rosengarten and Sons and Powers and Weightman in Philadelphia were destined to lose most of their market share.

By the late 1880s, the combination of the glut of cinchona and the abolition of tariffs on quinine imports into the United States sent the price of the drug spiraling downward.[67] Into the early 1880s, an ounce of quinine had brought two to three dollars on the U.S. retail market. In 1885, the price collapsed to a single dollar and to thirty cents by the end of the decade (Figure 4.2). A similar decline was reflected in prices in Europe.[68] European

[65] Karel Wessel Van Gorkom, *A Handbook of Cinchona Culture*, trans. B.D. Jackson (London: Trübner and Co., 1883), 268–269.

[66] As one late-nineteenth-century authority described the situation: "The adverse legislation in 1879 in this country, however, very seriously crippled the American manufacturers and for years past the foreign article has flooded this market, especially quinine of German manufacture, cheap labor giving them great advantage. The German manufacturers now control about three-fourths of the quinine sold in the United States, whereas, prior to 1879, almost all of the quinine sold in the United States was of American production." Letter from A.H. Jones to J.W. England dated January 8, 1898 in Joseph W. England, "The American Manufacture of Quinine Sulphate," *Alumni Report, Alumni Association of the Philadelphia College of Pharmacy* (March 1898), 58.

[67] The price of quinine in the United States of America had dropped precipitously during the early years of manufacture (as the quinine firms achieved economies of scale) and then showed considerable intraannual fluctuation, linked to the periods of malarial outbreaks, into the 1880s. Similar price series have not been developed for European quinine, with the exception of a few data from the Netherlands that suggest a similar drop from early years (see Jan Peter Verhave, "The Use of Quinine for Treatment and Control of Malaria in The Netherlands," *Tropical and Geographical Medicine*, vol. 47, no. 6 [1995], 253).

The Atlantic market for cinchona bark and quinine was integrated from the 1820s onward, however, and the U.S. price series probably reflect accurately the global trends in quinine prices. The United States was the largest national consumer of quinine in the world in the nineteenth century.

[68] In Europe, the price of quinine sulphate fell from 498 French francs in 1880 to 49 French francs in 1889 (Antoine Cloëtta, *Le problème économique et social de la Quinine* [Bâle: Impr. Kreis, 1928], 28–29).

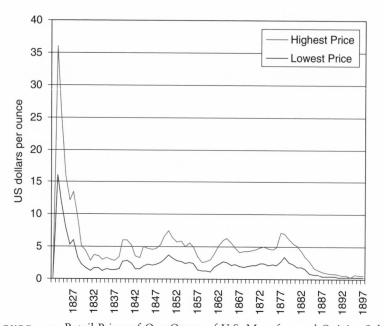

FIGURE 4.2. Retail Prices of One Ounce of U.S.-Manufactured Quinine Sulphate, 1823–1897
Source: Joseph W. England, "The American Manufacture of Quinine Sulphate," *Alumni Report* (Philadelphia: Philadelphia College of Pharmacy, March 1898), 60.

quinine, including a large volume from German factories, flooded into the United States. The United States remained the single largest national market, and in the late 1880s, the United States consumed some 40 percent of all the quinine produced.[69]

There was a decided benefit to this industrial turbulence. As the price of quinine plummeted around the North Atlantic basin, more sufferers could afford the medicine. Poor farmers in the United States who once had taken antimalarial medicines only sparingly began to self-medicate more regularly and with larger doses. This reduced the human reservoir of infection and undoubtedly played some role in the decrease in malaria in the United States.[70]

[69] D.C. Robbins, *Quinine and Our Tariff Policy: Quinine in Its Commercial Relations: Its Value Past and Present* (New York: Press of Drug Topics and Medical Abstract, 1888), 6.
[70] Marshall A. Barber, *A Malariologist in Many Lands* (Lawrence: University of Kansas Press, 1946), 11.

MALARIA AND THE FRONTIERS OF
EUROPEAN SETTLEMENT

During the nineteenth century, malarial infections spread more widely and at an accelerated pace around the world. There were three principal accelerators. The first was the migration of European and Euro-American settlers onto the world's great grasslands. The major malaria theaters were the grasslands of Eurasia and North America, as Europeans and Euro-Americans flooded into what had been the domains of the horse nomadic peoples. As we have seen, in central Eurasia, the culture of pastoral nomadism stretched back for several millennia. In North America, it was far more recent. The Sioux and a number of other Amerindian groups had adopted the Eurasian horse from contacts with Spanish ranchers and undergone their own "horse revolution" on the Great Plains of North America, beginning in the late seventeenth century in northern Mexico and expanding north into Canada by the early eighteenth century. The horse revolution had its own direct epidemiological consequences: it allowed for the rapid transmission of smallpox that ravaged the peoples of the Great Plains during the great epidemic of 1775 to 1782.[71]

Until the second half of the nineteenth century, the horse nomadic peoples on the steppes of Central Asia and the prairies of North America had suffered little ongoing exposure to malaria, owing to their low population densities and their mobility. However, in both continental heartland regions, from the mid-nineteenth century onward, farmers along a moving frontier ruptured their relative epidemiological isolation. Malaria, introduced by the infected immigrants, became established on the grasslands. In both Central Asia and North America, malaria spread to the indigenous peoples who, either through defeat in warfare, restrictions on their access to pasturelands, or economic inducements, gave up their nomadic ways of life and settled on the land.

Following the abolition of Russian serfdom in 1861, liberated agricultural workers flooded east, seeking farmland of their own, into the Central Asian grasslands. The Russian czarist government established a northern military perimeter around the Central Asian grasslands that restricted the seasonal migrations of the pastoralists. Under duress, from the expropriation of grasslands and the military cordon, the Central Asian pastoralists pared down their herds or lost them altogether and began to labor

---

[71] Elizabeth A. Fenn, *Pox Americana: The Great Smallpox Epidemic of 1775–1782* (New York: Hill and Wang, 2001), 196–233.

on the farms and in the mines controlled by the Russian immigrants. There they encountered the malaria parasites introduced by the immigrants. Both the former pastoralists and the former serfs were extremely poor, and it is unlikely that there was a single crystal of quinine among their possessions. They suffered as had millions before them.

A parallel process unfolded in North America. Following the military defeat of the Sioux and the other horse-nomadic peoples of the Great Plains, the victors forcibly relocated the conquered populations to reservations on marginal lands. There the societies of the defeated were torn asunder by depression, alcoholism, and disease. Malaria played a part in this destruction, although it probably ran a distant second to sexually transmitted disease. These major chapters in the collapse of pastoral nomadic societies were part of a global process of the forced settlement of nomadic peoples and a reduction in their numbers that accelerated during the course of the twentieth century.

By the end of the nineteenth century, the Euro-American settlement of the North American frontier was complete. In the Upper Mississippi Valley, the malarial environment became less intense and yielded to self-managed treatment. From the 1860s, cinchonine, known as the poor man's remedy, became widely available at a fraction of the cost of quinine. It was sometimes sold as a discrete product, and it also entered into use as an ingredient of patent medicines that had a reputation for curing agues and fevers. The major Philadelphia manufacturing chemical firm Powers and Weightman marketed both quinine and the other cinchona alkaloids and, in the 1870s, published pamphlets that promoted the use of cinchonine and cinchonidine.[72]

---

[72] William H. Van Buren referred to the other antimalarial alkaloids as amorphous quinine and noted, "Amorphous quinine is obtained from the 'mother-waters,' after the pure quinine has crystallized. It is to be obtained from the manufacturers of quinine, and enters into the composition of several patent medicines which have a reputation for curing agues. It is much cheaper than pure quinine, and a little more than half its strength" (Van Buren, "Quinine as a Prophylactic," see footnote on 104).

A similar bifurcation of the antimalarial market – for higher-priced quinine and less-expensive cinchona alkaloids – took place in Europe (Charles-Vital Brun, *Du sulfate de cinchonine, et de son emploi dans les fièvres intermittentes*. Thèse pour le doctorat en médecine. [Paris: Faculté de médecine de Paris, 1860], 6–7).

The price differentials were considerable. In the mid-1870s, when quinine was selling at two to three dollars per ounce, cinchonidine brought seventy-five to eighty cents per ounce and cinchonine in bulk a mere thirty-five cents per ounce. Physicians in the Midwest were counseled to treat the poor with the less expensive alkaloids, and research proved again and again that cinchonidine and cinchonine could be used effectively against malaria ([Anon.], *On the Use of Sulphate of Cinchonidia in Parts of the States of*

In regions where farmers' incomes were high enough to afford quinine or one of the other cinchona alkaloids, malaria could be effectively suppressed. A bottle of antimalarial medicine became a standard fixture on the fireplace mantle of the frontier cabin.[73] As the forestlands and grasslands were more fully converted to agricultural uses, mosquito habitat was lost, and the incidence of malarial infection gradually declined. This decline was punctuated by a spike in infections brought about by victorious northern veterans who returned home after war service in the southern states. They spread a plume of malaria throughout the northern states that took decades to subside. The U.S. South remained malarial into the twentieth century.

A variant of this process unfolded on the edges of the grasslands of South America, in the northwestern corner of Argentina. There, on the early-nineteenth-century pampas, European colonists defeated the indigenous populations who had embraced the cattle and horse revolutions in earlier centuries, and, in the aftermath of their defeat, new waves of European immigrants flowed into northwestern Argentina in the late nineteenth century. The prospect of new agricultural lands of the northwest beckoned the poor from Italy and Spain. They arrived with malaria in their blood. In short order, the region developed the reputation as the most backward and malarial within Argentina.[74]

MALARIA AND THE TRANSPORT REVOLUTION

A second major accelerator of the expansion of malaria in the nineteenth century was the dramatic improvements in travel across land and water known as the "transport revolution." The railroads, in particular, allowed overland migrants to reach more easily distant destinations with active

---

Illinois, Indiana, Missouri, Kentucky, and in the Mississippi Valley in 1875. From Medical Journals, Societies, and Individual Physicians [Philadelphia: James A. Moore, 1876], 5–10).

[73] The legacy of cinchona alkaloids also left its imprint on nomenclature. The town of Lima, OH is said to have taken its name from the marking "Lima" [Peru] on a box of cinchona bark that arrived during an epidemic of malaria. See the intervention of Dr. Richard S. Ross of Baltimore, in Thomas Findley, "Sappington's Anti-Fever Pills and the Westward Migration," *Transactions of the American Clinical and Climatological Association*, vol. 79 (1968), 44.

[74] Eric D. Carter, "Disease, Science, and Regional Development: Malaria Control in Northwest Argentina, 1890–1950" (PhD diss., University of Wisconsin–Madison, 2005). Carter emphasizes the cultural construction of the malaria problem and explores the political dimensions of the efforts at malarial control.

infections and to travel rapidly between malaria-ridden and malaria-free zones. In a sense, this was a simple, wholesale acceleration of the ancient processes of human migration that had brought about the extension of malaria across most of the globe. The important differences were in the speed of the expansion, and the fact that observers could sometimes link the movements with the infections. Malaria may well have been first introduced to the western coast of North America by pioneers who traveled west in wagons, or by visits from infected ship crews. But the westward flow of visitors accelerated with the completion of the transcontinental railroad in 1869. It allowed the parasites to ride the rails, leapfrog the Rocky Mountains, and bypass the relatively inefficient mosquito vectors in the arid western highlands. Malaria settled with the immigrants into the great agricultural valleys of California.[75]

Innovations in the nineteenth-century maritime sector such as the ocean-going steamships and clipper sailing ships also accelerated the advance of malaria. Here, again, the key was advanced speed. In earlier centuries of transoceanic commerce, parasites and mosquitoes (including *Aedes aegypti*, the vector for yellow fever) had been transferred across the Atlantic; but in the nineteenth century, the larger enclosed storage spaces onboard the fleeter ships allowed for mosquitoes to complete the voyages more easily. In the Indian Ocean, the effect was disastrous. Before the 1860s, malaria had already infected the islands of Mauritius and Réunion, whose plantation economies employed principally South Indian laborers who arrived burdened with parasites. However, the laborers were unable to transmit malaria because there were no competent mosquitoes on the islands. In the 1860s, however, the highly efficient *A. gambiae* mosquito, the bane of tropical Africa, was introduced from either Madagascar or mainland Africa and set off epidemics.[76]

Other regions were newly infected with malaria through maritime cross-cultural contact that was not enhanced by technological advances. Malay traders on their traditional seafaring vessels introduced malaria in 1843 to both Europeans and aboriginal peoples in northern Australia, and outbreaks reoccurred at intervals there over the next hundred years.[77]

---

[75] Linda Nash, *Inescapable Ecologies: A History of Environment, Disease, and Knowledge* (Berkeley: University of California Press, 2007).

[76] Erwin Ackernecht, "The History of Malaria," *Ciba Symposium*, vol. 7, nos. 3 and 4 (June–July 1945), 53–54.

[77] Margaret Spencer, *Malaria: The Australian Experience 1843–1991* (Townsville, Australia: Australasian College of Tropical Medicine, 1994), 10, 180–181.

MALARIA AND WAR

The third accelerator of the nineteenth-century expansion of malaria was war. One reason for the increase in malaria was the heightened exposure to infection, as troops slept on the open ground or under tents and moved through malarial environments on military campaigns. When military campaigns involved the movement of troops from one epidemiological zone to another, the effects of the infections became more deadly. This was likely the case during the Napoleonic Wars (1799–1815), when troops from the vivax zone were sent into the Mediterranean zone of mixed infections. When the infected troops returned from military service, some brought new malarial infections to their home communities. Major disasters also occurred when sending nonimmunes into vivax-rich environments. The British invasion of Walcheren in 1809 foundered in the polders of the Netherlands, when epidemic malaria devastated the British troops.[78]

The U.S. Civil War (1861–1865) provides a case study of what was certainly characteristic of other conflicts across malarial zones. In the Civil War, armies from the vivax zone of the northern states fought in the zone of mixed infections in the southern states. They suffered high rates of new infections. The armies of the Confederacy suffered badly from malaria as well, as a result of increased exposure. By contemporary accounting, malaria was figured to be second only to diarrhea and dysentery as a cause of morbidity during the war, reaching nearly 1.25 million cases. The number of deaths attributed to malaria was also significant, ranking fourth as a cause of death from disease. The category of malaria mortality was distinct from that of typhoid, typho-malaria, and continued fevers, and thus deaths from malaria were probably severely undercounted.[79] Moreover, the system of reporting did not allow for the recording of complications, and thus those who suffered complications of any sort – such as dysentery or pneumonia – were reported under the heading of the complication, without mention of malaria.[80]

During the early war years, the Confederate armies had little access to quinine.[81] After 1863 the price of quinine skyrocketed to four hundred to six

[78] Fiammetta Rocco, *The Miraculous Fever-Tree: Malaria and the Quest for a Cure That Changed the World* (New York: Harper Collins, 2003), 139–154.

[79] Paul E. Steiner, *Disease in the Civil War* (Springfield, IL: C.C. Thomas, 1968), 10.

[80] Charles Smart, "On the Paroxysmal Fevers," in *Medical and Surgical History of the War of the Rebellion (1861–65)*, vol. 5 (Washington, DC: Government Printing Office, 1870–1888; repr., Wilmington, NC: Broadfoot Publishing Co., 1991), 77.

[81] Ibid., 171.

hundred Confederate dollars an ounce, and the Confederate forces took recourse to the old formulas of dogwood and other local barks.[82] The Union forces were better provisioned because the quinine manufacturers were based in Philadelphia, and over the course of the conflict the Union dispensed some nineteen tons of quinine and nine and one half tons of cinchona bark to its troops.[83] Even so, it was difficult to get the quinine to the suffering troops in the fields. The Union quartermasters sometimes dispensed quinine in whisky to the troops as a prophylactic, but whisky, too, was often in short supply.

The U.S. Civil War had a profound influence on the distribution of malarial infection in the United States, because it exposed hundreds of thousands of northern troops to more intense malarial environments, and, in the aftermath of the war, the infected troops returned home. Malaria then opened a new historical chapter in North America, as regions of New England and the Mid-Atlantic States, largely free of the parasites in the prewar period, were reinfected.

After the war, malarial infections also multiplied in the U.S. South. There, the loss of manpower, owing to death and injury during the war and to the flight of freed African Americans, compounded the problem. The number of falciparum infections multiplied. As one commentator noted,

Before the war, the Southern States were in a high state of cultivation and the lands thoroughly drained; hence the malignant forms of malarial disease as a general rule were not known, except in very low, badly-drained swamp lands. Within the past eight years, owing to so much land lying waste, defective drainage and the general unsanitary condition of the country, the malarial poison has acted with intense virulence. . . . [84]

Similar processes may have taken place elsewhere in the world during the nineteenth century. In China, malarial infections increased in the mid-to-late nineteenth century, and it is possible that warfare played a significant role. Historians have not directly investigated this issue, and thus

---

[82] Alfred Jay Bollet, *Civil War Medicine: Challenges and Triumphs* (Tucson, AZ: Galen Press, 2002), 238–248.

[83] Smart, "Paroxysmal Fevers," 77, 167; Bollet, *Civil War Medicine*, 236.

[84] William A.B. Norcom, *Haemorrhagic Malarial Fever: An Address Delivered before the Medical Society of North Carolina at its 21st Annual Meeting* (Raleigh, NC: Edwards, Broughton, 1874), 12, cited by Charles A. Bentley, *Malaria and Agriculture in Bengal* (Calcutta: Bengal Secretariat Book Depot, 1925), 3 and J.A. Nájera, "Epidemiology in the Strategies for Malaria Control," *Parassitologia*, vol. 42 (2000), 10.

the role of war in the history of East Asian malaria must remain highly uncertain.

A few tentative observations, however, may be in order. The decline of the Qing Dynasty in China was likely a large-scale epidemiological disaster. From the 1770s onward, internal uprisings against the Qing dynasty brought extraordinary chaos and loss of life to some of the core areas of the Chinese Empire. The Taiping rebellion (1850–1864) is the best known of these cataclysmic events, resulting in some twenty to thirty million deaths and creating havoc among the survivors. The internal strife brought destruction and the displacement of peoples – and disease. The Taiping Rebellion, like the U.S. Civil War (although on a vastly larger scale), involved the movements of combatants and civilians between the zone of mixed infections and the zone of vivax infections. By contrast, the epidemiological consequences of the late-eighteenth-century British conquest of northern India, completed in 1805, and the brutal suppression of the 1857 to 1858 uprising in the native militaries against British colonial rule – known as the First War of Independence, the "Indian Mutiny," or the "Sepoy Mutiny" – took place within the zone of mixed infections. On the basis of British observations (that were concerned principally with the health of British troops and "native" troops under British command), the mid-nineteenth-century war does not appear to have involved large increases in malaria-related mortality. For the British colonial medical officers, cholera was apparently the main health threat to troops under their care unleashed in the aftermath of the conflict.[85]

DROUGHT, FAMINE, AND MALARIA

The far more significant demographic catastrophes for India – and perhaps even for China – were the devastating El Niño droughts from 1876 to 1878 and 1896 to 1900 that led to famine. In British India, these natural disasters were exacerbated by policies that insisted on the virtues of "market forces" and that inveighed against famine assistance. In British India, an estimated 12.2 to 29.3 million people starved to death in the two

---

[85] The epidemiological consequences of the 1857 to 1858 uprising for the Indian colonial subject populations have not been directly investigated. For general context, see Mark Harrison, *Climates and Constitutions: Health, Race, Environment and British Imperialism in India, 1600–1850* (New Delhi: Oxford University Press, 1999) and Mark Harrison, *Public Health in British India: Anglo-Indian Preventive Medicine, 1859–1914* (Cambridge: Cambridge University Press, 1994).

droughts. The El Niño droughts also struck China. There a fiscal crisis and the corruption of the Qing Dynasty in decline conspired to prevent effective famine relief. In China, an estimated 19.5 to 30 million people died famine-related deaths.[86]

In India, the 1870s also saw a dramatic increase in European investment in Indian agriculture that was predicated on the control of water supplies. The result was a decline in nutritional status and increased vulnerability to disease, including malaria. This had important implications for the spread of malaria. By the early 1880s, Indian laborers under British supervision had dug 12,750 miles of canals that irrigated 6.3 million acres – not counting the distributional canals and their watersheds. The Indian project was vast, and it held an enormous potential for the expansion of malaria. It is difficult to sort out just how many of the deaths from malaria were attributable to the expanded mosquito habitats, the new work patterns that required farmers to labor in the irrigated fields, the displacement of older rhythms of life, and the intensified struggle for access to the changed resources, but the physician Sir Joseph Fayrer, president of the India Officer Medical Board (1873–1895), estimated that of the 4,975,042 registered deaths in India in 1879, nearly 72 percent were attributable to fevers. The spike in mortality was horrifying. For Fayrer, in some years the extent of sickness and death was nearly so great as to challenge comparison with the Black Plague in fourteenth-century Europe.[87]

The aggravated disease environments of mid- and late-nineteenth-century India and China, exacerbated by general declines in nutritional status, created a heightened demand for treatments. Most sufferers, however, were poor – too poor to purchase "modern" medicines. In both India and China the expense of quinine or any of the cinchona alkaloids put them almost entirely out of the reach of the indigenous populations. The British Indian government, in the immediate aftermath of the First War for Independence (1857–1858), had launched cinchona plantations, but the volume of alkaloids produced was modest, and little of the output was destined for the "natives." One of the principal considerations of the colonial government was to defray the expense of quinine imports, rather than to achieve a broad improvement in public health or reduction in suffering among India's masses.

---

[86] Mike Davis, *Late Victorian Holocausts: El Niño Famines and the Making of the Third World* (London: Verso Press, 2001), 7, table P1.

[87] Sir Joseph Fayrer, *On the Climate and Fevers of India* (London: Churchill, 1882), 9, 13.

OPIUM AND MALARIA

The miracle of the cinchona alkaloids was largely unavailable to Indian sufferers. Many sought relief from opium, one of the common drugs used to ameliorate a range of maladies. In South Asia, opium was fully integrated into Islamic medicine, and it seems likely that its use was most common among Muslims, rather than Hindus or other non-Muslims, in northern India. Within the commercial nexus of British India, the Crown government controlled opium production for export. Another sizeable source of supply for internal consumption was grown within the independent princely states.

The nineteenth century saw a meteoric rise in opium production in India. Much of this opium was exported to China, where most was consumed in the burgeoning culture of opium smoking. This new method of using opium, which increased the opiate yields to the user by roughly fifty times more than the older methods of beating opium into solution for drinking, was addictive. The British colonial government was strongly supportive of the sale of opium to China because the trade made an important contribution to government revenues.[88]

There were major international consequences of the triangular opium trade that linked China (and Southeast Asia), India, and Great Britain. When the Qing government aggressively opposed the continued importation of Indian opium into China and confiscated chests of the drug in the late 1830s, the British retaliated militarily. During the conflicts known as the two Opium Wars (1839–1942 and 1856–1858), the Chinese dynasty lost control over its ocean ports and their hinterlands.[89] The expansion of opium production and consumption in India and China laid the foundation for the grand export of opium use throughout the Western world that eventually produced the illicit international heroin industry of the late twentieth century.[90]

Why did the Chinese and Indians increase their consumption of opium in the nineteenth century? In China, this increase was due, in part, to the fact that opium was held in high esteem as a medicinal drug that checked diarrhea and reduced fever.[91] During the summer months in the malarial

---

[88] John F. Richards, "The Opium Industry in British India," *Indian Economic and Social History Review*, vol. 39, no. 2 (2002), 149–180.

[89] David Edward Owen, *British Opium Policy in China and India* (New Haven: Yale University Press, 1934).

[90] Courtwright, *Forces of Habit*, 31–39.

[91] Jonathan Spence, "Opium Smoking in Ch'ing China," in ed. Frederic Wakeman Jr. and Carolyn Grant, *Conflict and Control in Late Imperial China* (Berkeley: University of California Press, 1975), 144.

regions, those who could afford it took opium daily as a prophylaxis against fevers. In 1879, an estimated 60 million men and 40 million women and, in 1906, an estimated 81 million men and 54 million women took opium for medicinal purposes.[92] In India, there are no comparable quantitative estimates. The core problem for historians is that the opium for internal consumption was grown largely within the independent princely states, whose recordkeeping was scant to nonexistent.[93]

Our contemporary perspectives on opium consumption have understandably focused on opium smoking and addiction. However, it is likely that this lens underplays the significance of opium as an inexpensive malarial medicine in both China and India. As the physician Fayrer in India put it:

The antipyretic [antifever] powers of opium are probably the chief reason why opium eating and smoking has become so widely spread a habit in China and India. There is little doubt that it does possess such a power, and that in the earlier stages of malarial fever it gives great relief; it relieves pain, soothes, breaks or stops the periodic return of fever, and seems to assist those exposed to malarial influences in resisting them.[94]

Many other physicians did not attribute such a "power" to opium, but in late-nineteenth-century British India, the colonial government adopted this view as a matter of expediency. The Royal Commission on Opium (1895) endorsed the use of opium to combat malaria in India, in the face of open challenge from moral reformers.[95]

THE EUROPEAN CONQUEST OF TROPICAL AFRICA

The late nineteenth century also saw a reprise of the confrontation between Europeans and the African falciparum zone that had played out earlier in the South Atlantic basin. The epidemiological barrier of

---

[92] R.K. Newman, "Opium Smoking in Late Imperial China: A Reconsideration," *Modern Asian Studies*, vol. 29, no. 4 (1995), 776, 784, 787.

[93] For testimony concerning the consumption of opium in Southeast Asia, India, and China to combat malaria, see Paul C. Winther, *Anglo-European Science and the Rhetoric of Empire: Malaria, Opium, and British Rule in India, 1756–1895* (Lanham, MD: Lexington Books, 2003), 345–348, app. B. John F. Richards has suggested that the internal consumption of opium in India is a rich topic to be explored (Richards, "Opium Industry," 154).

[94] Fayrer, *On the Climate and Fevers of India*, 114.

[95] Winther, *Anglo-European Science and the Rhetoric of Empire*, esp. 323–344.

falciparum malaria and yellow fever had long blocked European incursions into tropical Africa. Europeans were still immunologically naïve with regard to falciparum malaria. When unprotected by quinine and bed nets, they were as vulnerable as they had been in the early age of European exploration.

In the final quarter of the nineteenth century, European imperial powers launched a poorly considered "scramble" to colonize the African continent. This was driven principally by rivalry between European powers in the grip of competitive industrialization; Africa was thought to hold natural resources that might provide a decisive advantage in the struggle for industrial primacy. As a result of the scramble, European colonial powers staked their claims to lands that would constitute their African colonies.

By the 1880s, the dangers of African disease seemed more manageable to the Europeans than they had earlier in the nineteenth century. Knowledgeable observers thought that the malarial fevers of the African tropics were the same as the fevers of Europe, even if far more destructive.[96] The European and North American experiences with quinine thus had an immediate significance for the European imperial conquests of the African tropics. Quinine promised to reduce the military costs in suffering and troop deaths that had been an integral part of earlier imperial ventures into the tropical African environments.

In retrospect, it now is clear that the largest "savings" for European troops and administrators were reaped from innovations in public health and hygiene, rather than chemotherapeutic treatment.[97] The savings from quinine use, however, were real enough, but perhaps their even greater significance lies in the fact that they convinced the military decision makers that losses to malaria could be mostly controlled, and this in turn served as one of several supports that undergirded the imperial initiatives. In this respect, quinine was a key to human control over "natural" forces. It was a power that, at the time, only Europeans could wield.

* * *

In the late sixteenth century, the Spaniards "discovered" that cinchona bark from the Andes was a cure for malaria. Jesuit's Bark gradually gained acceptance in Western Europe. In 1820, Parisian pharmacists succeeded in

---

[96] Thomas Wilson, *An Enquiry into the Origin and Intimate Cause of Malaria* (London: Renshaw, 1858), 31; cited by Dobson, *Contours*, 319.

[97] Curtin, *Death by Migration*, passim.

isolating two of the medically active alkaloids in cinchona bark, and, within a few years, new chemical firms in the United States and Western Europe began to produce quinine for the market. Despite the new medicine, malarial infections multiplied during the nineteenth century and the zones of both vivax and mixed infections increased in extent. In both China and India, the use of opium as a palliative became widespread and constituted an alternative zone of malaria therapy.

5

Toward Global Public Health

For most of the nineteenth century, European and Euro-American physicians were in general agreement that quinine worked wonders against intermittent and remittent fevers. Quinine was thought to be able to prevent the eruption of fevers and, if administered after the onset of fevers, to "cure." The categories of intermittent and remittent fevers were vague, and in practice, specialists had difficulty distinguishing between different diseases, particularly yellow fever and malaria. Thus, there was considerable confusion about the therapeutic range of quinine and the other cinchona alkaloids. At times, physicians employed quinine to treat typhoid, typhus, erysipelas, scarlatina, pneumonia, cynanche trachealis, delerium tremens, acute rheumatism, chronic rheumatism, cholera infantum, cerebro-spinal meningitis, and surgical shock, in addition to yellow fever and malaria.[1] Even as late as 1882, Otis F. Manson, the author of a lengthy volume on the physiological and therapeutic action of quinine, noted, "Although nearly two-thirds of a century has elapsed since the introduction of quinine into the *materia medica*, yet perhaps there is no agent in its vast catalogue concerning whose properties such opposite opinions are held, or which has elicited more discussion."[2]

Even in the treatment of intermittent and remittent fevers, physicians disagreed over the size and the timing of the appropriate dosage and as to whether or not the alkaloids should be combined with more standard treatments, such as bleeding and purging. Most physicians considered these actions necessary to adjust the humoral balances within the patient's body. The doctors administered quinine because they were tonics that

[1] Otis F. Manson, *A Treatise on the Physiological and Therapeutic Action of the Sulphate of Quinine* (Philadelphia: J.B. Lippincott and Co., 1882), 115, 117, 128–152.
[2] Ibid., 3.

could strengthen the body to resist disease, particularly malaria that rose out of the miasmatic swamps.[3] Quinine's efficacy against malaria eventually won it the medical distinction as the first disease-specific drug in the Western *materia medica*. Beyond the medical communities, however, the notion that quinine was a general tonic gained in currency through the first decades of the twentieth century, as manufacturers added the inexpensive cinchona alkaloids to "chill tonics" and quinine to a wide range of consumer products such as perfumes, teeth-strengthening pastes, laxatives, cold medicines, and hair tonics.

In the 1880s, "germ" theory slowly began to displace "humoral" theory as a disease paradigm among medical practitioners. In 1880, Alphonse Laveran, a French military physician in Algeria, made an important discovery under the microscope. He noticed motile, spherical bodies in the blood of patients suffering from "marsh fever." He identified these bodies correctly as protozoal parasites, and he deduced that he had found the cause of malaria.[4] Laveran traveled to Italy to search for the parasite in the air, water, and soils, without success. By 1884, he suspected that the parasite might be found within mosquitoes.

His discovery of falciparum parasites, however, did not at first do much to displace the miasmatic theory. After all, it seemed perfectly plausible to many that the "germs" emerged from the marshes. In the latter half of the 1880s, the parasitic origin of malaria became accepted in some, but not all, scientific circles. The death knell for miasmatic theory began to toll only later in the next decade, ringing out first from one of the British hill stations in southern India that had been established to offer relief to government officials from the oppressive heat of the plains.

A TRIO OF DISCOVERIES IN 1897

On August 20, 1897, Ronald Ross, a medical doctor in British India, who had spent years dissecting mosquitoes and squinting through a primitive

---

[3] As Manson noted in 1882: "By many – we may say by the large majority of writers – cinchona had been regarded as the first and most valuable of tonics, possessing excitant and stimulant properties, which rendered its use hazardous in the presence of fever and inflammation; whilst on the other hand, in the opinion of a numerous and powerful minority, it was held to be endowed with sedative and even antiphlogistic virtues in the same conditions of the organism. The controversy has therefore been renewed in our day, with as much zeal and earnestness as in the famous discussion between Ramazzini and Torti in the past century" (ibid., 8).

[4] Gordon Harrison, *Mosquitoes, Malaria and Man: A History of the Hostilities since 1880* (New York: E.P. Dutton, 1978), 7–16.

microscope looking for physical evidence of malaria parasites, concluded that the mosquito was the vector for bird malaria. He then argued, by extension, that the mosquito must also be the vector for human malaria. During the same eventful year, Giovanni Battista Grassi and other Italian scientists who had been hot on the trail of malaria conclusively proved that the female *Anopheles* mosquito was the vector for human malaria.[5] Also in 1897, Robert Koch, the German bacteriologist, was at work in Dar es-Salaam in German East Africa, seeking an answer to the malaria problem that threatened to derail plans for German colonization in tropical Africa. He discovered in his laboratory that quinine destroyed malaria parasites in human blood. These three epochal discoveries struck a destabilizing blow to miasmatic theory. In the years after 1897, among the fraternity of scientists devoted to the emerging field of malariology, the theory of miasmas was dead in the water.

DIVERGENT PATHS TO MALARIA CONTROL

The trio of discoveries promised an entirely new set of possibilities for treating malaria. Now, physicians and public health specialists had two robust approaches to the problematic disease. Koch's research had validated the older chemotherapeutic approach, proving that quinine worked as a parasiticide, and because of the dramatic decline in the price of quinine, it now seemed feasible to use it broadly in the service of public health. Those treated with quinine would have "cleansed" blood and would no longer be able to act as reservoirs of infection, putting others at risk. The metaphor fit well with the mid-nineteenth-century paradigm that filth was the principal cause of disease.

The discoveries of Grassi and Ross opened up a new possibility for the control of malaria. Perhaps it would be possible to destroy the mosquito populations in badly stricken areas and "sanitize" the local landscapes. In a sense, the idea was not strictly novel; the Romans had drained swamps as early as the late first millennium BCE in an attempt to destroy miasmatic disease, and the Abbasid Caliphate (750–1258) had drained the swamps around Baghdad and reduced malaria in the city. However, armed with the new understanding that the female *Anopheles* mosquito was the

---

[5] The Culex mosquito transmitted bird malaria. The significance of Ronald Ross's discovery would be bitterly contested by Italian scientists who were also on the trail of the vector for human malaria, and who would prove only months later that the culprit was the *Anopheles* mosquito. See ibid., 64–108.

malaria vector, the epidemiological rationale for the destruction of mosquito habitat was new and seemed indisputably sound. As the first generation of malariologists learned more about mosquitoes, they discovered that many anopheline vectors did not breed in swamps or even in still waters, and that they would have to tailor their interventions to the local *Anopheles* mosquito species.

The virtues of each approach – at least on a large scale – were untested. Here the national ambitions and injured pride of Ronald Ross and his Italian competitors played large. Small-scale experiments were undertaken, and bold claims were made. Ross championed an assault on the mosquitoes – and the creation of mosquito brigades to wage these malaria wars. Ross's opposition to the large-scale administration of quinine put him at odds with many of the most talented malariologists – particularly the Italians, whose leading scientist, Grassi, felt he had been denied the glory of the discovery of the role of the mosquito in human malaria.[6] The Italians tacked in the opposite direction, drawing inspiration from breakthroughs in the field of bacteriology, pioneered by Koch, and committed themselves to the chemical therapy approach, wagering that it would be possible to "sanitize" the bloodstreams of afflicted populations through the mass administration of quinine.

A die was cast. Ross held that mass quinine therapy would not repay the expense and would not work to control malaria, although he was in favor of the free distribution of quinine to schoolchildren who were suffering from fever or enlargement of the spleen. Ross had the ear of the British Colonial Office, and in 1899 the British sent a mission to Sierra Leone to attempt to eradicate the local mosquito vector in Freetown. The attempt fell short, in part because of a lack of funds and because the difficulty of destroying the mosquito habitat in a sprawling urban settlement with heavy rainfall proved overwhelming. The *Anopheles gambiae* could breed in a tin can or in puddles as small as that made by a boot heel.

The idea of mosquito eradication in Africa, however, was not immediately washed up. The British launched a broader sanitation effort for the larger, and more important colonial settlement in Lagos in southern Nigeria. It, too, failed. The British had stumbled onto one of the intractable problems in the transmission of falciparum malaria in tropical Africa: the highly efficient mosquito vectors, with their strong preference for human blood and their ability to breed in high rainfall microenvironments.

---

[6] Ibid., 102–108; Frank M. Snowden, *The Conquest of Malaria: Italy, 1900–1962* (New Haven: Yale University Press, 2006), 38–52.

RACIAL HYGIENE

Not all the British experts, however, had their eyes on the mosquito. Some were taking blood smears and counting blood parasites, and they discovered that African children had a lot of them. The children also had extremely high rates – up to 90 percent – of a distension of the spleen (splenomegaly), which could be palpated and measured as an index of infection.[7] In infected adults, the spleen rates dropped to 40 or 30 percent or less. The children rather than the mosquitoes were identified as the actionable threat.[8] The "scientific" understanding took hold that the Africans, and in particular African children, were the source of greatest danger to the Europeans. Infected African children were found to have very high levels of gametocytes in their blood, and from this evidence it was presumed that infected children would be the most effective transmitters of disease. (The current understandings are that the level of gametocytes in the blood is not a reliable indicator of the infectivity of the individual. Adults with low levels of gametocytes have been shown to be highly effective transmitters.)[9]

With these presuppositions, the solution to the malaria problem in the tropical colonies became race specific. The Europeans should separate themselves from the native reservoirs of disease by establishing all-white residential zones.[10] Malaria in colonial British West Africa, at least along

[7] A man by the name of Dempsey is credited with the first use of a spleen rate in 1845 in his mapping of the distribution of malaria in the Eastern Jumna Canal in India (Brevet Colonel S.R. Christophers, "Note on Malaria Research and Prevention in India," League of Nations, C.H./Malaria/135 [Geneva, November 1929], 3).

[8] During the interwar period, the Dutch zoologist Nicolaas Hendrik Swellengrebel found that there were major differences in malaria endemicity between the Dutch East Indies and tropical Africa. In the Dutch East Indies, the spleen index (the percentage of people with an enlarged spleen) was high among all age groups; in tropical Africa it was lower among adults and adults' spleens were also less enlarged (J.P. Verhave, "Malaria: Epidemiology and Immunity in the Malay Archipelago," in ed. G.M. van Heteren, A. de Knecht-van Eekelen, and M.J.D. Poulissen, *Dutch Medicine in the Malay Archipelago* [Amsterdam: Rodopi, 1989], 98–100).

[9] Interestingly, evidence concerning this issue was produced as early as the 1930s, but did not fit in with the thinking about malaria at that time. R.C. Muirhead-Thomson, "Where Do Most Mosquitoes Acquire Their Malarial (Plasmodium Falciparum) Infection? From Adults or From Children?," *Annals of Tropical Medicine and Parasitology*, vol. 92, no. 8 (1998), 891–893.

[10] S.R. Christophers and J.W.W. Stephens, "The Segregation of Europeans," in *Reports to the Malaria Committee of the Royal Society*, 3rd series (London: Harrison and Sons, 1900), 21–24; Philip D. Curtin, "Medical Knowledge and Urban Planning in Colonial Tropical Africa," *American Historical Review*, vol. 90, no. 3 (1985), 594–613; Harrison, *Mosquitoes, Malaria and Man*, 121–129.

the coast, became less a matter of mosquitoes and parasites than race. Europeans were to live apart from the natives.[11] The malaria problem was how to keep Europeans free from the disease, not how to limit or treat the infections of the Africans. As two of the foremost British malariologists put it, "The question that is of the most urgent necessity, then, is not so much how large towns with sometimes 40,000 native inhabitants can be freed from anopheles, but how the comparatively small number (at most 200) of Europeans can be protected."[12]

Thus, by the early twentieth century, both mosquito sanitation and mass quinine therapy in tropical Africa seemed highly impractical to the British. Even an individual European's efforts to avoid or treat malaria seemed fraught with problems. Investigators from the Liverpool School of Tropical Medicine and Medical Parasitology noted that the Europeans who resided in West Africa roundly misused their "mosquito curtains" and incompetently medicated themselves with quinine. There seemed to be only one logical conclusion:

Segregation of Europeans at a distance from all natives offers itself now as the only measure by which absolute freedom from the disease can be guaranteed, and all the scientific evidence that has been collected respecting the cause of malarial fever and the manner in which infection among Europeans is brought about, markedly points to the adoption of the segregation principles as the only way in which absolute protection from the disease can be assured.[13]

In practice, the impulse toward residential segregation was fragmented by realities on the ground. Only some local terrains lent themselves to effective separation of the races. Some colonial governors argued that residential segregation was impractical, and that if the Africans were the reservoir of malarial infections they should be treated with quinine. Some were concerned that the residential segregation might harm race relations. The result was a heterodox pattern of tropical African colonial urban planning that produced European residential neighborhoods that were distinct, if not always entirely separate, from those of Africans.[14]

---

[11] S.R. Christophers and J.W.W. Stephens, "The Native as the Prime Agent in the Malarial Infection of Europeans (With Map)," in *Further Reports to the Malaria Committee of the Royal Society* (London, 1900), 3–19.

[12] Christophers and Stephens, "The Segregation of Europeans," 23.

[13] H.E. Annett, J. Everett Dutton, and J.H. Elliott, *Report of the Malaria Expedition to Nigeria of the Liverpool School of Tropical Medicine and Medical Parasitology*, vol. I (Liverpool: University Press of Liverpool, 1901), 47–49; quotation from vol. I, 54–55.

[14] Philip D. Curtin, "Medical Knowledge and Urban Planning in Colonial Tropical Africa," *American Historical Review*, vol. 90, no. 3 (1985), 594–613.

The idea of residential segregation was an old idea, one that harkened back to the "double towns" that separated Muslim and non-Muslim trading groups, particularly in North Africa and Sub-Saharan Africa. It had been put into practice more thoroughly in tropical western Africa than anywhere else in the world, perhaps in part because the dangers from falciparum infections were most intense there. Later, a similar pattern repeated itself in European colonial empire. Outside of tropical Africa, the notion of "safe" residential segregation was honored more in the breach; Europeans developed a dependence on native servants, who for convenience generally were encouraged to live either in the employer's house or nearby the compound.

Residential segregation in tropical Africa supplemented an older practice of avoiding the worst heat and seasons of disease. In the first half of the nineteenth century, the British established colonial "hill stations" in India and Ceylon that were at elevations above the local mosquito disease vectors. These stations were conceived of as "healthy," convalescent retreats in the mountains. The tropical "hill station" put the British at least temporarily "above" the anopheline mosquito line and away from the worst heat.[15] In the early twentieth century, British settlers in tropical Africa brought with them the same appreciations of the relative safety of high elevations. Three thousand feet above sea level, the absence of tsetse flies, and an annual minimum of twenty inches of rainfall were considered the *sine qua non* of settlement.

CAMPAIGNS OF CHEMICAL THERAPY

The chemotherapeutic approach to malaria was given its first trial in tropical Southeast Asia. The German government dispatched Robert Koch, whose pathbreaking work on the disease agents that caused anthrax and tuberculosis had brought him international acclaim, to "Kaiser-Wilhelms-Land" (the German colony on New Guinea) to study endemic malaria. Koch stopped along the way in Italy and the Dutch East Indies, learning about the local malarial environments and talking about the possibility of mass quinine therapy.

In Kaiser-Wilhelms-Land, German colonial doctors deplored the high rate of morbidity and mortality among the small European population. The situation was grave. Malaria had forced the Germans to abandon

---

[15] Dale Kennedy, *The Magic Mountains: Hill Stations and the British Raj* (Berkeley: University of California Press, 1996).

Finschafen, their administrative center. The devastation extended to the imported laborers: of the 273 Chinese "coolies" who arrived in Stephansort in 1898, 125 died within a year, most from malaria. The continued existence of the German colony was in question.

Koch carried out mass blood screenings, and he discovered that the indigenous inhabitants often had no clinical symptoms of malaria, even though their blood tests were positive for infection. This led Koch to two important understandings: (1) that immunities to malaria could be acquired, and (2) that the localities to be treated should be selected on the basis of a general blood survey. Koch launched a small, controlled quinine regimen for seven hundred plantation workers, and the local progress of malaria ground to a standstill.

Koch's plantation success suggested the need for a general scale-up, to address the malaria problem on a colony-wide basis. Koch asked for more specialized doctors and parasitologists to be sent out to "Kaiser-Wilhelms-Land," but few were sent. The costs were deemed prohibitive, compared to the unimportance of the colony.

Koch also proposed a large-scale chemical therapy program for Dar es-Salaam in German East Africa. Here the potential political significance of the project was greater. The extent of malaria in German East Africa – even on the slopes of Mount Kilimanjaro up to 1,500 meters – seemed to preclude European settlement, and in the frantic international competition of the 1890s, there was concern that the failure of colonization in Africa might have dire implications for Germany's survival as a great power.

The chief German medical officer in Dar-es-Salaam, Dr. Freidrich Plehn, however, had a different view of the malaria situation. Plehn was convinced that Africans with acquired immunity did not need to be treated with quinine, Europeans and Africans should have separate residential areas, and only Europeans should be provided protection from mosquitoes. Koch's quinine mass therapy program foundered, in good measure because many inhabitants and visitors went entirely untreated.[16]

The Germans came to the view, as had the British in West Africa, that the separation of the European community from the "native" community was the appropriate public health strategy. Within a few years, a medical pattern asserted itself: quinine for the European community and racially

---

[16] Ann Beck, "Medicine and Society in Tanganyika, 1890–1930: A Historical Inquiry," *Transactions of the American Philosophical Society*, vol. 67, pt. 3 (1977), 14–15; David F. Clyde, *History of the Medical Services of Tanganyika* (Dar es Salaam, Tanzania: Government Press, 1962), 24–25; David F. Clyde, *Malaria in Tanzania* (London: Oxford University Press, 1967), 31.

segregated residential patterns. In the German colonies, the separation of the races was conceptualized as an "ideal malaria therapy": If the Germans could keep the local Africans at least 1,200 meters away, Europeans would eventually be able to dispense with "quinine prophylaxis." Within a few years, the notion of malaria prevention was dropped, and the policy came to be known simply as "racial hygiene." The program of quinine therapy for the indigenous population and the imported workers came to an end in 1912.[17] Malaria did not.

The idea of racial segregation was contagious. The French and the Belgians also adopted it as standard colonial practice in their African colonies. The Russians did the same on the steppes of Russian-controlled Central Asia, identifying the malarial danger as emanating from the natives and keeping the settlements of Central Asian peoples at a safe distance from their own.[18]

During the years that the mass quinine campaign in German East Africa was faltering, the Italians launched a national chemotherapeutic war against malaria. The south of Italy, and in particular the environs of Rome, had been among the most malaria-infested areas in Europe for more than two millennia and lay squarely with the zone of mixed infections. Many of the infections, although not the majority, were falciparum. An estimated ten to twenty thousand Italians died every year, and annual infections probably totaled somewhere between 300,000 and two million. The modernizing Italian state began to calculate the economic costs of malaria. Millions of labor days were lost each year, and perhaps two million hectares of fertile land were left uncultivated.[19]

The Italian scientists had experienced enormous success in proving that only the females of *some* species of anopheline mosquitoes were implicated in the transmission of malaria and that malaria could be transmitted only by mosquito, rather than through the emanations of miasmatic vapors. Grassi and his colleague Angelo Celli were convinced that it would be possible to undertake a campaign of mass quinine treatment, although they differed as to whether the quinine should be given as a prophylaxis or cure. In principle, both men thought that a mass quinine campaign would be much less expensive than the destruction of mosquito habitat.

---

[17] W.U. Eckart, "Malaria and Colonialism in the German Colonies New Guinea and the Cameroons. Research, Control, Thoughts of Eradication," *Parassitologia*, vol. 40 (1998), 83–90.

[18] C.W. Daniels, "Prophylaxis," in *Reports to the Malaria Commission of the Royal Society*, 3rd series, 43.

[19] Louis F. Amoroso Jr., Gilberto Corbellini, and Mario Coluzzi, "Lessons Learned from Malaria: Italy's Past and Sub-Sahara's Future," *Health and Place*, vol. 11 (2005), 68.

During the first phase of the state-sponsored quinine campaign (1904–1914), the Italian state constructed rural health stations from which officials undertook local health censuses and distributed quinine. The campaign sought to overcome the chasm between the state and the peasantry, who were suspicious of state medicine and long accustomed to suffering from malarial infections. The Italian state responded by establishing schools for peasants; these schools had staff living on the school premises, interacting with the rural communities, and distributing quinine. During the same years, the swamplands in the Po Valley were drained as part of the large-scale land-reclamation projects for intensified agriculture.

The quinine campaign achieved mixed results: Deaths from malaria dropped dramatically but sickness from malaria did not. Many social reformers and malariologists came to the conclusion that education and an improvement in the material conditions of life were critical for improving the health of the population. Malaria was understood as a marker of depressed economic conditions and a result of a lack of access to education. It ultimately gave birth to a new malarial paradigm. Malaria was launched on a new career as a social problem, a marker of depressed economic conditions, and a result of a lack of access to education.[20] Later in the twentieth century, this argument would be radically reconfigured as a rhetorical strategy. The extension of rural health care and education would be downplayed. Instead of "malaria is the result of the lack of development," the argument was recast as "malaria blocks development," with its corollary that antimalaria programs – rather than education and rural health care – would promote development.[21]

LANDSCAPE SANITATION AND MOSQUITO BRIGADES

As the experiments in racial segregation and mass quinine therapy began in European tropical colonies in Asia and Africa, the United States scored remarkable "successes" in mosquito control in the South Atlantic Basin. Following the war with Spain in 1898, the United States took possession of Cuba in 1899. There, the major public health problem was yellow fever, rather than malaria. U.S. scientists unraveled a maze of evidence that led to the conclusion that the mosquito was the vector for yellow fever,

---

[20] Snowden, *Conquest of Malaria*, 53–114.
[21] Randy Packard has explored the history of this argument in a forthcoming essay "Roll Back Malaria, Roll in Development" (personal communication).

thereby confirming the hypothesis of the Cuban physician Carlos Finlay, who first proposed the idea in the 1860s.

Unlike the *Anopheles* mosquito, the yellow fever mosquito, *Aedes aegypti*, bred in domestic contexts – in tin cans and water barrels. The United States created "sanitation squads" to destroy the mosquito's urban microhabitats, by flushing out the larvae and by laying down poisons. The results were salubrious: the incidence of yellow fever in Havana dramatically declined. Toward the end of the Havana yellow fever campaign, the sanitation squads began to push out from the urban center into the suburbs, and there they took aim at malaria, as well. Here, the techniques were far less successful. However, a major lesson was drawn nonetheless from the Havana campaign: An aggressive attack on mosquito habitat could reap enormous health benefits or, put differently, reduce the economic costs of disease.

This lesson was transferred to the Panama Canal Zone, where once again the principal disease was yellow fever, and this time the mosquito warriors enjoyed double successes. At great expense, the United States eliminated yellow fever from the narrow Panama Canal Zone, and the incidence of malaria also declined dramatically. The malaria campaign was in fact something of a hybrid: Not only was the mosquito habitat destroyed, but the "sanitation" workers who fell ill with malaria were treated with quinine. The question for the future was: Could this success be replicated elsewhere? After initial enthusiasm, it was realized that the great expense in the Panama Canal Zone could only be justified by the economic benefits that were expected to flow through it.[22] With the exception of the Suez Canal, there probably was not another piece of real estate on earth with such economic potential.

In India, the British launched a major effort in sanitation engineering at Mian Mir, near Lahore in present-day Pakistan. This initiative was in part a response to the forceful advocacy of Ross that a program to destroy mosquito-breeding habitat would greatly reduce mosquito density and that these efforts would significantly reduce malaria. In Ross's view, the key to effective malaria control was the willingness of government to take on the challenge and for government to concentrate on the most densely populated areas.[23]

Over the period 1902 to 1909, roughly coincident with the first expansion of the mass quinine therapy program in Italy, mosquito brigades sought

[22] Harrison, *Mosquitoes, Malaria and Man*, 157–168.
[23] Ronald Ross, "The Best Antimalarial Organization for the Tropics," *Separat-Abdruck aus Malaria*, Band I, Heft 2 (Leipzig, 1909), 89–94.

out the mosquito habitats and destroyed them. Much of this work was aimed at relatively small areas that surrounded groups of houses or military barracks. The results were extremely disappointing. The overall rates of sickness were even higher in 1908 than they had been in 1904. Some observers concluded logically enough that antimosquito habitat interventions were the wrong approach. Ross thought that the trial had been badly botched; but the lessons of Mian Mir survived his wrath. The small-scale work of mosquito brigades was judged a waste of resources. The poor results seemed to point up the significance of the different mosquito species' behavioral patterns: What had been successful against the *Aedes* mosquito in Havana apparently would not work against the *Anopheles*. They also suggested a problem of scale. If environmental interventions were to be successful in malaria control, they might have to involve major engineering projects.[24] This would mean great expense, and such efforts to destroy anopheline habitat might run directly afoul of the large-scale British water control and irrigation projects, particularly in the Punjab, that aimed at increasing export revenues for the British Raj.

If the severity of the malaria problems were the principal criterion for a large-scale intervention, the Punjab projects would have been a prime candidate. These projects had been fraught with tragic malaria epidemics, which were compounded by famine that struck the local populations repeatedly in the late nineteenth century. The scale of suffering remained enormous into the early twentieth century. In 1900, more than 254,000 Punjabis lost their lives, and, in 1908, the number of deaths was estimated at more than 300,000.[25] The British finally altered their doctrinaire opposition to food relief, and after 1908, the intertwined waves of famine and epidemic malaria in northwestern India began to subside, largely because the new policies of "drought relief" brought food to the starving.[26]

---

[24] William F. Bynum, "An Experiment That Failed: Malaria Control at Mian Mir," *Parassitologia*, vol. 36 (1994), 107–120.

[25] As early as 1869, things began to go badly awry. More than 116,000 Punjabis died from fever that year. Malaria epidemics broke out again in 1878, 1879, 1884, 1890, 1892, and 1900. Major S.R. Christophers, *Malaria in the Punjab* (Calcutta: Superintendent Government Printing, 1911), 9, 24.

[26] Major S.R. Christophers investigated the relationship between famine and epidemic malaria in his book *Malaria in the Punjab*. The statistical relationships and causal links between starvation and malaria have been reinvestigated and reconfirmed by Sheila Zurbrigg in "Re-Thinking the 'Human Factor' in Malaria Mortality: The Case of Punjab, 1868–1940," *Parassitologia*, vol. 36 (1994), 121–135. Elsewhere, Zurbrigg has successfully challenged the view that starvation protected against malaria by starving the parasite as well as the host (Sheila Zurbrigg, "Did Starvation Protect from Malaria?," *Social Science History*, vol. 21, no. 1 [1997], 27–58).

Food relief policies, however, only indirectly addressed the issue of malaria. Deadly fevers still remained a major problem. If large-scale landscape sanitation was out of the question, chemical therapy might be possible. The ongoing experience in Italy with mass quinine therapy seemed promising. However, the malaria problem in India was of a larger order of magnitude. The annual number of malaria deaths in Italy before the quinine campaign was estimated at ten to twenty thousand. In India, an estimated 1.3 million died every year. The problem was worse in some areas, such as the Punjab, but when the difficulties were summed, malaria loomed as the greatest problem that confronted the government and populations of British India. The politics of the Italian malaria problem were also vastly different from India. The Italian campaign was an attempt to build the state by extending its reach into the countryside. In India, the British had no such aspirations with its colonial populations of subjects.[27] Ever parsimonious, the British administrators adopted the use of quinine to medicate the native troops' children who were thought to pose a threat to the British.[28]

WORLD WAR I AND ITS AFTERMATH

The Italian mass quinine treatment program had made good progress in reducing malaria deaths but not sickness. The outbreak of World War I

[27] Nonetheless the Italian campaign to defeat malaria among the working poor was something of a challenge to British imperial sensibilities. In British India, S.P. James wrote defensively of the British program to make quinine available to the poor by selling single doses of quinine for the lowest denomination coin in general daily use, through the Post Office. This program had been initiated in various provinces between 1890 and 1894 – and thus well before the Italian experiment – but the quantities of quinine were tiny in comparison with the need (S.P. James, "A Note on Some of the Measures That Have Been Taken to Make Quinine Available to the Poor in India," in ed. S.P. James and S.R. Christophers, *Paludism, Being the Transactions of the Committee for the Study of Malaria in India* [Simla, India: Government Central Branch Press, 1911], 10–14). W.F. Bynum, "'Reasons for Contentment': Malaria in India, 1900–1920," *Parassitologia*, vol. 40, nos. 1–2 (1998), 19–27.

In 1906, during an epidemic in the colony of Ceylon, off the southeastern coast of India, the British colonial government there extended a program of free quinine distribution throughout the island but with disappointing results. The chief medical officer concluded that the money would have been better spent fighting the mosquitoes (Margaret Jones, *Health Policy in Britain's Model Colony Ceylon (1900–1948)* [New Delhi: Orient Longman, 2004], 174–175).

[28] S.P. James, "A Report of the Anti-Malarial Operations at Mian Mir (1901–1902)," in *Reports to the Malarial Committee of the Royal Society*, 8th series (London: Harrison and Sons, 1903), 76.

(1914–1918) reversed this success. The state mobilization of resources for war starved the antimalarial campaign in Italy of personnel, funds, medicine, and public attention. It became a casualty of war. Infections skyrocketed. Malaria mortality and morbidity returned to precampaign levels. Tens of thousands died, millions sickened.[29] In the wider theaters of the conflict, malaria reaped new harvests.

World War I, like so many wars before it, was a grim multiplier of malarial infections. The deployment of armies to the battlefronts entailed the movement of nonimmunes into malarial environments, and, as in the case in the U.S. Civil War, access to quinine became critical to the military effort. The demand for quinine soared, and the forces of the Allied Powers (Great Britain, France, Russia, and later Italy and the United States) were largely successful in blocking the flow of cinchona bark and alkaloids to the opposing Central Powers (Germany, the Austro-Hungarian Empire, Bulgaria, and the Ottoman Empire). On the Turkish front and in the Balkans, the impact of malaria on the combatants was particularly severe.[30]

The desperate epidemiological circumstances of troops mired in trench warfare and the transfer of troops between theaters of war and the home fronts spilled malaria into old haunts. In the English marshlands, troops from Greece and India who were stationed there provoked a reinfection of the local vector, and several hundred deaths were reported during the years 1917 to 1919.[31] After the war, when the troops returned home, many were infected carriers. New waves of malaria broke out in parts of England, France, and Germany from which it had previously been eliminated. This was true in the Middle East as well. Baghdad, formerly free of malaria, became reinfected (Maps 5.1 and 5.2).[32]

In terms of malaria morbidity and mortality, the larger malarial consequences of the Great War came in the form of aftershocks. Following the breakup of the Ottoman Empire and the Greek-Turkish war of 1921 to 1922, 1.5 million refugees, mostly from malaria endemic regions, flooded into Greece. This set off epidemics in Macedonia and Thrace. The Greek

[29] Snowden, *Conquest of Malaria*, 115–141.

[30] The malaria caseload in the Balkans was 92.6 per 1,000 troops in the third year of the war and rose to 232.4 per 1,000 in the fourth year. On the Turkish front, the caseload skyrocketed to 651.2 per 1,000 in the third year and then dropped to 183.7 per 1,000 in the final year of the war (Bureau for Increasing the Use of Quinine, *Malaria and Quinine* [Amsterdam: Bureau for Increasing the Use of Quinine, 1927], 27).

[31] Mary J. Dobson, *Contours of Death and Disease in Early Modern England* (Cambridge: Cambridge University Press, 1997), 349.

[32] Bureau for Increasing the Use of Quinine, *Malaria and Quinine*, 27–28.

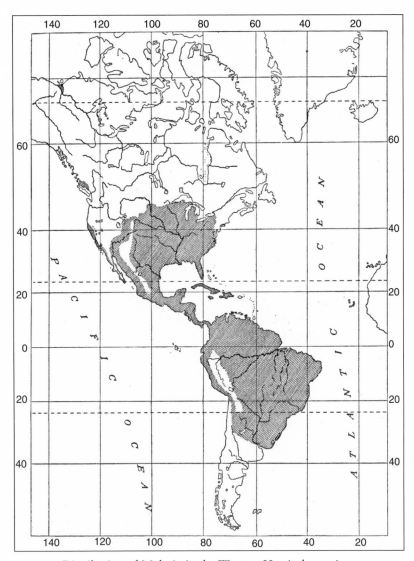

MAP 5.1. Distribution of Malaria in the Western Hemisphere, circa 1920
Source: Adapted from S.P. James and S.R. Christophers, "Malaria," in W. Byam
and R.G. Archibald, eds., *The Practice of Medicine in the Tropics*, vol. 2 (London:
H. Frowde and Hodder and Stoughton, 1922), 1503.

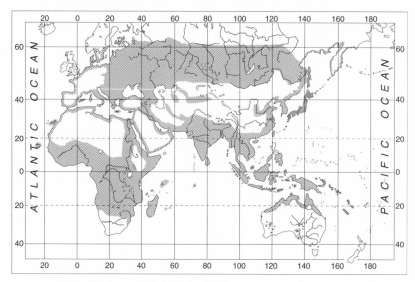

MAP 5.2. Distribution of Malaria in the Eastern Hemisphere, circa 1920
Source: Adapted from S.P. James and S.R. Christophers, "Malaria," in W. Byam
and R.G. Archibald, eds., *The Practice of Medicine in the Tropics*, vol. 2 (London:
H. Frowde and Hodder and Stoughton, 1922), 1502.

government imported substantial quantities of quinine to treat the sick
and began major drainage works in 1928.[33]

The largest consequences unfolded in Russia. The Bolshevik Revolution
(1917) and the subsequent civil war (1918–1921) destroyed the system of
public health services that had been created in czarist times and sowed
disorder and disruption throughout the regional economy. Ecological
disaster ensued. In the immediate postwar period, irrigation programs
created vast swamps on the Caucasus and in Central Asia that served as
mosquito breeding habitat. Famine weakened the peasantries.[34] In 1922 to
1923, the greatest European malaria epidemic of modern times struck the
middle Volga basin.[35] The Red Cross estimated that there were three
million cases of malaria in the Russian Republic to the west of the Ural

[33] Gregory A. Livadas and John C. Sphangos, *Malaria in Greece (1930–1940)* (Athens: Pyrsos
Press, 1941), 50.
[34] L. Tchesnova, "Socio-economic and Scientific Premises for Forming the Strategies
against Malaria in Russia under Soviet Power," *Parassitologia*, vol. 40 (1998), 104.
[35] Lewis W. Hackett, *Malaria in Europe: An Ecological Study* (London: Oxford University
Press, 1937), 222–223; L. Tarassevich, "Expansion pandémique de la malaria en Russie,"
Bulletin de la Société de Pathologie Exotique, vol. 16 (1923), 71–74.

Mountains. Half of the population of Georgia was infected, and in southeast Russia, approximately 60 to 70 percent of the population suffered from malaria, with the percentage in some districts as high as 90 to 100 percent.[36] This first wave of postwar infections peaked at 2.8 million cases in 1928.

A second wave hit the Soviet Union as a result of Stalin's compulsory collectivization of farmers and forced industrialization. During the 1930s, malarial infections soared. The forced relocation of peoples sent non-immunes into malarial environments, and infected individuals into areas without malaria. During the state-created famine in the Ukraine in the early 1930s, epidemic malaria broke out among the starving peasants.[37] The second malarial epidemic peaked in 1934 with some nine million cases.[38]

World War I marked a watershed in the understandings of the limitations of quinine as a prophylaxis. Quinine was medically rationed, despite the fact that the Cinchona Department in India ramped up its drug production by cutting down the cinchona trees to harvest the bark and driving the price down by 75 percent.[39] Perhaps because of the heightened exposure of soldiers stationed in malarial areas and confined to trenches, in addition to rationed quantities, quinine given as prophylaxis frequently failed. Malarial infections immobilized the armies involved in the Macedonian campaign. There the daily prophylactic dose of five grains of quinine did not stop relapses of vivax and did

---

[36] Bureau for Increasing the Use of Quinine, *Malaria and Quinine*, 29

[37] Marshall A. Barber, *A Malariologist in Many Lands* (Lawrence: University of Kansas Press, 1946), 108–109.

Malaria was widely distributed in nineteenth-century Russia. According to Mary Schaeffer Conroy, "Malaria was particularly prevalent in Russia in the provinces bordering the Volga River, in the Black Sea area of the southern Ukraine, in the Caucasus, and in Central Asia. However, it existed all over Russia. Epidemics of malaria reportedly broke out every ten years between 1832 and 1880 in Viatka province located in the northeastern part of European Russia. Epidemics occurred in the city of Kiev in the 1850s, 1860s, and 1870s; in the late 1880s, malaria supposedly accounted for eighty percent of illness recorded annually in the city, although it was often confused with cholera and typhus. Malaria was endemic in Volhynia province to the west of Kiev; in the mid-1880s, 300 of the 2,000 troops stationed there were stricken annually with 'marsh fever.' In 1826, malaria was reported in Siberia; in 1905 it was quite common in Irkutsk near Lake Baikal; it flared up in Tomsk in western Siberia in the 1890s." (Mary Schaeffer Conroy, "Malaria in Late Tsarist Russia," *Bulletin of the History of Medicine*, vol. 56, no. 1 [1982], 42).

[38] Tchesnova, "Strategies against Malaria in Russia under Soviet Power," 105.

[39] League of Nations, O.H./Malaria/32 (Geneva, December 5, 1924). Dr. Martinotti, "La production de l'ecorce de quinquina et le prix de revient du sulfate de quinine," 4.

not appear to prevent new infections, and a very large proportion of the soldiers got malaria.[40]

A loss of confidence in quinine percolated throughout the British medical establishment.[41] If quinine could only suppress but not prevent malaria, the implications were clear: Landscape sanitation and mosquito control were the path to malaria control, rather than mass quinine treatment. In a conceptual sense, it was a major victory for Ross and his mosquito brigades, although because interventions in the British colonies until the end of World War II were extremely limited, it was a victory honored in the breach. It was also one based on a misunderstanding. Quinine could be an effective prophylaxis, in that it could kill all four types of malaria parasites in their asexual blood stages and thus largely prevent the eruption of disabling symptoms. However, quinine could not reach the vivax parasite in its dormant liver stage, and thus relapses of vivax infections were common when troops did not take their quinine on a continuous basis. As late as the outbreak of World War II, most British army medical officers held the view that quinine could suppress, but not prevent, malarial infection.[42]

The role of quinine and the other cinchona alkaloids in the treatment of malaria remained uncontested. In British India, in particular, where malaria was the largest single cause of death, it was clear that there was a potentially enormous demand for cinchona alkaloids for treatment. One idea was to scale-up cinchona cultivation in order to produce enough medicines in India to meet the internal treatment demand and perhaps to supply the needs of the rest of the British Empire. A survey undertaken in 1918 threw cold water on this idea. It found, following extensive land surveys, that there was little suitable land for cinchona plantations, apart

---

[40] W.G. Willoughby and Louis Cassidy, *Anti-Malarial Work in Macedonia among British Troops* (London: H.K. Lewis, 1918), 59; Editorial, "Quinine in the Treatment and Prevention of Malaria," *The Lancet* (February 23, 1918), 301–2.

Paul Russell noted that the wartime reports from Macedonia in 1915 to 1917 about prophylactic quinine were contradictory. See Paul F. Russell, "Lessons in Malariology from World War II," *American Journal of Tropical Medicine*, vol. 26 (1946), 9, citing J.W. Field, *Notes on the Chemotherapy of Malaria* (Kuala Lumpur: Institute for Medical Research, 1938).

[41] As R.N. Chopra noted: "After the Great War there was a feeling against the use of cinchona alkaloids, especially quinine, and it was said that this drug was not effective against certain forms of malaria. Further investigation, however, showed that this was not due to any fault of the drug but due to its improper use" (R.N. Chopra, "Present Position of Anti-Malarial Drug Therapy in India," *Indian Medical Gazette* [July 1938], 419).

[42] Mark Harrison, "Medicine and the Culture of Command: The Case of Malaria Control in the British Army during the Two World Wars," *Medical History*, vol. 40 (1996), 437–452.

from one site in Bengal.[43] Without the ability to expand cinchona production greatly, and convinced that large-scale engineering works were impractical, the British Indian government consoled itself in the fact that fewer epidemics seemed to be breaking out. By the 1920s, the reigning view was that the principal constraint to treating malaria in India was financial – the high cost of importing quinine. Malaria cases were estimated at between eighty and one hundred million per year, and the potential annual demand for quinine was thought to be as high as 750 tons.[44]

THE LEAGUE OF NATIONS MALARIA COMMISSION AND THE ROCKEFELLER FOUNDATION

The League of Nations formed in the immediate aftermath of the Paris Peace Conference in 1919. In 1924, as epidemics of malaria swept through Greece and the Soviet Union, the League of Nations established a Malaria Commission under the aegis of its Health Organisation to address the critical challenge of malaria. As the commission surveyed the malaria interventions among member nations, as well as the projects of the Rockefeller Foundation in the United States (which did not join the League of Nations), it strove to make sense of the lessons to be drawn from contradictory experiences around the globe.

Within Europe, the Italian experiences were extremely important. World War I had undone the successes of the Italian malaria campaign, and not until 1923 would malaria be reduced to its prewar levels. The postwar program initially involved microenvironmental sanitation of mosquito breeding sites, in combination with quinine therapy. It soon evolved into a multifaceted approach, and with Mussolini's ascension to power it became focused on the "bonification" of the notoriously malarial Pontine Marshes.

In parts of Southeast Asia, mosquito control had proven successful at modest cost. As early as the first decade of the twentieth century, Malcolm Watson had embarked on a mosquito reduction program in Malaya, first in the port of Swettenham and the town of Klang and then on the rubber plantations in the interior. Watson succeeded in dramatically reducing the incidence of malarial infection in Swettenham and Klang, and he came to

[43] Lt.-Col. A.T. Gage, *Report on the Extension of Cinchona Cultivation in India* (Calcutta: Government Printer, 1918).

[44] Major-General Sir Patrick Hehir, *Malaria in India* (London: Oxford University Press, 1927), 290, 427.

appreciate the utility of methods that allowed for the manipulation of the breeding environments of different mosquito species. This opened up the possibility of reducing vector breeding to the point where it reduced malaria transmission, an approach known as "species sanitation." Watson aligned himself with Ross as one of the major spokesmen for mosquito control.[45]

In Argentina, the government took a hybrid approach in the malaria-ridden northwestern corner of the country. Many of the late-nineteenth-century immigrants to Argentina from southern Italy and Spain had flowed into the northwestern corner of Argentina, where there were good prospects to secure title to agricultural land. Malaria became deeply ensconced, and it soon became known as the unhealthiest region of the country. By 1911, the Argentinian government, echoing important elements of the Italian approach, launched a multidimensional, state-building program of free quinine and an educational campaign. It also undertook major sanitary engineering projects to drain swamps and spread larvicides.[46] Argentina relied on imported quinine until it created its own industry in the 1920s.[47]

Other positive results came from the United States. The Rockefeller Foundation, fresh from the success of its inaugural health program in hookworm eradication (1909–1914), had embarked in 1915 on a series of experiments in the U.S. South to determine if, by what means and at what cost, it might be possible to control malaria. The foundation's experiments focused on "cleaning up" anopheline breeding grounds in slow-moving or stagnant waters, the classic breeding grounds of *A. quadrimaculatus*, tilting strongly toward mosquito control rather than quinine therapy. The Rockefeller Foundation analysis suffered from serious statistical shortcomings; nonetheless, by 1918 the foundation confidently expressed its conclusions: malaria "elimination" was scientifically and economically feasible (Map 5.3).[48]

Beginning in the 1920s and 1930s, the Rockefeller Foundation extended its landscape sanitation approach into the Caribbean. Its engineers

---

[45] Socrates Litsios, *The Tomorrow of Malaria* (Karori, NZ: Pacific Press, 1996), 47–48.

[46] Frederick L. Hoffman, *The Malaria Problem in Peace and War* (Newark, NJ: Prudential Press, 1918), 65–68.

[47] Eric D. Carter, "Disease, Science, and Regional Development: Malaria Control in Northwest Argentina, 1890–1950" (PhD diss., University of Wisconsin–Madison, 2005), 159–161.

[48] J. Farley, "Mosquitoes or Malaria? Rockefeller Campaigns in the American South and Sardinia," *Parassitologia*, vol. 36 (1994), 165–173.

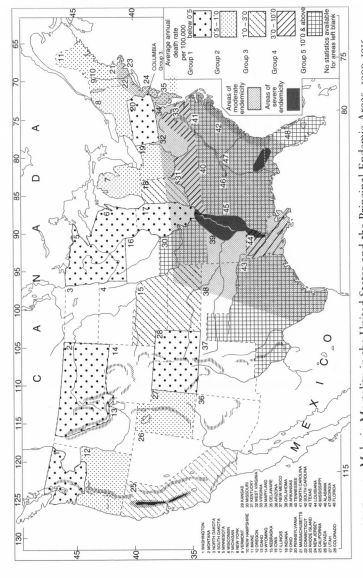

MAP 5.3. Malaria Mortality in the United States and the Principal Endemic Areas, 1900–1915

Source: Adapted from S.P. James and S.R. Christophers, "Malaria," in W. Byam and R.G. Archibald, eds., *The Practice of Medicine in the Tropics*, vol. 2 (London: H. Frowde and Hodder and Stoughton, 1922), 1505.

undertook environmental engineering projects on several of the islands and achieved high levels of malaria control, if not eradication.[49] In Puerto Rico, the Rockefeller Foundation embarked on a mosquito control program using Paris Green as a larvicide,[50] and by 1925 had declared that quinine was not indispensable to antimalarial work. This argument was based on the finding that quinine did not eliminate the vivax parasite from the human host (owing to the parasite's dormant liver stage).[51] This understanding was extended incorrectly to other forms of malaria, including falciparum.

The Rockefeller Foundation's approach promised the possibility of mosquito control at an affordable cost. The foundation's malariologist Lewis Hackett traveled to Italy in 1924 and convinced Mussolini to support a countrywide malaria survey. The interwar Italian programs combined landscape engineering to drain swamps and social programs to improve housing and education with quinine therapy. In the reworked Pontine Marshes, malarial infections plummeted. This success, cast as the Fascist strengthening of the Italian race, was attributed to the iron will of *Il Duce*.[52]

The broader European experience with malaria from the late nineteenth century onward, however, suggested a different approach to malaria control. Western Europeans in the vivax zone had seen malaria recede in the late nineteenth century. The driving forces were almost certainly a complex blend of rising incomes that allowed for screening and the purchase of quinine, increased urbanization (with less exposure to the local vectors), and the expansion of mixed farming systems in which more farmers kept a larger number of livestock penned and thus provided some degree of zooprophylaxis. It may have been very roughly comparable to the decrease in malaria along the agricultural frontier in the U.S. Midwest.

---

[49] Darwin H. Stapleton, "Lessons of History? Anti-Malarial Strategies of the International Health Board and the Rockefeller Foundation from the 1920s to the Era of DDT," *Public Health Reports*, vol. 119 (March–April 2004), 206–215; Darwin H. Stapleton, "Technology and Malaria Control, 1930–1960: The Career of Rockefeller Foundation Engineer Frederick W. Knipe," *Parassitologia*, vol. 42 (2000), 59–68.

[50] The U.S. malariologists also pioneered the use of insecticides to control mosquitoes, transferring lessons drawn from the chemical poisoning of agricultural pests such as grasshoppers and potato beetles. The first insecticide was copper aceto-arsenite, a common color pigment used in paints and wallpaper known as Paris Green. On the early history of Paris Green, see Thomas R. Dunlap, *DDT: Scientists, Citizens, and Public Policy* (Princeton: Princeton University Press, 1981), 19–20.

[51] Stapleton, "Lessons of History?," 207.

[52] Snowden, *Conquest of Malaria*, 142–180.

These different understandings of how to go about addressing the "malaria problem" reverberated in the League of Nations Malaria Commission. The early core debate within the commission was over whether malaria was a "social disease" that could be treated by "bonification," as well as with quinine to relieve suffering, or whether malaria should be understood principally as an entomological problem that could be solved by enlightened engineering. The two main camps were the "mitigators" and the "eradicators," and these also fell out along hemispheric lines: the Europeans versus the Americans. The Americans, however, had refused to join the League of Nations, and although they offered professional counsel, the eradicators were not central to the deliberations.

The mitigators embraced a key role for quinine. This was made possible by a postwar arrangement between the two major Dutch manufacturers and a cinchona growers' manufacturing plant on Java. The collaboration allowed the Dutch firms to set prices for the cinchona growers and established Dutch hegemony in the quinine industry. The markets for cinchona bark became centralized in Amsterdam under the aegis of a private organization known in Dutch as the Kina Bureau.[53]

In most respects, the Kina Bureau served its own interests well and stabilized the notoriously erratic cinchona sector. The vertical integration allowed the growers and manufacturers to establish healthy profit margins for themselves, assuring the continuity of production and manufacture, at a time when the global potential demand for antimalarial medicines was strong and growing. Soon, however, one of the central problems of the "market" for global public health reared its head. The number of malaria

---

[53] From 1892 until the eve of World War I, the cinchona planters and the quinine manufacturers had sparred for financial advantage. The quinine manufacturers formed a cartel in 1892, and as prices for cinchona continued to drop, the Java planters countered in 1896 with the establishment of their own manufacturing plant, Bandoengsche Kinine Fabriek (B.F.K.), on Java that produced quinine and paid the growers a set price. Within a few years, however, the B.F.K. was drawn into the large manufacturers' camp, and prices for growers again dipped below production costs. A number of manufacturers' further efforts to form cartels failed. Finally, in 1913, a solution seemed to be at hand. The cinchona bark producers in the Dutch East Indies forged an agreement with the principal quinine manufacturers, in an effort to bring the supply of bark into a rough balance with demand. The core principle was that manufacturers would buy a supply of bark that would yield a quantity of quinine equal to the quantity of quinine sold in the previous year. Shortly after the agreement was made, World War I erupted.

For the details of these arrangements, see Antoine Cloëtta, *Le problème économique et social de la Quinine* (Bâle: Impr. Kreis, 1928), 88–135.

sufferers was enormous, but most were too poor to pay for medicine. In the North Atlantic basin, many sufferers could afford the occasional therapeutic dose. Beyond the North Atlantic basin, the consumption of quinine and other cinchona alkaloids was restricted to an elite class.

The provision of medicines to the sick would require subsidization by the state. In the colonies, during the interwar period, the imperial powers had other, pressing concerns. The lion's share of their budgets went for defense expenditures, and the colonial public health structures were too weak to support the distribution of antimalarials had they been made available. Missionaries, too, played a significant role in therapeutic treatment, dispensing quinine to their congregants and native students in missionary-run schools. For those outside of these networks, the poor had recourse to only their indigenous pharmacopoeia, and were often without the means to relieve their own suffering. Their children died, generation after generation.[54]

By the early 1920s, the scale of the global malaria disaster began to be calculated. Professor Reiner Müller in Cologne estimated that 800,000,000 people suffered from malaria on an annual basis. Ronald Ross calculated that there were two million deaths per annum. Most of the deaths were thought to occur in India: the British malariologist S.P. James estimated that in an ordinary year 1,300,000 Indians died of the disease.[55]

In 1927, the second general report of the League of Nations Malaria Commission was issued. The experts were reframing the issues. The new paradigm posited "direct" action versus "indirect" action. Direct action was twofold: the provision of quinine to sufferers and the killing of engorged mosquitoes inside of houses. Indirect action constituted the general improvement of the economic and social conditions of populations exposed to malaria and often included the drainage of swamps. The report explicitly did not endorse the antilarval approaches to mosquito control. The entomological findings that some regions were rife with anopheline mosquitoes but not malaria argued against a broad anti-anopheline mosquito campaign as a poorly focused waste of time and money. Only in the 1930s did entomologists discover that the European vector *A. maculipennis* was not, as had been thought, a homogenous

---

[54] M. Kerbosch, "Some Notes on Cinchona Culture and the World Consumption of Quinine," *Bulletin of the Colonial Institute of Amsterdam*, vol. 3, no. 1 (1939), 49–51.
[55] Bureau for Increasing the Use of Quinine, *Malaria and Quinine*, 29.

species; it was a complex of similar species, some of which were unable to transmit malaria.[56]

In principle, the direct action program hinged on the availability of quinine. How much quinine was needed? What were the dimensions of the global malaria problem? The Malaria Commission embarked on studies to estimate the global demand for quinine. In short order, it became apparent that the demand for cinchona alkaloids far outstripped the supply.

CINCHONA PLANTATIONS AND IMPERIAL PUBLIC HEALTH

Any program of regular quinine therapy depended on a stable supply of the drug at a predictable price. Seedlings of cinchona took several years to mature into trees with sufficient bark to be stripped, and this lag, along with the inability to forecast demand and price, created great uncertainty for the quinine manufacturers as well as the cinchona planters. By the early twentieth century the plantations on Java produced approximately 90 percent of the quinine that made its way onto the world market.[57] The quinine yields per tree were approximately four times those in British India, and the production costs were far lower in the Dutch East Indies than anywhere else.[58]

As malarial infections increased in the post–World War I years, therapies that relied only on quinine began to seem exceedingly wasteful. Shouldn't better use be made of the other cinchona alkaloids? In British India, the nonquinine alkaloids had been prepared since the late nineteenth century as a nonstandardized mixture known as "cinchona febrifuge" and later as "quinetum."[59] Quinetum prepared on an industrial scale had virtually all the benefits of quinine at lower cost. The "multialkaloid" nature of the preparation thus anticipated the success of the multidrug therapies of the mid-twentieth century – most famously for tuberculosis and HIV. (One supposed downside was that the proportions

---

[56] Hughes Evans, "European Malaria Policy in the 1920s and 1930s," 40–59.
  For a history of the conceptualization and solution to the problem, see also B. Fantini, "Anophelism without Malaria: An Ecological and Epidemiological Puzzle," *Parassitologia*, vol. 36 (1994), 83–106.

[57] Émile Prudhomme, *Le Quinquina: Culture, Préparation, Commerce* (Paris: Challamel, 1902), 8.

[58] Kerbosch, "Some Notes on Cinchona Culture," 38–40, 44.

[59] The preparation of quinetum was "brought to notice" by the Dutch scientist Dr. De Vrij (Sir Joseph Fayrer, *On the Climate and Fevers of India* [London: Churchill, 1882], 113).

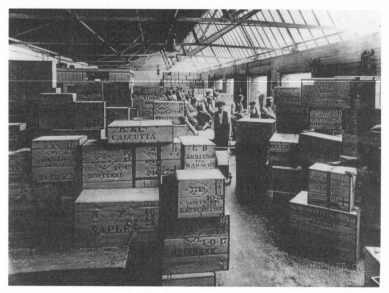

FIGURE 5.1. British Quinine to the World: The Warehouse of Howards and Sons.
Source: London Borough of Redbridge, Local Studies and Archives.

of the cinchona alkaloids varied in each batch of bark. In retrospect, it appears that the varying composition may have inhibited the evolution of parasite resistance.) The League of Nations made plans to carry out experiments with the other cinchona alkaloids in Italy, Spain, Yugoslavia, Romania, and Algeria.[60]

Should cinchona production be sharply increased? In 1929, the British forester J.M. Cowan called for an expansion in cinchona production within the British Empire. Cowan bolstered his case with the economic arguments made by Dr. Andrew Balfour who estimated that the direct annual loss sustained by the British Empire owing to malaria was on the order of £52 to £62 million pounds. In India, the current demand for antimalarial medicines was at least eighteen times the current level of production. The constraint was financial.[61] The British and French started up new cinchona plantations in their tropical colonies, but these efforts were modest in scope (Figure 5.1).[62]

[60] League of Nations, O.H./Malaria/41, Malaria Commission, "Cinchona Alkaloids Enquiry."
[61] J.M. Cowan, "Cinchona in the Empire," *Empire Forestry Journal*, vol. 8, no. 1 (1929), 45–53.
[62] J.L. Gramont, "Le Paludisme," *Marchés Tropicaux* (November 1947), 1679–1683.

As the great economic depression of the 1930s struck, the prospects for more aggressive mosquito vector control projects in Europe and in the imperial colonies receded. The Third Report of the Malaria Commission (1933) focused on quinine and quinine derivatives, and the final, Fourth Report of the Malaria Commission (1937), too, only discussed drug therapy.[63]

INCOMMENSURATE LESSONS

In the Americas, there were different lessons to be drawn. The successes of the U.S. government in the Panama Canal Zone and the Rockefeller Foundation projects in the U.S. South and the Caribbean provided a model for malaria control that was mosquito based. Beginning in 1933, during the first months of the first administration of Franklin D. Roosevelt, the U.S. Congress created the Tennessee Valley Authority (TVA) to undertake large-scale public works engineering schemes to bring electricity to new areas of the U.S. South. The TVA played a significant role in reengineering problematic malarial environments by moving populations to higher elevations, flooding swamps to create reservoirs for hydropower production, and putting the rural unemployed to work draining lowlands. Many private landowners also undertook wetland drainage, primarily to increase the prospects for agriculture. By the 1940s, it is estimated that the United States had drained an area as large as the British Isles.[64]

A major decline in malarial infections took place between 1938 and 1942, and the government claimed success for its efforts at swamp drainage and ditch digging. From 1942 to 1950, the government began to spend more money at home than ever before on malaria, fueled in part by the anxiety

---

[63] The League of Nations Health Organization remained interested in the possibility of mass prophylaxis, and the Pasteur Institute of Algiers undertook comparative experiments on Algerian subjects who lived in a highly malarial area.

These experiments took place during 1935 and 1936, when the weather was so hot that it prevented the development of the local vectors (*A. maculipennis* and *A. hispaniola*). The results, thus, were concerned only with the effect of the drugs on residual malaria. Quinine proved more effective than either atabrine (known then as quinacrine) alone or in combination with praequine [pamaquine], although the investigators attributed the partial failure of atabrine to insufficient doses (L. Parrot, A. Catanei, and R. Ambialet, "Comparative Experiments in Mass Prophylaxis by Means of Quinine and of Synthetic Drugs (Quinacrine and Praequine)," *Bulletin of the Health Organisation [League of Nations]*, vol. 6, no. 5 [1937], 683–765).

[64] M.A. Farid, "The Malaria Programme – From Euphoria to Anarchy," *World Health Forum*, vol. I, nos. 1–2 (1980), 12.

over the viciousness of malaria in the Pacific war theater. These expenditures – and the ecological transformations of the U.S. South wrought by the TVA – probably were not determinative. Margaret Humphreys has argued convincingly that the larger influence responsible for the decline of malaria in the U.S. South was the southern migration of rural workers to southern towns or to northern cities.[65] The lesson drawn by the malariologists at the time was quite different: environmental engineering that targeted mosquito habitat would sharply decrease the incidence of malaria.

Another major lesson for the U.S. malariologists was learned in Brazil. In 1930, an entomologist working with the Rockefeller Foundation in Brazil on the problem of yellow fever discovered that the highly efficient African vector, *Anopheles gambiae*, had survived a passage across the South Atlantic and was colonizing the floodlands near Natal. It seemed likely that the nightmarish intensity of malarial infections in tropical Africa would be transferred to Brazil. An outbreak of malaria hit Natal in 1930, and a full-blown epidemic followed in 1931.

Spurred to action, the Brazilian government teamed up with the Rockefeller Foundation in the late 1930s to wage a war of extermination against the tropical African mosquito. Fred Soper, the Rockefeller Foundation malariologist who lobbied for the program and led it toward full success, narrowly framed the campaign as a struggle against the *Anopheles gambiae* mosquito rather than against malaria.[66] After years of broad applications of larvicidal sprays – "victory" against *A. gambiae* was declared in the mid-1940s.

It was not a general victory over malaria in Brazil. Malaria remained the principal health obstacle to the colonization of the Amazon and

---

[65] Margaret Humphreys, "Water Won't Run Uphill: The New Deal and Malaria Control in the American South, 1933–1940," *Parassitologia*, vol. 40 (1998), 183–191; Margaret Humphreys, *Malaria: Poverty, Race, and Public Health in the United States* (Baltimore: Johns Hopkins University Press, 2001).

[66] There was little, if any, consideration of the regional ecological dynamics – e.g., of the drought conditions that apparently drove larger than usual numbers of "dry season" migrants to the Atlantic coast in search of work during the 1930s. It is likely that the immunological status of the migrants was far less robust than that of the regular workers on the sugar plantations in the northeast of Brazil, and that these dry season immigrants were in part responsible for the increase in infections along the coast, and when they fled the epidemic, already parasitized, in their home villages (see Randall M. Packard and Paulo Gadehla, "A Land Filled with Mosquitoes: Fred L. Soper, the Rockefeller Foundation, and the Anopheles Gambiae Invasion of Brazil," *Parassitologia*, vol. 36, nos. 1–2 [1994], 197–214).

the principal "source of terror" in the region.[67] The victory against *A. gambiae*, however, was important in its own right. The malariologists' success was real enough, and the possibility of eradicating an introduced vector – if it were to be identified before it became broadly established – was a lesson that could be applied elsewhere. The even larger significance of the eradication campaign in Brazil was that it gave new life to the vector control movement. It was a profoundly different paradigm from that of "bonification," progressive social policy, and therapeutic treatment. For Soper, and the Rockefeller Foundation, the principal actors in the *A. gambiae* drama were the mosquitoes and the eradicators.

The Rockefeller Foundation developed an almost exclusive focus on mosquito control as the key to malaria control. It carried out antilarval work in Italy, India, and Mexico on an experimental basis, hoping to develop a methodology that could be funded by national governments. By the early 1940s, the foundation had launched antilarval research projects that were increasingly focused on the use of insecticides in North America, South America, the Caribbean, southern and eastern Europe, and the Indian subcontinent.[68] There the benefits were generally strongly positive, although they never offered the hope of full eradication of the local vectors, and the emphasis was on control, rather than eradication, of the disease.[69]

Another major lesson in malariology was delivered through epidemic. Although during the 1920s and 1930s, malaria continued to take a massive toll in the zones of mixed infections in Asia and of falciparum in tropical Africa, much of the suffering was attributed to endemic infections that were considered largely beyond the abilities of the colonial regimes to address. Then epidemic malaria shattered this complacency in one of the "model" colonies. In 1934 to 1935, an epidemic broke out in Ceylon that infected up to 1.5 million people and killed on the order of 100,000 people.[70]

---

[67] Before the large-scale deforestation of the Amazon that opened the region to colonization by new vectors, gold miners working in the interior Amazon forests experienced epidemic malaria. The mystery of "forest malaria" was untangled by the ecological insights of Brazilian scientists who discovered that an anopheline vector bred in the small water pockets formed by the leaves of the bromeliad climbing plant. The bromeliad also bred in cityscapes, and as the ecology of this malaria infection became understood, it was reconceptualized as "bromeliad malaria" (see P. Gadelha, "From 'Forest Malaria' to 'Bromeliad Malaria': A Case-Study of Scientific Controversy and Malaria Control," *Parassitologia*, vol. 36 [1994], 175–195).

[68] Stapleton, "Lessons of History?," 210.

[69] Darwin H. Stapleton, "Technology and Malaria Control, 1930–1960: The Career of Rockefeller Foundation Engineer Frederick W. Knipe," *Parassitologia*, vol. 42 (2000), 59–68.

[70] Jones, *Health Policy in Britain's Model Colony*, 187.

Here the immediate cause was "natural" drought, rather than state-sponsored irrigation or recent biome conversion. A series of low annual rainfalls in the normally highly malaria-ridden dry zone of Ceylon had greatly reduced the mosquito density and the number of malarial infections. Many people became parasite free – and consequently had a lowered immunological status. When the droughts became increasingly severe, the decreased stream flow in some of the major rivers in the island's wet zone left pools of water in which the local anopheline vector could multiply. Catastrophe ensued throughout the island. The epidemic exposed the vulnerability of even a "model colony" of the British Empire. The medical services ordered and dispensed quinine in quantity, but the large number of dead repudiated the pretensions of colonial government control.

MALARIA AND WORLD WAR II

During World War II, the movement of large numbers of nonimmune combatants into regions of endemic malaria challenged the abilities of the opposing militaries to wage war. This was the case for both the Japanese and the Allied troops who were sent into Southeast Asia and for the Axis and Allied soldiers who fought in North Africa. The war also created more intense patterns of infections as a result of the movement of troops and war material between malarial regions. For the civilian populations, the strictures imposed by the war, such as the shortages of food and medicine, increased the incidence and severity of the infections.

Following the Japanese invasion of Manchuria in 1931, natural disasters and civil war in China produced enormous suffering and great losses to malaria. The overall picture remains difficult to document, but there are limited glimpses into the scope of the disaster. In 1932, for example, when the lower Yangzi Valley flooded, about 60 percent of the population became infected with malaria, and the death toll reached some 300,000. In 1933, in a single county in Yunnan Province, thirty thousand malaria deaths were recorded.[71] From the Japanese invasion of China in 1937 through the internal civil war that culminated in the foundation of the People's Republic of China in 1949, little evidence about malaria can be collected, although it is certain that the destruction, human suffering, and forced

---

[71] Tang Lin-Hua, Qian Lui-Lin, and Xu Shu-hui, "Malaria and Its Control in the People's Republic of China," *Southeast Asian Journal of Tropical Medicine and Public Health*, vol. 22 (1991), 467.

population movements contributed to a colossal increase in malarial infections. By 1950, an estimated thirty million cases were reported in China and of these cases, perhaps 1 percent died. Seventy percent of the counties in China were endemic for malaria.[72]

Following the Japanese attack on Pearl Harbor in December 1941 and the U.S. declaration of war, the Japanese invaded the Dutch East Indies in January 1942 and seized control of the cinchona plantations on Java.[73] They cut off the Allies' supply, and the Allied troops in the Southwest Pacific contracted malaria and were unable to fight. Malaria soon mushroomed into a larger problem than the enemy hostilities. Military historians have estimated that in the Southwest Pacific from October 1942 to April 1943, there were ten Allied soldiers admitted to hospital with malaria for every battle casualty.[74] The U.S. government requisitioned all supplies of quinine within the United States to redirect to the troops overseas and coordinated a growing range of research initiatives to find a way to make synthetic quinine or to find a substitute for quinine that would work. This antimalarial program was one of the formative models for the postwar National Institute of Health.

Over the course of the war, more than fourteen thousand compounds were screened for antimalarial activity. Many were dye compounds that had originally been discovered by German scientists earlier in the century. In 1943, one of these dye compounds – atebrine – was selected as the antimalarial drug of choice. From 1944, in the Burma and North-East India theater of the war, the British medical services provided prophylactic doses of atebrine to British troops and markedly reduced the incidence of malaria. There, by 1945, the British medical advantage became more decisive, as the medical services of the Japanese began to

---

[72] K. Yip, "Antimalarial Work in China: A Historical Perspective," *Parassitologia*, vol. 40 (1998), 29, citing D.T. Jameson et al., *China: The Health Sector* (Washington, DC: The World Bank, 1984), 33.

[73] In an act of wartime daring, just before the Japanese conquest of the Philippines in May 1942, cinchona seed from the Philippines was evacuated to Australia and then to the U.S. Department of Agriculture in Beltsville, MD. The seed was then shipped off to the American tropics – Puerto Rico, Costa Rica, Guatemala, and Peru – in an effort to restimulate production in the western hemisphere. The Americans also relaunched the collecting of bark in the Andes on a large scale. The quinine yields from the Andean barks, however, were very low, and the U.S. government adopted an old formula of the League of Nations Malaria Commission and began to produce "totaquina," from the total alkaloids of the bark (Norman Taylor, *Quinine: The Story of Cinchona* [New York: Cinchona Products Institute, 1952], 10–12).

[74] C.W. Hays, "The United States Army and Malaria Control in World War II," *Parassitologia*, vol. 42 (2000), 49.

collapse.[75] U.S. troops in the Southwest Pacific theater also used atebrine to great effect, dramatically reducing troop morbidity.[76] Then late in the war chloroquine was identified as the superior compound. It provided complete protection to the troops, without the yellowing of the skin that was one of the hallmarks of atebrin use.[77]

In the North African theater, during the peak years of the Allied military campaigns in the desert of western Egypt, the tropical African vector, *Anopheles gambiae*, invaded Egypt from the south. This set off an epidemic that killed more than 180,000 Egyptians between 1942 and 1943. Ultimately, the malaria threat to the Allies led to the creation of an Egyptian national, autonomous Gambiae Eradication Service that mobilized a large number of workers and succeeded in eradicating the vector within eleven months. The lesson from Brazil was apt: species eradication, at least within a subregion, could work.[78]

Within the European theater of war, malaria surged. In the Soviet Union, malaria control efforts completely collapsed. Mass migrations from Nazi-occupied regions of Russia and the destruction of hydraulic structures created new epidemics.[79] In Italy, the new understandings of the malariologists were put to devastating use. As the Nazis withdrew from Italy in May 1944, they dynamited the bonification works constructed during the 1930s that had drained eighty-one thousand hectares of swampy mosquito habitat, and malaria flooded back into the central lowlands. This act of biowarfare reestablished the horrors of malaria in Italy, as in the years before the era of bonification and land reclamations.[80]

In the aftermath of World War II, understandings about malaria were profoundly different than at the conclusion of World War I. Malariologists had succeeded with programs of "species eradication" in Brazil and in Egypt, and many specialists now thought of malaria principally as an entomological problem. A new and inexpensive antimalarial drug,

[75] Mark Harrison, *Medicine and Victory: British Military Medicine in the Second World War* (Oxford: Oxford University Press, 2004), 213–214, 231.

[76] Hays, "The United States Army and Malaria Control," 50.

[77] On antimalarial research during the war, see Leo B. Slater, "Malaria Chemotherapy and the 'Kaleidoscopic' Organisation of Biomedical Research During World War II," *Ambix*, vol. 51, no. 2 (2004), 107–134; Leo B. Slater, "Malarial Birds: Modeling Infectious Human Disease in Animals," *Bulletin of the History of Medicine*, vol. 79 (2005), 286–290.
    Choloroquine was first synthesized in 1924 in Germany. It was marketed under the name plasmochin (Slater, "Malaria Chemotherapy," 115).

[78] Farid, "Malaria Programme," 9.

[79] Tchesnova, "Strategies against Malaria in Russia under Soviet Power," 106.

[80] Snowden, *Conquest of Malaria*, 181–197.

chloroquine, opened the prospect of wider mass prophylaxis and treatment. Despite the successes in drastically reducing the burden of malarial infections in the United States, parts of the Caribbean, Argentina, and northwestern Europe, malaria remained very much a global problem.

* * *

From the late nineteenth century onward, malaria prophylaxis and control had made considerable strides. Some were attributable to broader economic forces that raised living standards; some to the use of quinine and the other cinchona alkaloids; some to entomological interventions with larvicides. The League of Nations Malaria Commission had attempted to assay for the first time the global malaria situation, although the prospects for interventions in global public health remained poor through the Great Depression and World War II. Following the creation of the WHO in 1948, the possibility of interventions in global public health once again came under consideration, and this time there were new tools at hand.

6

Africa Redux

In the spring of 1944, the Allied Control Commission in Italy invited a Rockefeller Foundation team to determine what could be done to cope with the malaria epidemics that the Nazis had unleashed. Their answer was surprisingly simple and effective: In two trials on flooded lands, the Rockefeller group showed that a single spraying of a new insecticide known by its initials DDT could stop the spread of malaria for an entire season. DDT worked so well that by 1945 the Health Division of the UN relief organization decided to undertake a comprehensive DDT campaign to drive malaria out of Italy. In the immediate postwar period, DDT campaigns were also launched in Greece, Venezuela, and Ceylon. In 1946, the Rockefeller Foundation, inspired by its successful participation in the eradication of *A. gambiae* in Brazil, decided on an experimental program on Sardinia to eradicate the sole mosquito vector, *A. labranchiae* – and thus malaria – from the island.[1]

DDT seemed like a miracle. The venerable Paris Green worked well as a larvicide, but it could not kill adult mosquitoes. The natural insecticide pyrethrum made from the dried flower heads of the chrysanthemum plants (*Chrysanthemum cinerariaefolium* and *Chrysanthemum coccineum*) was effective against adult mosquitoes, but it was highly unstable and quickly lost its potency. DDT killed adult mosquitoes, *and* it was a residual killer. It could stop mosquito transmission dead. In most areas of seasonal malaria transmission, two applications per year were enough. Where DDT was laid down, the number of new malarial infections plummeted toward zero. Here was an approach that had broad appeal. DDT sprayers reduced mosquito populations vastly more effectively than had Ross's

---

[1] Gordon Harrison, *Mosquitoes, Malaria and Man: A History of the Hostilities since 1880* (New York: E.P. Dutton, 1978), 223–224.

mosquito brigades, and DDT cost far less than chemical therapy. Because DDT got rid of other nuisance insects and crop pests, it initially had a broad popular constituency.

In the midst of these early momentous victories, however, distressing news began to filter in from the killing fields. In Greece, in 1947, common houseflies began to show a surprising resistance to the killer insecticide. Then, on the island of Sardinia, houseflies also demonstrated resistance to DDT. By 1951, some anopheline mosquitoes in the Greek islands had become impervious to the insecticide treatments, alighting on DDT-treated walls and flying off again to bite.

The early successes with DDT inspired malaria specialists to think more broadly than ever before about the control of malaria – not only in Europe, the European colonies in Asia, and the Americas but also in Africa. The conclusion of World War II heralded not only the victory of the Allies over the German, Italian, and Japanese fascists, but it also precipitated the great movement for decolonization of European empires in Asia. As India, Ceylon, and Burma began to move toward independence in the immediate postwar period, it was clear that the continuing claim of the European empires to rule other tropical peoples would have to include greater provisions for the health and welfare of colonial subjects, particularly if they were to be inoculated from the revolutionary rhetoric of Marxist-Leninism that championed the movements for national self-determination of colonized peoples. What could be done about African malaria?

THE CONUNDRUM OF ACQUIRED IMMUNITY IN TROPICAL AFRICA

In 1948, the newly created WHO took over the work of the Malaria Commission of the now-defunct League of Nations. The first major conference on African malaria took place in Kampala, the capital of the British protectorate of Uganda, in 1950. There expert malariologists clashed over the issue of tropical Africans' acquired immunity to falciparum malaria. What could and should be done to combat malaria in tropical Africa? Was it financially practical and morally sound to bring chemical insecticides to bear on African malaria? The debates at Kampala reprised issues that the League of Nations had grappled with two decades earlier.

During the interwar years, the daunting realities of malarial infections in the imperial tropics had impressed themselves on the European colonizers. It was clear that most Africans suffered from malaria, and that the death rates, particularly for children, were very high. It also seemed to be the case that many tropical Africans were functionally immune to falciparum malaria. The core paradox was that the rates of malarial infection – as measured by the spleen index and the presence of blood parasites – remained high in adults, although most adults appeared to suffer few, if any, ill effects from malaria.[2] Given this acquired immunity, what types of treatment were appropriate? How should scarce resources be spent? During the early 1930s, the League of Nations Malaria Commission had suggested a strategy aimed to promote the acquisition of "relative immunity" through a "nonradical" treatment of severe symptoms that did not attempt a full and complete "cure" of infected peoples living in highly endemic areas. Critics attacked this position as heartless, and it was abandoned as an official strategy.[3] The shift in official strategy, however, had limited practical significance for African colonial subjects because, with the exception of laborers who worked on colonial plantations or in mines and were treated by hired doctors and of those within the orbit of Christian medical missions, most Africans had little or no access to Western antimalarial medicine in the period before 1950.

The issue of mosquito control in tropical Africa was largely moot: The near ubiquity of breeding sites and the fact of year-round transmission in regions of high rainfall seemed to rule out environmental engineering interventions. Malaria specialists had long recognized that the tropical African malarial situation was more difficult than in other regions. Until the immediate postwar years, mosquito control had been practiced principally outside of tropical Africa, and the body of knowledge about mosquito control was based principally on experiences outside the continent. Most regional programs had been in the United States, Central America, South America, and Western Europe, where the infections were primarily vivax. Sickness, rather than death, was the principal hazard. Drawing on the successes of the Rockefeller Foundation programs and the regional malaria control efforts in the vivax and mixed infections zones, and now armed with the miracle insecticide DDT, many malariologists endorsed the accepted wisdom that any degree of endemic malaria was harmful. How could this be reconciled with the broad experience of acquired immunity in tropical Africa?

In 1950 at Kampala, the experts discussed for the first time the possibility of a full-scale assault on malaria. The sheer inexpensiveness and residual

---

[2] D. Bagster Wilson, "Implications of Malarial Endemicity in East Africa," *Transactions of the Royal Society of Tropical Medicine and Hygiene*, vol. 32, no. 4 (January 1939), 435–465.

[3] G. Corbellini, "Acquired Immunity against Malaria as a Tool for the Control of the Disease: The Strategy Proposed by the Malaria Commission of the League of Nations in 1933," *Parassitologia*, vol. 40 (1998), 109–115.

killing power of DDT suggested the new possibility of attacking mosquito transmission in tropical Africa. The conference chairman, Dr. N.H. Swellengrebel, had conducted malariological research in the Dutch East Indies, traveled widely in Africa, and published seminal work on levels of immunity to falciparum malaria. He raised strong cautions about the idea of eradication and was deeply concerned that incomplete or unsuccessful epidemiological interventions could compromise individual or collective immunities and leave entire communities worse off than they had been before.[4] This was far from a purely theoretical position. The British antimalarial campaign in Bombay in the early twentieth century, for example, had been curtailed as soon as the incidence of malaria began to fall. This had paved the way for a disastrous recrudescence of the disease.[5] What would be the health impact of the loss of immunity to falciparum malaria?[6]

The question of acquired immunity was so difficult to address because the scientific understandings were so incomplete. Moral certainties about the need to protect human populations collided with realistic assessments of the possibilities for intervention. There were two extremely thorny issues. First, the "costs" – in terms of sickness and death – for parasitized adults to acquire "relative immunity" were extremely high. If large-scale mosquito control or eradication efforts failed, the acquired immunities might deteriorate and populations might be at greater risk than before. The maintenance of relative immunity appeared to depend on continuous infection. Second, the carriers who had achieved an acquired immunity remained infectious and thus were a health threat to nonimmunes. Relative immunity referred to absence of malaria symptoms, not to the absence of malaria parasites, which remained in the blood.[7]

The experts also grappled with the fact that there were different degrees of acquired immunity. Those who had a fully functional acquired immunity lived in what were termed areas of *holo-endemicity*. These

[4] J.P. Verhave, "Malaria: Epidemiology and Immunity in the Malay Archipelago," in ed. G.M. van Heteren, A. de Knecht-van Eekelen, and M.J.D. Poulissen, *Dutch Medicine in the Malay Archipelago* (Amsterdam: Rodopi, 1989), 98–100.

[5] Gordon Covell, *Malaria Control by Anti-Mosquito Measures*, 2nd ed. (Calcutta and London, 1941), 119–120; Gordon Covell, *Malaria in Bombay* (Bombay: Government Press, 1928).

[6] World Health Organization, Afr/Mal/Conf/25, Geneva, February 27, 1953; Malaria Conference in Equatorial Africa, November 27–December 9, 1950; Town Hall, Kampala, Uganda, Summary Records of the Meetings, 48.

[7] The fact that quinine did not destroy the gametocytes of falciparum was recognized as early as 1900 (Harrison, *Mosquitoes, Malaria, and Man*, 173).

populations, however, were interspersed with others whose immunities were less complete because they lived in areas of *meso-endemicity* in which transmission was less intense, and who were thus at greater risk as adults from additional infective bites. Populations in both epidemiological environments were thought of as isolated from one another.[8]

At the Kampala conference, Swellengrebel posed the moral challenge that cut to the heart of the "eradicationist" activities under discussion for tropical Africa. Did Europeans have the moral right to take away the immunological status of Africans? Did they have the right to bring workers from less endemic regions into more endemic regions, if this represented greater risk to those workers? Should the imported workers be protected if this meant compromising the immunological status of others?[9] There were no easy answers.

The eradicationists argued that the idea of allowing Africans to suffer infections in order to acquire a functional immunity was a repudiation of the pretensions of the scientific community in general and the malariologists in particular. In their view, malaria should be considered in the same light as other communicable diseases, and African populations should be relieved of this pressure. There was no higher morality in allowing poorer and less technologically sophisticated peoples to suffer.

At the Kampala conference, the divisions among experts were protracted and bitter. The eradicationist school of thought prevailed and established malaria as a health problem in Africa to be tackled with the modern weapons of DDT and chloroquine.[10] The acquired immunity school of thought argued for a pilot study to test the efficacy of mosquito control interventions and to monitor the health of the populations. The Kampala participants threw a sop to the losers and agreed that a long-term study of the impact of the antimalarial campaigns should be undertaken, and in the event that the antimalarial campaign was shown to have not brought about an improvement (or had brought about a decline) in the health of the populations, the study would continue to track these results over time.

---

[8] N.H. Swellengrebel, "Reflections à propos de la Conference sur le paludisme de Kampala (1950)," *Annales de la Société Belge de Médicine Tropicale*, vol. 31 (1950), 113.

[9] Ibid., 114.

[10] M.J. Dobson, M. Malowany, and R.W. Snow, "Malaria Control in East Africa: The Kampala Conference and the Pare-Taveta Scheme: A Meeting of Common and High Ground," *Parassitologia*, vol. 42 (2000), 149–166; World Health Organization, Afr/Mal/ 67, February 19, 1965, "The Malaria Eradication Programme in the African Region," 1.

One of the malariologists most concerned about the health consequences of the potential loss of immunity, D. Bagster Wilson, along with his wife Margaret, a parasitologist, undertook a longitudinal study to track the health impacts of malaria control measures in the highlands of East Africa. This study at Pare-Taveta in northeastern Tanganyika and southeastern Kenya (1954–1966) produced frustratingly ambiguous data. The use of insecticides and larvicides, in combination with medical treatments, reduced the incidence of malaria, particularly among infants under the age of one and small children between the ages of one and four. At the end of the project, mortality among small children returned to preproject levels, but mortality among infants did not, for reasons that were not understood then and are not understood now.[11]

While the Pare-Taveta study was in progress, government authorities and malaria experts began to back away from the commitment to push for aggressive malaria control in Africa. The costs of these interventions – owing to the pervasiveness of the infections and the near-ubiquity and efficiency of the vectors – seemed prohibitively high and unable to be funded. Some pilot projects in some regions of tropical Africa enjoyed small-scale successes, seeming to block the transmission of malaria in high-plateau regions in southwestern Uganda and in forest areas of Liberia and southern Cameroon. In the southern Cameroonian city of Yaoundé, in 1958, the interventions completely interrupted malaria transmission.[12] However, in other regions the results were disappointing. The pilot projects in the savannah areas of northern Cameroon, Upper Volta, Senegal, Ghana, Nigeria, and southern Dahomey failed to interrupt transmission.

Then a malaria disaster struck populations in the northeastern highland frontier of tropical Africa. An epidemic of falciparum malaria broke out in the Ethiopian highlands between June and December of 1958. Unusually wet conditions, along with abnormally high temperatures and humidity pushed the *A. gambiae* vector into elevations above 1,600 meters, where the communal immunity of the population was very low. Food shortages, owing to crop failures the previous year, eroded the health status of the highlanders. Some three million people came down with malaria during the epidemic, and more than 150,000 are thought to have lost their lives.[13]

---

[11] Ibid., 160–166.
[12] Jean-Paul Bado, "La lutte contre le paludisme au Cameroun des années 1950 aux années 1960," in *Colloques internationaux. Milieux de vie et santé. Quelques pratiques inter-disciplinaires* (Aix-en-Provence, France: Edisud, 2008), forthcoming.
[13] Russell E. Fontaine, Abdallah E. Najjar, and Julius S. Prince, "The 1958 Malaria Epidemic in Ethiopia," *American Journal of Tropical Medicine and Hygiene*, vol. 10, no. 1 (1961), 803.

The epidemic underscored the vastness of the challenge in controlling malaria in Africa.

The upshot was that the great "global" eradication program was never cleared for takeoff in tropical Africa. The paradigm of the global eradication campaign focused on the interruption of transmission,[14] and the African project reports took the same approach, highlighting the efficient vector (*A. gambiae*), the long transmission season, the extremely high levels of endemicity, the poor communications infrastructure, and the weak administrative structures. The issue of acquired immunity to falciparum lay dormant.

By 1960, the malaria problems of tropical Africa began to slip quietly off the global health agenda.[15] During the 1960s, the WHO and the United Nations Children's Fund helped to fund a few pilot projects in tropical Africa. Considerable tension arose over whether or not public health monies should be poured into basic health services or into a program to build a public health infrastructure to support a malaria eradication program.[16] The initiatives threw into bold relief the differential impacts of malaria on different age cohorts. Outside of tropical Africa, in the zone of mixed infections, malaria imposed high costs in suffering and death across the generations. In tropical Africa, malaria principally killed and sickened children under the age of five. Was the model designed for the zones of vivax and mixed infections appropriate for tropical Africa? Was there only one model of global public health? What was the proper use of scarce public health monies? Who should decide?

THE GLOBAL ERADICATION CAMPAIGN, 1955–1969

During the late 1940s and early 1950s, the antimosquito campaigns to interrupt the transmission of malaria achieved important successes outside of tropical Africa. The aggressive interventions in Venezuela, Ceylon, Greece, and Italy and the many other national programs of DDT use in their early stages spurred the optimism of eradicationists in the early 1950s,

---

[14] The Sixth Session of the Expert Committee defined *malaria eradication* as "the ending of the transmission of malaria and the elimination of the reservoir of infective cases in a campaign limited in time and carried to such a degree of perfection that when it comes to an end, there is no resumption of transmission." Cited by J.A. Nájera, "Malaria Control: Achievements, Problems and Strategies," *Parassitologia*, vol. 43, no. 1–2 (2001), 35.

[15] Tropical Africa's exclusion from the global eradication campaign went unmentioned in the WHO resolution that started the campaign or in subsequent assemblies (ibid., 35).

[16] World Health Organization, Afr/Mal/67, February 19, 1965, "The Malaria Eradication Programme in the African Region," 6.

even as the problem of DDT resistance spread. The eradicationists' argument was simple: It was logical, necessary, and prudent to move toward total eradication before mosquito resistance to DDT became more widespread and before parasite resistance to chloroquine began to emerge. The core questions about the potential loss of acquired immunity in tropical Africa were sidelined.

The enthusiasms of the eradicationists proved infectious. The Eighth World Health Assembly of the WHO in 1955 endorsed a global campaign to eradicate malaria. The global eradication program would be organized by national campaigns. The campaigns would progress in successive phases – preparation, attack, consolidation, and maintenance. Each national eradication campaign would be a building block, and phase-by-phase this building block approach would yield a stable architecture of global public health.

There were significant problems with the model. It largely ignored the realities of transnational labor migration. This was an important issue within the tropics of Southeast Asia and between Southeast Asia and China. If Burma could achieve eradication within its national borders, this condition would be difficult to maintain, given the flows of parasitized migrants from the wider region. It was an even larger issue in tropical Africa. During the era of the eradication campaigns, it was conservatively estimated that five million people were involved in migrant labor movements within Africa south of the Sahara. The model also overlooked the importance of religious pilgrimage to Mecca for Africa's Muslim populations. The Sudan, for example, embarked on an eradication campaign in 1962, even though it was the region through which most Sub-Saharan Muslim pilgrims traveled on their way to Mecca.[17]

Even apart from nonparticipation of most of tropical Africa, there was another potentially enormous lacuna in the global program: mainland China. The People's Republic of China was not a member of the United Nations, and it was one of the great malarial expanses of Eurasia. In 1956, the Chinese Communist Party launched a national program for agricultural development and convened a special antimalarial conference with a goal of eliminating malaria within seven years. At the beginning of this campaign, some thirty million Chinese were sick with malaria.[18]

---

[17] R. Mansell Prothero, *Migrants and Malaria* (London: Longmans, 1965), 41.

[18] The Chinese antimalarial campaign did not have to start from scratch. During the 1930s, the Nationalists, with the assistance of the Rockefeller Foundation, had carried out some antimalarial work in the southern falciparum zone. The Chinese Communists integrated the malariological findings of the Nationalists into a vertically organized system.

Little detail is available on the Chinese campaign from the mid-1950s until the late 1970s, a period in which the successive calamities of the Great Leap Forward (1958–1960) and the Cultural Revolution (1966–1976) severely disrupted the health care system. It is clear, however, the Chinese program was two-pronged and involved extensive destruction of mosquito breeding habitat – as part of the national campaign to eliminate the "four pests" of rodents, flies, mosquitoes, and bedbugs – and the mass treatment of patients with modern antimalarial drugs, herbal remedies, and even acupuncture. By the late 1970s, China reported that it had made enormous strides against malaria, and the infection rate had been cut by almost 97 percent. The Chinese government had succeeded in mobilizing the masses of the Chinese peasantry and in constructing a rural primary health care infrastructure staffed by barefoot doctors. At the same time, the top-down system created regional antimalarial alliances with strategies tailored to regional conditions.[19]

From a geographical perspective, the major successes in China were in the zones of what had been vivax infections. The Chinese medical interventions made less progress in the zone of mixed infections in the south, where falciparum malaria remained a major problem. In part, this was owed to the large-scale movement of populations across the Chinese border in Yunnan province with Burma, Vietnam, and Laos. Even today, the south of China retains its epidemiological affinities with the larger malarial zone of Southeast Asian mixed infections.[20]

The other Eurasian behemoth, the Soviet Union, had also suffered an enormous expansion of malarial infection in addition to the vast human losses of World War II. The Soviet Union had developed an expert antimalaria service during the 1930s, and in the postwar period (1945–1960) it undertook its own, self-styled program of malaria control, based on Soviet scientists' concepts of "landscape epidemiology." Soviet scientists developed new synthetic antimalarial medicines and revived their network of research institutes and treatment facilities. A major focus was on the destruction of mosquitoes through the large-scale use of DDT and hexachlorane. In 1950 and 1951, 236 million square kilometers were doused with these insecticides. Before the emergence of resistance, the Soviet Union was able to reduce the number of infected persons to less than two per

---

[19] K. Yip, "Antimalarial Work in China: A Historical Perspective," *Parassitologia*, vol. 40 (1998), 35–37.

[20] In the 1990s, these population movements were estimated at ten to twenty million person crossings per year. C. Kidson and K. Indaratna, "Ecology, Economics and Political Will: The Vicissitudes of Malaria Strategies in Asia," *Parassitologia*, vol. 40 (1998), 41–43.

ten million. But by the mid-1960s, malaria was breaking out in pockets once again, this time fueled by imported infections and by massive deforestation, large irrigation projects, and the creation of massive reservoirs for hydropower production that provided new habitats for the mosquito vectors.[21]

The global eradication campaign was launched during the height of a global cultural movement known to historians of science as "scientific modernism." The core belief was that there was to be great progress in the resolution of old problems through the application of science. The science was to be universal. The model of malaria eradication by successive stages seems remarkably naïve in retrospect, an analog to the models of development that were going to allow for universal economic progress in the 1960s. It was blind to the social and political landscapes on which the malaria eradication programs would have to work and overly optimistic in its estimates of the time and money that would be required.

It also proved unexpectedly costly to the field of malariology. Until the immediate post–World War II years, the sheer diversity of malarial ecologies had earlier argued for the importance of local epidemiological studies – the need to understand the local topography, the species composition of the local mosquito populations, the behaviors of those species, and the types and distributions of malarial infections. This was time-consuming and expensive. The complexities of the local ecologies were sidelined by this belief in universal science, in particular by the delivery of a brilliant, unitary mathematical model of malarial dynamics by George MacDonald, a professor of tropical hygiene at the University of London and director of the Ross Institute.[22] During the course of the global eradication campaign, local epidemiological studies fell out of favor, and the prestige of malaria specialists was significantly downgraded. They were no longer considered necessary.[23] The universal model of antimalarial activities foreclosed the role of local epidemiological studies in favor of a broad antimosquito focus. The ironic result was that the field of malariology dried up. As the retiring malariologists would later joke bitterly, the global campaign had succeeded in eradicating malariologists rather than malaria.

The belief that one approach fit all circumstances soon ran into difficulties. Problem areas began to be reported – particularly in areas of extensive agriculture with large temporary work forces. The fields were

---

[21] L. Tchesnova, "Socio-Economic and Scientific Premises for Forming the Strategies against Malaria in Russia under Soviet Power," *Parassitologia*, vol. 40 (1998), 103–108.

[22] George MacDonald, *The Epidemiology and Control of Malaria* (London: Oxford University Press, 1957).

[23] Nájera, "Malaria Control: Achievements, Problems, and Strategies," 42–43.

larded with huge doses of DDT and other pesticides to reduce agricultural losses, and this multiplied the evolution of mosquito resistance to these chemicals. Moreover, the in- and out-migrations meant that workers could contract malaria *in situ* and then return to their sending communities. Other problem areas were those of new colonization – such as new mines in "jungle" areas and slash-and-burn agriculture or charcoal-making pits in forest areas. Others were in regions with dispersed populations or in zones of conflict that prevented the operation of antimalarial services.[24] The realities of malaria were more complicated than had been suggested by MacDonald's model. The conceptual chessboard on which the global eradication campaign was played had been artificially simplified. Other problems were encountered with the "maintenance" part of the plan. The continued surveillance of infections required a health service that in some countries simply did not exist. Should malaria eradication properly wait for the development of basic health services?

Despite all of these problems, in many areas outside of tropical Africa the early eradication campaigns made large initial strides. This was true in India, Taiwan, the Philippines, and Ceylon. These strides were so large that as early as 1959, the directors of these national programs moved to implement the general policy of the global eradication campaign, to pass from the attack phase that focused on the mosquito to the consolidation phase that identified and treated the sick. From the point of view of the entomologists, this spelled a potential catastrophe. The redoubtable Fred Soper visited the national programs and sounded the alarm. In his view, the costs and logistical difficulties of surveillance of the populations for evidence of infection were impractical, and the shift of resources away from mosquito destruction could be disastrous.[25]

One full success was achieved in Asia. Taiwan followed the WHO guidelines for malaria eradication closely and developed a program that progressed from the preparatory stage through the attack, consolidation, and maintenance stages. In 1965, the WHO certified Taiwan as free of malaria – a status that it has maintained up to the present day. It was by any measure a grand achievement in a region that had been plagued by malaria at least since its colonization by settlers from mainland China in the seventeenth century.[26] In the Mediterranean basin, the eradication

---

[24] Ibid., 45.
[25] Socrates Litsios, "Criticism of WHO's Revised Malaria Eradication Strategy," *Parassitologia*, vol. 42 (2000), 167–172.
[26] The successes of the Taiwanese nationalist government built on the antimalarial program of the colonial Japanese administration (1895–1945). By the late 1930s, more than

campaigns scored additional full successes in Portugal, Spain, France, Italy, and Greece. In the Americas, malarial infections were extinguished in Chile and on five small islands in the Lesser Antilles of the Caribbean. Measured on a national scale, these were highly impressive victories. Measured by the ambitious goals of the global eradication campaign, the full victories appeared few.

There were also indications that the partial successes might not be permanent. On one of the larger islands in the Caribbean, for example, the ongoing work of eradication proved highly vulnerable to uncontrollable acts of nature. In October 1963, Hurricane Flora smashed ashore in Haiti and undid the gains from two years of DDT spraying. The massive storm destroyed housing, driving most of the population either out into the open or, at best, into temporary shelters, where mosquitoes feasted on them. The heavy rainfall and extensive flooding brought about an explosive increase in mosquito breeding. Two or three months later, a malaria epidemic swept through Haiti, causing seventy-five thousand cases, and the malaria eradication program there was set back to the beginning.[27]

Elsewhere, the best that could be achieved was a substantial reduction in infections. In South Asia, the Indian antimalarial program had to deal with a bewildering complexity of environments and a vast landscape. The problems had been daunting, and some of the efforts had been plagued by incompetence at various levels. The antimosquito DDT teams cleared out malaria from rural and urban areas. The areas where malaria had been endemic were in the zone of mixed infections, where general immunities to falciparum had not been achieved. The overall result of the Indian campaigns was a substantial improvement in health. Even when the vector

---

three million people underwent routine blood examinations for parasites every year, and the Japanese succeeded in preventing any large-scale epidemics during their rule. The Chinese nationalist government had received assistance from the Rockefeller Foundation as early as the 1930s, and after the transfer of the nationalist government to the island in 1949, the foundation supported a malarial laboratory that undertook entomological and epidemiological studies that were crucial to the planning of the eradication campaign. Confounding our ability to understand the cause-and-effect relationships that led to success in malaria eradication was the fact that Taiwan was under martial law, received financial and technical backing from international agencies, and was in the midst of carrying out other public health initiatives, all the while undergoing a process of economic growth in both agricultural and industrial sectors (K. Yip, "Malaria Eradication in Taiwan," *Parassitologia*, vol. 42 [2000], 117–126).

[27] John Mason and Phillipe Cavalie, "Malaria Epidemic in Haiti Following a Hurricane," *American Journal of Tropical Medicine and Hygiene*, vol. 14, no. 4 (1965), 533–539.

rebuilt its strength and malaria returned at lower levels, the new infections were principally of vivax.

Malaria cases declined dramatically. In a mere decade, India reduced its malarial burden by several orders of magnitude – from perhaps seventy-five million cases in 1951 to some fifty thousand by 1961. In the early 1960s, India seemed on the verge of slamming the door shut on malaria. Then, the number of malaria cases started to rise, to 350,000 by the end of the 1960s and then precipitously from 1973 to 1976 when 6.5 million cases were reported. Vigorous attack then brought the number of cases down to 1.5 to 2 million per year. Sri Lanka had edged even closer to full eradication, reducing the number of malaria cases to a mere handful by 1954 and verging on complete eradication in the early 1960s. The final steps proved illusive (Map 6.1).[28]

In retrospect, the campaign for the global eradication of malaria had serious conceptual shortcomings, and it was also grossly underfunded. The major donor, the United States, had initially committed funds to global eradication, predicated on the notion that global eradication could be accomplished in three to five years. In 1960, the International Cooperation Administration of the United States projected the need for a tenfold increase in funding, but none was forthcoming, and the U.S. Congress closed off any further appropriations for malaria eradication after 1961. In 1963, the flow of antimalaria funds to the WHO Malaria Special Account (but not to the Pan-American Health Organization or selected country programs) stopped cold. Of the forty-four countries that had made some financial contribution between 1956 and 1963, the United States had contributed 86.1 percent. Without U.S. support, the costs of the eradication effort were shunted to the governments of developing nations. When the malaria eradication funds dried up, the WHO emphasized the need to expand basic health services globally as a prerequisite for malaria eradication.[29]

Although the global eradication campaign fell far short of its goals, it had a profound effect on the global distribution of malaria. By the 1970s, in the Americas and in Asia, endemic malaria had been driven out of most urban areas and largely restricted to frontier areas and regions of political instability. In tropical Africa, malaria continued to exact an enormous toll in human sickness and death, although the expanding use of chloroquine and other synthetic antimalarial drugs reduced the extent of the suffering.

---

[28] Harrison, *Mosquitoes, Malaria and Man*, 253–255.
[29] J.A. Nájera, "Tropical Diseases and Socioeconomic Development," *Parassitologia*, vol. 36 (1994), 17–33.

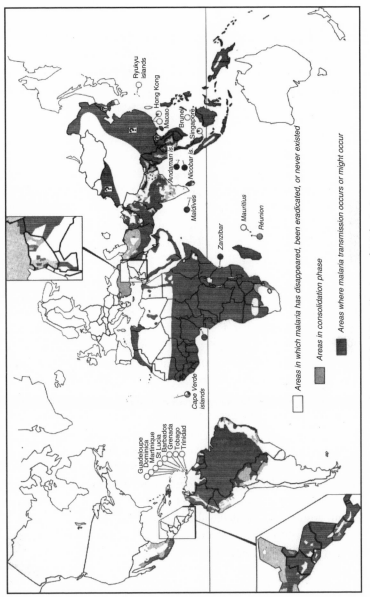

Labels on map:
Ryukyu islands
Hong Kong
Macao
Brunei
Singapore
Andaman is.
Nicobar is.
Maldives
Mauritius
Réunion
Zanzibar
Cape Verde islands
Guadeloupe
Dominica
Martinique
St Lucia
Barbados
Grenada
Tobago
Trinidad

Legend:
☐ Areas in which malaria has disappeared, been eradicated, or never existed
▨ Areas in consolidation phase
■ Areas where malaria transmission occurs or might occur

MAP 6.1. Global Distribution of Malaria in 1970
Source: World Health Organization.

THE VEXED CAREER OF DDT

The eradication campaigns ended with an array of full-blown permanent successes, partial and temporary successes, and a malaria problem in tropical Africa whose full extent had never been addressed. The banner of the great antimalarial insecticide – DDT – was frayed. DDT had produced resistance in anopheline mosquitoes, and its future effectiveness was in doubt.

Concurrently, the broad ecological problems caused by the profligate use of DDT began to come to light. In the United States, the vast majority of the DDT had been spread in the agricultural sector to reduce insect infestation. The emergence of DDT resistance in the United States appeared slowly in response to intensive DDT agricultural use – particularly in the cotton sector – rather than in response to antimalarial activities.[30] (This was likely the case throughout most of the rest of the world, although global DDT use is underdocumented.) The wholesale applications produced DDT resistance in the targeted agricultural pests and killed birds, fish, and small animals – a kind of unanticipated collateral damage in the war against insects.

In 1962, Rachel Carson published a devastating and highly literate critique of the biological costs of large-scale use of the insecticide. Her book, *Silent Spring*, won a wide audience. It helped to found the modern environmental movement in the United States and served as a call to arms, rallying activists against DDT use. Many scientists and environmentalists suspected that DDT posed fundamental threats to human health and the broad web of life. The biological chaos, including thinned eggshells and dead birds, fish, and rodents, certainly suggested that DDT might have grave and incalculable long-term consequences.

The development of new alternative insecticides led to a decrease in DDT agricultural use in the 1960s, and in the 1970s, many industrialized countries, including the United States (1972), banned the agricultural use of DDT. The environmental concerns about DDT were gradually extended into malarious countries, and as the global public health paradigm shifted toward the creation of primary health care systems, the efforts at vector control in many countries languished.

---

[30] In the United States, malaria was in retreat before DDT arrived in the chemical arsenal, and it had only a small role in malaria control. See Margaret Humphreys, "Kicking a Dying Dog: DDT and the Demise of Malaria in the American South, 1942–1950," *Isis*, vol. 87, no. 1 (1996), 1–17.

The deleterious impact of DDT use on birds, fish, and small animals raised alarms about the consequences for human health of the use of DDT for malaria control. A sizeable body of scientific literature argued that there was no evidence that DDT caused cancer in human beings or affected human reproduction, and that in the communities in which the highest amounts of DDT have been found in human tissues and human milk, there have been no confirmed ill effects.[31] Other researchers found evidence of statistical associations between DDT exposure and breast cancer, and, in recent years, some researchers have expressed concern that DDT may be an endocrine disrupter – a compound that interferes with normal hormone functioning.[32]

CHLOROQUINE: THE WONDER DRUG

The other great arm of the global eradication campaign was chemical therapy. The grand success of atebrine during World War II was followed by the even grander success of chloroquine in the postwar period. Chloroquine promised the prospect of inexpensive and safe chemical therapy, and it did not have atebrine's undesirable side effect of producing a yellow cast to the skin.

Initially, the eradication campaigns were based principally on DDT use, but as resistance to DDT began to emerge, planners envisioned a greater role for mass chemical therapy administered by the state. Some projects that included mass drug administration along with DDT fared better than those that used DDT alone. However, the results were not positive enough to justify their broad extension. One of the main problems – as had been the case during the era of quinine use – was that those who were infected but asymptomatic were notoriously reluctant to take the drugs.[33] One possible solution was to distribute medicated cooking salt that was laced with synthetic antimalarial medicines. Malariologists had launched an early trial in Brazil in the late 1940s and subsequent small-scale projects in The Netherlands, New Guinea, and Cambodia, but soon pyrimethamine

---

[31] Peter F. Beales and Herbert M. Gilles, "Rationale and Technique of Malaria Control," in ed. David A. Warrell and Herbert M. Gilles, *Essential Malariology*, 4th ed. (New York: Arnold Press, 2002), 170.

[32] For other health concerns, see Kathleen R. Walker, Marie D. Ricciardone, and Janice Jensen, "Developing an International Consensus on DDT: A Balance of Environmental Protection and Disease Control," *International Journal of Hygiene and Environmental Health*, vol. 206 (2003), 425–426.

[33] World Health Organization, Afr/Mal/67, February 19, 1965, "The Malaria Eradication Programme in the African Region," 20–21.

resistance was reported. Chloroquine-medicated salts were also tried, including a large-scale trial in Guyana that had the most success, but this method of mass drug administration produced wide variations in the levels of the ingested drug.[34] In the 1970s, the WHO shifted its focus back to control of the mosquito vector. The official view was that mosquito control was the only way to effectively reduce endemic levels of malaria.[35]

Chloroquine, however, remained the drug of choice for malaria treatment. Chloroquine allowed for many of the tropical African poor to self-medicate, just as North American pioneers had done with quinine and other cinchona alkaloids in the nineteenth century. The difference was one of scale. The sheer inexpensiveness of chloroquine saved many millions of lives. In tropical Africa, sufferers could purchase chloroquine by the pill in the local market. This pattern of incomplete treatment probably sped up the evolution of parasite resistance, although the exact details of this process will likely never be known.[36]

Chloroquine was effective throughout the 1960s and much of the 1970s and 1980s. Resistance, though, began to be reported as early as 1960 in Colombia, Venezuela, and Brazil; in the early 1960s in Southeast Asia; and, during the 1970s, more widely in South America and Eastern and Central Africa. By 1988, chloroquine-resistant parasites had been reported all across tropical Africa. Even so, chloroquine continued to be used as the frontline treatment for malaria into the mid-1990s.[37]

In tropical Africa and in parts of Asia, choloroquine had a major impact on the health of the populations. In tropical Africa, the rapid expansion of basic health services to some large sectors of the population also made a significant contribution, but it is likely that choloroquine was probably most responsible for the marked trend toward fewer malaria deaths and

---

[34] U. D'Allesandro and H. Buttiëns, "History and Importance of Antimalarial Drug Resistance," *Tropical Medicine and International Health*, vol. 6, no. 11 (2001), 846.

[35] World Health Organization, Afr/RC25/7, June 9, 1975, "Development of the Antimalarial Programme in Africa," 18.

[36] In 1993, Malawi became the first African state to replace chloroquine with sulfadoxine and pyrimethamine for the treatment of malaria. In 2005, randomized clinical trials in Blantyre of 210 children with uncomplicated falciparum infections who were treated with chloroquine indicated that chloroquine had regained its efficacy. Miriam K. Laufer et al., "Return of Chloroquine Antimalarial Efficacy in Malawi," *New England Journal of Medicine*, vol. 355, no. 19 (November 9, 2006), 1959–1966.

For early and promising research on the reversal of chloroquine resistance, see Maud Henry et al., "Chloroquine Resistance Reversal Agents as Promising Antimalarial Drugs," *Current Drug Targets*, vol. 7 (2006), 935–948.

[37] Jean-François Trape, "The Public Health Impact of Choloroquine Resistance in Africa," *American Journal of Tropical Medicine and Hygiene*, vol. 64, nos. 1–2 (2001), 12.

lower morbidity from the 1960s until the mid-1980s, when the efficacy of chloroquine broadly declined. From the early 1980s, the International Monetary Fund and the World Bank imposed "structural adjustment" programs in exchange for new loans, in an effort to shrink the public sector of African economies. By the 1990s, all of the antimalarial gains from chloroquine use and the expansion in basic health services had been lost, and malaria reaped a toll in childhood mortality comparable to that in the 1930s, in the era before effective interventions for colonial subjects.[38]

During the global deployment of both DDT and chloroquine, malarial infections had been greatly reduced. In some regions, where DDT agricultural uses had been heavy, the mosquito vectors had outsmarted DDT and developed resistance. In some regions where chloroquine use had been pervasive and incomplete, the malaria parasites had outsmarted the antimalarial drug and developed resistance. In the process, a major shift in the geography of malarial infections had taken place: Malaria was all but eliminated from the Western nations and the wealthier Asian tiger economies and was greatly reduced in India, China, Latin America, and the Caribbean. Africa became indisputably the center of global malaria. Early in the twenty-first century, an estimated 80 to 90 percent of contemporary infections and 90 percent of malaria deaths occur in tropical Africa.[39]

THE REDISCOVERY OF NATURAL THERAPIES

By the 1990s, the prospects for reliable chemical therapy were tenuous. The emergence of chloroquine resistance, and then resistance to the next generation of antimalarial drugs including sulfadoxine-pyrimethamine, suggested a potential crisis.

Help came from an unexpected quarter. During the Chinese cultural revolution, the Chinese rediscovered the efficacy of an ancient antimalarial drug, an alkaloid that could be extracted from a common plant known as sweet wormwood (*Artemisia annua*). The drug, known as artemisinin, extended a new lease on life to the chemical therapy approach. Artemisinin-based drugs could be produced in quantity, but

---

[38] Robert W. Snow, Jean-François Trape, and Kevin Marsh, "The Past, Present, and Future of Childhood Malaria Mortality in Africa," *Trends in Parasitology*, vol. 17, no. 12 (2001), 593–597.

[39] Nájera, "Malaria Control: Achievements, Problems, and Strategies," 52.

they cost much more to produce than chloroquine, even if the annuals were grown on plantations in Africa, close to their markets and using local labor. Would the higher price of artemisinin put it beyond the means of the very poor?

There was trouble, too, on the biological front. Experts agreed that it was only a matter of time before artemisinin-based drugs provoked parasite resistance. As of the early twenty-first century, quinine – the venerable alkaloid from the nineteenth century that was never used in large enough quantities to provoke significant resistance – remained the drug of last resort for the treatment of multi-drug-resistant falciparum malaria.

The fact that another natural alkaloid was effective against malaria, though, provoked a broad and ongoing reassessment of other natural antimalarial remedies. There were, however, literally thousands of possibilities, and the early findings were positive if not overly hopeful. Those natural remedies that did have antimalarial properties (and this was a small fraction of the total investigated) were less efficacious than the cinchona alkaloids or the artemisinin-based drugs. The acceptance of the (partial) efficacy of these natural remedies, however, was a retrenchment and part of the growing acceptance that the complex realities of malarial infection would have to be addressed through a multitude of means.

In the early twenty-first century, more than 1,200 plant species from 160 plant families are used to treat malaria and fever. Perhaps one-fifth of all patients use traditional herbal remedies for malaria in endemic countries. There are few data, however, on safety and efficacy. Even among traditional healers, there is no consensus on the plants, preparations, and dosages that are the most effective; and the concentrations of active ingredients in a plant species varies considerably.[40] The positive side is that the lack of standardization impedes the evolution of parasite resistance.

Another hopeful development is the reevaluation of the ancient techniques of using oils on skin to repel mosquitoes. A recent survey of forty-one essential oils found that five utterly repelled the three species of *Aedes*, *Culex*, and *Anopheles* mosquitoes submitted to trial for a period of eight hours.[41]

---

[40] Merlin L. Willcox and Gerard Bodeker, "Traditional Herbal Medicines for Malaria," *Clinical Research*, vol. 329, no. 7475 (2004), 1156–1159.

[41] Abdulkrim Amer and Heinz Mehlhorn, "Repellency Effect of Forty-One Essential Oils against *Aedes*, *Anopheles*, and *Culex* Mosquitoes," *Parasitology Research*, vol. 99 (2006), 478–490.

THE NEW HIGH TECHNOLOGIES: MALARIA
VACCINES AND TRANSGENIC MOSQUITOES

Even during the era of chloroquine efficacy, malaria remained the primary focus of a few groups of biomedical researchers. They were keen to find a "solution" to falciparum malaria, and they sought it at the laboratory bench. Perhaps a vaccine could slay malaria. Over the course of the 1970s, 1980s, 1990s, and deep into the first decade of the twenty-first century, vaccine researchers have labored away. They have encountered enormously complex problems, sought more funds, and assured their patrons that one or more malaria vaccines would be forthcoming. The vaccine makers have made considerable progress, and yet a fully protective malaria vaccine is not thought to be a near-term prospect.[42]

Another initiative came from molecular entomologists who focused on the mosquito vectors.[43] They announced the first "transgenic" mosquito in the year 2000. Their hopes were that through the manipulation of the mosquito's genes it would be possible to control the disease by disrupting the mosquito's interaction with the malaria parasite, altering its choice of blood target from man to animal, or selectively creating sterile male mosquitoes. At present, the researchers' hopes for a sterile male mosquito are high, and plans are on hold for a massive release of sterile mosquitoes into the wild.[44] Another approach is to engineer a malaria-resistant mosquito that has a survival advantage over a malaria-tolerant mosquito. Researchers at Johns Hopkins University in 2007 published encouraging results, although they cautioned that the release of transgenic mosquitoes into the wild might not occur for ten to twenty years, and that it was extremely difficult to anticipate what would happen in the event that a release took place.[45]

---

[42] For a survey of these efforts over the course of the twentieth century, see R.S. Desowitz, "The Malaria Vaccine: Seventy Years of the Great Immune Hope," *Parassitologia*, vol. 42 (2000), 173–182.

[43] For an overview of the field, see A.M. Handler, "An Introduction to the History and Methodology of Insect Gene Transformation," in ed. A.M. Handler and A.A. James, *Insect Transgenesis: Methods and Applications* (Boca Raton, FL: CRC Press, 2000), 3–26.

[44] David Adam, "Scientists Create GM Mosquitoes to Fight Malaria and Save Thousands of Lives," *The Guardian*, October 10, 2005. This article is available online at http://www.guardian.co.uk/science/2005/oct/10/infectiousdiseases.medicineandhealth. On earlier sterile mosquito releases, see Mark Q. Benedict and Alan S. Robinson, "The First Releases of Transgenic Mosquitoes: An Argument for the Sterile Insect Technique," *Trends in Parasitology*, vol. 19, no. 8 (2003), 349–355.

[45] Mauro T. Marelli et al., "Transgenic Malaria-Resistant Mosquitoes Have a Fitness Advantage When Feeding on Plasmodium-Infected Blood," *Proceedings of the National Academy of Sciences*, vol. 104, no. 13 (March 27, 2007), 5580–5583.

MALARIA RESURGENT

When the global eradication campaign ended in 1969, the military metaphor of the "war against malaria" backfired. With "victory" beyond reach, public health officials were saddled with the metaphor of "defeat." The field-tested methods of environmental management, allowed to languish during the global eradication campaign, did not return to favor.[46] Antimalarial services were either disbanded or had their funding cut. A new global public health model arose in the 1970s that stressed integrated health services and community health care rather than single-disease-control programs.[47] This model carried the day during the 1980s and into the late 1990s.

Following two decades out of the spotlight, malaria began to reemerge as a global health concern during the late 1990s (Figure 6.1; Map 6.2). Malarial infections multiplied in South America from the late 1970s to the late 1980s. Some increases were owing to the agrarian reforms of the military government of Brazil that opened the Amazon for internal colonization. Others appeared to result from a reduction in DDT use in house spraying. Ecuador increased its DDT use in 1993 and was the only South American state to report a large reduction in malaria.[48] In Southeast Asia, the countries of Vietnam, Laos, and Cambodia targeted malaria as a major public health problem and achieved progress in vector control, except in the hilly, forested regions and a few coastal areas.[49] Malaria continued to be a significant problem in the Western Pacific, South, and Southwest Asia.[50] Throughout the zone of mixed infections, where malaria control efforts improved, the mix shifted toward a higher percentage of vivax infections.[51]

---

[46] A recent study of the effectiveness of environmental modifications that included drainage, the filling of marshes, cleaning of anopheline breeding environments, and vegetation management reviewed forty studies, ranging from 1902 to the present, which reported clinical malaria outcomes. Most took place before the Global Eradication Campaign (1955–1969). During the era of the campaign, not a single study relied on applied environmental management as the central tool (Keiser et al., "Reducing the Burden of Malaria," 701–706).

[47] Brown, "Global Resurgence of Malaria," 122.

[48] Donald R. Roberts et al., "DDT, Global Strategies, and a Malaria Control Crisis in South America," *Emerging Infectious Diseases*, vol. 3, no. 3 (1997), 295–302.

[49] H.D. Trung et al., "Malaria Transmission and Major Malaria Vectors in Different Geographical Areas of Southeast Asia," *Tropical Medicine and International Health*, vol. 9, no. 2 (2004), 230–237.

[50] R. Carter and K.N. Mendis, "Evolutionary and Historical Aspects of the Burden of Malaria," *Clinical Microbiology Reviews*, vol. 15 (2002), 579, table 3.

[51] Kamini Mendis et al., "The Neglected Burden of *Plasmodium Vivax* Malaria," *American Journal of Tropical Medicine and Hygiene*, vol. 64, nos. 1–2, suppl. (2001), 97–106.

Time Years	Global Population n	Land Area Malarious square kilometers	Countries at Risk percent	Countries at Risk n	Population Exposed n	Population Exposed percent
1900	1,158,409,472	77,594,480	53–16	140	892,373,056	77–03
1946	2,391,400,960	58,565,752	40–12	130	1,635,815,808	68–40
1965	3,363,417,344	53,492,988	36–65	103	1,924,360,320	57–21
1975	4,085,759,488	48,075,780	32–93	91	2,121,086,592	51–91
1992	5,419,255,808	43,650,812	29–90	88	2,565,702,144	47–34
1994	5,582,432,256	39,537,020	27–08	87	2,570,555,136	46–05
2002	6,204,095,488	39,758,172	27–24	88	2,996,419,584	48–30
2010	6,807,085,056	39,758,172	27–24	88	3,410,862,080	50–11

FIGURE 6.1. Global Population at Risk from Malaria from Preintervention to 2010 (approx. 1900–2010)[65]

Source: Simon I. Hay, Carlos A. Guerra, Andrew J. Tatem, Abdisalan M. Noor, and Robert W. Snow, "The Global Distribution and Population at Risk of Malaria: Past, Present, and Future," *Lancet Infectious Diseases*, vol. 4, no. 6 (2004), 328. Reprinted with permission from Elsevier.

[65] The area totals were generated using the maps of all-cause malaria risk distribution through time (Figure 6.1). The percentage of Earth malarious was calculated from a total global land surface area of 145,975,899 square kilometers. To estimate countries at risk territorial designations for 2002 were used throughout (Environmental Systems Research Institute, Inc., Redlands, CA). Country-specific medium "variant" population growth rates from the World Population Prospects database (http://esa.un.org/unpp) between 1950 and 2010 were applied to the Gridded Population of the World v2.025 to generate population distribution maps for 1900, 1946, 1965, 1975, 1992, 1994, and 2002 to match with the malaria risk distribution maps (Figure 1) and were also projected to 2010 to enable evaluation of potential future changes in global malaria risk. Global summary counts of these population distribution maps give accuracy to within 5% of the United Nations Development Program global population estimate (http://esa.un.org/unpp) for all calculated years. All area and population summaries from these polygons were processed in Idrisi Kilimanjaro (Clark Labs, Clark University, Worcester, MA).

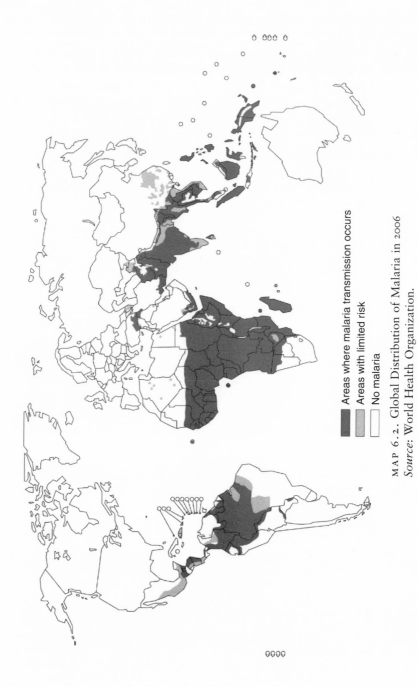

MAP 6.2. Global Distribution of Malaria in 2006
Source: World Health Organization.

Areas where malaria transmission occurs

Areas with limited risk

No malaria

Within tropical Africa, the impact of malaria from the 1960s onward is difficult to assess. The African data are not robust, and thus the interpretations cannot be definitive. As mentioned in the preceding text, some researchers found that in areas of stable transmission, widespread chloroquine use had reduced malaria mortality over the period 1960 to 1989. The data gathered by the WHO indicated a dramatic increase in African malaria from an estimated 300,000 deaths in 1970, to 787,000 in 1990, and 990,000 in 1997.[52] (Much of the increase in malaria into the 1980s may have been a result of rapid population growth – i.e., the absolute numbers of Africans with malaria increased, but the rates of infection did not increase as rapidly.) In any event, the point of broad agreement was that malaria had increased sharply at least since 1990.

Faced with this resurgence, African scientists led the fight to renew the battle against malaria. The WHO launched its "Roll Back Malaria" initiative in 1998, and in 2000 at the Abuja Summit, African heads of state set goals to achieve large improvements in malaria treatment and prevention. To date, the initiative has not met its goals, and the number of malarial infections both within and outside of tropical Africa continues to rise.[53]

What caused the resurgence of malaria in tropical Africa? Climate change did not appear to be an important factor. Time-series analysis of a climate-driven model of malaria showed only limited evidence for an increase in environmental suitability during the last century across the African continent. In those areas where positive trends could be determined, the increase in infections seemed to be related to increased precipitation rather than temperature. The overall study suggested that nonclimatic factors were the drivers of increased malaria transmission across the continent.[54]

In some highland regions subject to unstable malaria, the cessation of antimalarial interventions laid the groundwork for future epidemic

---

[52] Carter and Mendis, "Evolutionary and Historical Aspects," 579, table 3.

[53] In 2005, a group of malaria experts estimated that in 2002 a total of 515 million clinical cases of falciparum malaria occurred worldwide. Their data suggested that one-third of the global incidence occurred outside of Africa (Robert W. Snow et al., "The Global Distribution of Clinical Episodes of Plasmodium Falciparum Malaria," *Nature*, vol. 434 [March 10, 2005], 214–217).

[54] Jennifer Small, Scott J. Goetz, and Simon I. Hay, "Climatic Suitability for Malaria Transmission in Africa, 1911–1995," *Proceedings of the National Academy of Sciences*, vol. 100, no. 26 (2003), 15341–15345.

outbreaks. The most devastating case took place in the central plateau region of the island of Madagascar. The large island is inhabited by the highly efficient tropical African vector, *Anopheles funestus*, and is very much part of the zone of falciparum malaria. There the antimalarial campaigns of the 1940s and 1950s that used DDT house spraying had succeeded in ridding the highlands of malaria. When the vector reestablished itself in the mid-1980s, malarial infections increased sharply, and most highlanders were defenseless as nonimmunes. Informed estimates of the number of people who died in the 1986 to 1988 outbreaks range from fifteen thousand to thirty thousand up to one hundred thousand.[55]

The increase in malarial infections, centered in tropical Africa, did not appear to be a result of "man-made" malaria. This term was coined in the mid-twentieth century, to refer to malaria that was intensified by development projects and the aggregation of laborers at the work sites. In tropical Africa, a recent survey found that irrigation projects played an extremely small role in malarial infections, and, in some regions, irrigation suppressed rather than intensified the problem.[56]

Recent evidence suggests that the agroeconomic changes of the "green revolution" may have had a significant effect on the transmission of malaria in highland regions. In 1998, in the Ethiopian highland district of Burie, farmers suffered an outbreak of epidemic malaria for the first time ever. It appears to be related, in part, to their adoption of hybrid maize that produces abundant pollen that in turn allows for the survival of more mosquito larvae and thus greater vector density. If this association is confirmed by ongoing research, a new field of malariological issues will open up. Hybrid maize is on the leading edge of an agrarian transformation throughout eastern and southern Africa, and public health programs will need to reintegrate environmental management techniques to control this unanticipated accelerant of malaria.[57]

The interaction of disease agents in the broader epidemiological environment is also implicated in the increase in malarial infections. This

---

[55] Jean Mouchet et al., "Evolution of Malaria in Africa for the Past 40 Years: Impact of Climatic and Human Factors," *Journal of the American Mosquito Control Association*, vol. 14, no. 2 (1998), 124–125.

[56] Jennifer Keiser et al., "Effect of Irrigation and Large Dams on the Burden of Malaria on a Global and Regional Scale," *American Journal of Tropical Medicine*, vol. 72, no. 4 (2005), 392–406.

[57] James C. McCann, *Maize and Grace: Africa's Encounter with a New World Crop* (Cambridge, MA: Harvard University Press, 2005), 174–196.

is particularly true of the HIV pandemic. HIV-1 infection (the most common form in tropical Africa) increases the risk and severity of endemic malarial infections. In both high- and low-intensity HIV transmission zones, observers have noted the increased severity and case fatality rates from malaria, and in high-transmission zones, HIV-1 also increases the incidence of symptomatic malaria among adults.[58] The diseases have an awful synergy. Malarial infections in HIV-infected individuals boost the HIV viral load, and, in this respect, malaria seems to be an important factor in promoting the spread of HIV in tropical Africa.[59]

APPROACHES OLD AND NEW

During the first decades after World War II, indoor residual house spraying with DDT in tropical Africa had a limited trial. The early pilot projects had shown that spraying the interior house walls could not effectively stop transmission in areas of stable malaria, and thus there was little incentive to scale up. There were some exceptions: on the small islands of Réunion, Mayotte, Zanzibar, Cape Verde, and São Tomé DDT spraying effectively reduced transmission. There were some other successes in regions of unstable malaria. In South Africa and Swaziland, on the fringe of the falciparum zone, and in some highland regions, indoor house spraying achieved significant reductions in malarial infections, although after a hiatus in spraying, malaria in these regions was again on the rise by the mid-1980s.[60] In the aftermath of the 1986 to 1988 outbreaks in the highlands of Madagascar, DDT house spraying resumed there in 1993, and malaria declined by more than 90 percent after two annual spray cycles.[61]

During the 1990s, political pressure to expand the use of DDT for malaria control gained momentum, and in 2001, the DDT provision to the Stockholm Convention on Persistent Organic Pollutants preserved access

[58] E.L. Korenromp et al., "Malaria Attributable to the HIV-1 Epidemic, Sub-Saharan Africa," *Emerging Infectious Diseases*, vol. 11, no. 9 (2005), 1410–1419.

[59] Laith J. Abu-Raddad, Padmaja Patnaik, and James G. Kublin, "Dual Infection with HIV and Malaria Fuels the Spread of Both Diseases in Sub-Saharan Africa," *Science*, vol. 314 (December 8, 2006), 1603–1606.

[60] Musawenkosi L.H. Mabaso, Brian Sharp, and Christian Lengeler, "Historical Review of Malarial Control in Southern Africa with Emphasis on the Use of Indoor Residual Spraying," *Tropical Medicine and International Health*, vol. 9, no. 8 (2004), 846–856.

[61] D.R. Roberts, S. Manguin, and J. Mouchat, "DDT House Spraying and Re-Emerging Malaria," *The Lancet*, vol. 356, no. 9226 (July 22, 2000), 330–332.

to the use of DDT for WHO-approved disease-control programs.[62] By the first decade of the twenty-first century, DDT house spraying came back into favor in selected areas where DDT resistance was not a problem and where malaria transmission was unstable. The advocates of DDT use for indoor residual spraying argued that the health benefits strongly outweighed the risks. The current WHO judgment is that DDT does not pose a major risk to human health when used within approved guidelines for the sole purpose of spraying the inside walls of houses, and in 2006, the WHO began to promote the wider application of indoor residual spraying in highly endemic areas in tropical Africa.

Since the mid-1990s, insecticide-treated bed nets (ITNs) have been championed as the most powerful malaria control tool since DDT and chloroquine.[63] As of the first decade of the twenty-first century, coverage in Africa has been weak. Only 3 percent of African children sleep under ITNs, and only 20 percent sleep under any net at all. Although the ITNs are more effective than untreated nets in reducing the number of infective bites, the untreated nets are far more widely used, and thus they make a larger contribution to the reduction of malaria. A "global consensus" is emerging about the need to scale-up ITN usage in tropical Africa, although some fundamental questions about the impact of ITNs on acquired immunity have not been addressed. One of the worst case scenarios – that ITNs reduce acquired immunities and, in the case of interrupted use, result in increased vulnerability to malaria and greater morbidity and mortality – does not seem to be borne out by the few studies that have addressed these questions.[64]

In the first decade of the twenty-first century (in 2002 with the creation of the Global Fund to Fight AIDS, Tuberculosis, and Malaria and in 2007 with an additional financial commitment by the Bill & Melinda Gates Foundation), a new era in malaria research and control appeared to be dawning. The malariologists at the WHO wisely counseled against a reprise of the eradication campaigns of the 1950s and 1960s, because the tools at hand were still inadequate to the task. One or more laboratory breakthroughs were possible. But the most tangible prospects for the

---

[62] Walker, Ricciardone, and Jensen, "Developing an International Consensus on DDT," 423–435.

[63] Christian Lengeler, Jacqueline Cattani, and Don de Savigny, eds., *Net Gain: A New Method for Preventing Malaria Deaths* (Ottawa, ON: International Development Research Centre/World Health Organization, 1997).

[64] Jenny Hill, Jo Lines, and Mark Rowland, "Insecticide-Treated Nets," *Advances in Parasitology*, vol. 61 (2006), 77–128, esp. 90–92, 116–117.

reduction of human suffering from malaria seemed to rest upon the expansion of malaria control activities, the improvement of the standards of living of those afflicted by the disease, and the strengthening of primary health care systems in some of the poorest and most parasitized regions of the world.

* * *

In the aftermath of World War II, the miraculous insecticide DDT and wonder-drug chloroquine emboldened malariologists to advocate programs to eliminate rather than to control malaria. The WHO embarked on a global eradication campaign (1955–1969) that had mixed success. Tropical Africa was largely excluded from the "global" campaign. By the 1990s, malarial infections were rising in several parts of the world, and most malaria deaths were within tropical Africa.

7

Conclusion

Malaria is an ancient affliction of humanity, and over deep time malaria parasites and human beings coevolved. Some human populations developed genetic mutations to mitigate the burden of malaria. In tropical Africa, an early genetic mutation to vivax infections known as Duffy antigen negativity was dominantly successful: It dramatically reduced the incidence of vivax malaria and produced no deleterious health consequences for those who carried it. By contrast, a later genetic mutation to falciparum infections known as sickle cell hemoglobin reduced morbidity and mortality for those who inherited the sickle cell gene from only one parent but caused early death for those who inherited the sickle cell gene from both. Both Duffy negativity and sickle cell are molecular testimonies to humanity's struggle to expand our domain in early tropical Africa. They constitute the first chapter in the history of human infectious disease, and they unveil the profound depth of our African past, dissolving the artificial boundary between the supposed timelessness of "prehistory" and the chronology of "history."

Our immune systems also responded to the burden of malaria. Few individuals infected by vivax parasites achieved immunities, even after extensive suffering, probably because the rates of vivax transmission with less efficient vectors were low compared to those in the falciparum zone.[1] By contrast, most falciparum sufferers in areas of intense transmission, who survived their early childhood infections, remained parasitized but achieved partially or fully functional immunities.

Our genetic and immunological responses to vivax and falciparum parasites challenge the conventional wisdom in parasitology and epidemiology

[1] Kamini Mendis et al., "The Neglected Burden of *Plasmodium Vivax* Malaria," *American Journal of Tropical Medicine and Hygiene*, vol. 64, nos. 1–2, suppl. (2001), 97–106.

that assumes that parasites evolve toward benign coexistence with their hosts. Neither vivax nor falciparum parasites seem to have done so. In the case of vivax, in west and west-central tropical Africa the wide expression of Duffy negativity virtually foreclosed the possibility of infection and thus coexistence with the parasite. Elsewhere, throughout the vivax-ridden regions of the world, vivax did not decrease in virulence. In the falciparum zone, those infected in areas of high transmission acquired functional immunities only after surviving multiple crises. Falciparum took an extraordinarily deadly toll there.

Explanations of why some parasites have not evolved toward benignness have begun to emerge from a new discipline known as evolutionary epidemiology that takes nonhuman hosts such as anopheline mosquitoes into consideration.[2] A broad observation from the new discipline is that vector-borne pathogens are generally more virulent than directly transmitted pathogens. One line of explanation is that evolution to benignness cannot occur easily in both the vector and the primary host, and that benign adaptation in the vector is more important.[3]

From the perspective of evolutionary epidemiology, the virulence of the malaria parasites can be understood as a function of their adaptation to human beings. Paul Ewald, a pioneer in the field, has expressed this as the hypothesis of adaptive severity. The logic here is that healthy human immune systems can control nearly all organisms that have not had a history of adaptation to human beings. From this perspective, it seems likely that falciparum parasites – and most other vector-borne parasites – have evolved *toward* greater virulence. It may be that the virulence of early childhood falciparum infections is a consequence of the adult acquisition of functional immunities.[4]

* * *

Over the long run of human history, human communities have had only partial understandings of malaria. Many communities successfully mobilized their understandings in an effort to reduce their suffering. Many societies discovered natural plant therapies, and some societies adopted

---

[2] Paul W. Ewald, *Evolution of Infectious Disease* (New York: Oxford University Press, 1994), 3–13.
[3] William H. McNeill first advanced this idea in his seminal work in historical epidemiology, *Plagues and Peoples* (Garden City, NY: Anchor Press, 1976).
[4] Margaret J. MacKinnon and Andrew F. Read, "Immunity Promotes Virulence Evolution in a Malaria Model," *PLoS Biology*, vol. 2, no. 9 (2004), 1286–1292.

practical measures such as the use of insect repellents, screening and nets, and the draining of swamps. Some developed nuanced understandings of landscapes and environments that posed malarial threats.

The momentum of human expansion out of Africa into Eurasia, and much later the thickening of the webs of global intercommunication in the post-Columbian period that included the Americas, eventually created a global distribution of malarial infections in three great zones that was at its maximum extent during the nineteenth century. During the twentieth century, malaria was banished from approximately a quarter of the earth's surface, roughly half of its nineteenth-century domain. However, owing to massive population growth, particularly on the African continent, by the end of the twentieth century the number of people exposed to malaria had increased dramatically, by more than 300 percent. Early in the twenty-first century, the malarial areas remaining are mostly those of intense transmission, and falciparum infections constitute a far larger percentage of infections than a century earlier. Malaria has come full circle. From its origins in tropical Africa, through lengthy arcs of Eurasian and New World expansion and retraction, malaria is again recentered in tropical Africa.

Bibliography

Dissertations and Unpublished Manuscripts

Bado, Jean-Paul. "Malarial Campaigns in Francophone Africa from the 1940s: A Challenge for Medicine," presented at the conference on Health and Medicine in Africa, Bryn Mawr and Haverford Colleges, April 2005.

Carter, Eric D. "Disease, Science, and Regional Development: Malaria Control in Northwest Argentina, 1890–1950" (unpublished PhD diss., University of Wisconsin–Madison, 2005).

Pérez, Carlos. "Quinine and Caudillos: Manuel Isidoro Belzu and the Cinchona Bark Trade in Bolivia, 1848–1855" (unpublished PhD diss., University of California, Los Angeles, 1998).

Books and Articles

Abel, Laurent and Jean-Laurent Casanova. "Genetic Predisposition to Clinical Tuberculosis: Bridging the Gap between Simple and Complex Inheritance," *American Journal of Human Genetics*, vol. 67, no. 2 (2000), 274–277.

Abu-Raddad, Laith J., Padmaja Patnaik, and James G. Kublin. "Dual Infection with HIV and Malaria Fuels the Spread of Both Diseases in Sub-Saharan Africa," *Science*, vol. 314 (December 8, 2006), 1603–1606.

Ackernecht, Erwin H. "The History of Malaria," *Ciba Symposium*, vol. 7, nos. 3 and 4 (June–July 1945), 53–54.

———. "Aspects of the History of Therapeutics," *Bulletin of the History of Medicine*, vol. 36 (1962), 387–419.

———. *History and Geography of the Most Important Diseases* (New York: Hafner Publishing, 1965).

———. *Malaria in the Upper Mississippi Valley, 1760–1900*. Supplement to the *Bulletin of the History of Medicine*, no. 4 (Baltimore: Johns Hopkins University Press, 1945; repr., New York: Arno Press, 1977).

Adam, David. "Scientists Create GM Mosquitoes to Fight Malaria and Save Thousands of Lives," *The Guardian*, October 10, 2005. Available online at http://www.guardian.co.uk/science/2005/oct/10/infectiousdiseases.medicineandhealth.

Adams, David P. "Malaria, Labor, and Population Distribution in Costa Rica: A Biohistorical Perspective," *Journal of Interdisciplinary History*, vol. 27, no. 1 (1996), 75–85.

Ambrose, Stanley H. "Late Pleistocene Human Population Bottlenecks, Volcanic Winter, and Differentiation of Modern Humans," *Journal of Human Evolution*, vol. 34 (1998), 623–651.

———. "Did the Super-Eruption of Toba Cause a Human Population Bottleneck? Reply to Gathorne-Hardy and Harcourt Smith," *Journal of Human Evolution*, vol. 45 (2003), 231–237.

Amer, Abdulkrim and H. Mehlhorn. "Repellency Effect of Forty-One Essential Oils against *Aedes, Anopheles,* and *Culex* Mosquitoes," *Parasitology Research*, vol. 99, no. 4 (2006), 478–490.

Amoroso Jr., Louis F., Gilberto Corbellini, and Mario Coluzzi. "Lessons Learned from Malaria: Italy's Past and Sub-Sahara's Future," *Health and Place*, vol. 11 (2005), 67–73.

Andah, Bassey W. "Identifying Early Farming Traditions of West Africa," in ed. Thurston Shaw, Paul Sinclair, Bassey Andah, and Alex Okpoko, *The Archaeology of Africa: Food, Metals and Towns* (London: Routledge, 1995), 240–254.

Anderson, J.B. "Malaria in India," *Journal of the Royal Army Medical Corps*, vol. 14 (1910), 50–60.

Anderson, Warwick. "Immunities of Empire: Race, Disease, and the New Tropical Medicine, 1900–1920," *Bulletin of the History of Medicine*, vol. 70, no. 1 (1996), 94–118.

Andrade-Neto, V.F., M.G.L. Brandão, J.R. Stehmann, L.A. Oliveira, and A.U. Krettli. "Antimalarial Activity of Cinchona-like Plants Used to Treat Fever and Malaria in Brazil," *Journal of Ethnopharmacology*, vol. 87 (2003), 253–256.

Annett, H.E., J. Everett Dutton, and J.H. Elliott. *Report of the Malaria Expedition to Nigeria of the Liverpool School of Tropical Medicine and Medical Parasitology*, 2 vols. (Liverpool: University Press of Liverpool, 1901).

[Anon] *On the Use of Sulphate of Cinchonidia and Other Cheap Alkaloids of Cinchona Barks* (Philadelphia: James A. Moore, 1876).

———. *On the Use of Sulphate of Cinchonidia in Parts of the States of Illinois, Indiana, Missouri, Kentucky, and in the Mississippi Valley in 1875. From Medical Journals, Societies, and Individual Physicians* (Philadelphia: James A. Moore, 1876).

———. "Manufacture of Quinine in India," *Kew Bulletin*, no. 38 (February 1890), 29–34.

———. "Mosquitoes and Malaria: A Campaign That Failed," *The Lancet*, vol. I (1909), 1012–1014.

———. "Quinine in the Treatment and Prevention of Malaria," *The Lancet* (February 23, 1918), 301–302.

———. *A Century or Longer in Business* (Philadelphia: Insurance Company of North America, 1922).

———. "Malaria," in W.G. MacPherson, W.P. Herringham, T.R. Elliott, and A. Balfour, eds. *History of the Great War Based on Official Documents. Medical Services. Diseases of the War*, vol. I (London: H.M.S.O., 1923), 227–293.

———. "Malaria Control," *Indian Medical Gazette* (December 1930), 701–706.

———. "The Romance of Cinchona," *Indian Medical Gazette* (April 1931), 211–214.

———. "The Quinine Policy," *Indian Medical Gazette* (April 1931), 519–522.

———. "Cinchona Policy," *Indian Medical Gazette* (July 1932), 391–394.

———. "The First of the Rosengartens," *Chemical Industries*, vol. 37, no. 3 (September 1935), 221–226.

———. "Report and Recommendations on Malaria: A Summary," *American Journal of Tropical Medicine and Hygiene*, vol. 10, no. 4 (1961), 451–503.

———. "Rediscovering Wormwood: Qinghaosu for Malaria," *The Lancet*, vol. 339 (March 14, 1992), 649–651.

Arnold, David. "Introduction: Disease, Medicine, and Empire," in ed. David Arnold, *Imperial Medicine and Indigenous Societies* (Manchester: Manchester University Press, 1988), 1–26.

Austen, Ralph. *African Economic History* (Portsmouth, NH: Heinemann, 1987).

Bado, Jean-Paul. "La lutte contre le paludisme en Afrique centrale. Problèmes d'hier et d'aujourd'hui," *Enjeux*, no. 18 (January–March 2004), 10–13.

———. "La traque du paludisme en Afrique. Leçon d'hier, perspectives d'aujourd'hui," *Enjeux*, no. 31 (April–June 2007), 40–45.

———. "La lutte contre le paludisme au Cameroun des années 1950 aux années 1960," in *Colloques internationaux. Milieux de vie et santé. Quelques pratiques interdisciplinaires* (Aix-en-Provence, France: Edisud, 2008), forthcoming.

Baker, George. "Observations on the Late Intermittent Fevers; To Which Is Added a Short History of the Peruvian Bark," *Medical Transactions* (1785), 141–216.

Baker, Major W.E., T.E. Dempster, and H. Yule. "Report of a Committee Assembled to Report on the Causes of the Unhealthiness Which Has Existed at Kurnaul, and Other Portions of the Country along the Lane of the Delhie Canal and Also Whether Any Injurious Effect on the Health of the People of the Dooab Is, or Is Not, Likely to Be Produced by the Contemplated Ganges Canal, with Appendices on Malaria by Surgeon T.E. Dempster [1847]," in ed. J.A. Sinton, *Records of the Malaria Survey of India*, vol. 1, 1929–1930 (Calcutta: Thacker, Spink and Co., n.d.), 1–68.

Barber, M.A. "The History of Malaria in the United States," *Public Health Reports*, vol. 44 (1929), 2575–2587.

Barber, Marshall A. *A Malariologist in Many Lands* (Lawrence: University of Kansas Press, 1946).

Beales, Peter F. and Herbert M. Gilles. "Rationale and Technique of Malaria Control," in ed. David A. Warrell and Herbert M. Gilles, *Essential Malariology*, 4th ed. (New York: Arnold Press, 2002), 107–190.

Beauchamp, Chantal. "Fièvres d'hier, paludisme d'aujourd'hui. Vie et mort d'une maladie," *Annales ESC*, vol. 43, no. 1 (1988), 249–275.

Beck, Ann. "Medicine and Society in Tanganyika 1890–1930: A Historical Inquiry," *Transactions of the American Philosophical Society*, vol. 67, pt. 3 (1977), 5–59.

Becker, F.T., L.I. Kaplan, H.S. Read, and M.F. Boyd. "Variations in Susceptibility to Therapeutic Malaria," *American Journal of Medical Science*, vol. 21 (1946), 680–685.

Beier, John C. "Malaria Parasite Development in Mosquitoes," *Annual Review of Entomology*, vol. 43 (1998), 519–543.

Bello, David A. "To Go No Where No Han Could Go for Long: Malaria and the Qing Construction of Administrative Space in Frontier Yunnan," *Modern China*, vol. 31, no. 2 (2005), 1–35.

Benedict, Mark Q. and Alan S. Robinson. "The First Releases of Transgenic Mosquitoes: An Argument for the Sterile Insect Technique," *Trends in Parasitology*, vol. 19, no. 8 (2003), 349–355.

Bentley, Charles A. *Malaria and Agriculture in Bengal* (Calcutta: Bengal Secretariat Book Depot, 1925).

Besansky, Nora J., Catherine A. Hill, and Carlo Costantini. "No Accounting for Taste: Host Preference in Malaria Vectors," *Trends in Parasitology*, vol. 20, no. 6 (2004), 249–251.

Bettini, S. and R. Romi. "Zooprofilassi: un problema vecchio e attuale," *Parassitologia*, vol. 40 (1998), 423–430.

Biswas, K. "Cinchona Cultivation in India," *Journal of the Asiatic Society*, vol. 3 (1961), 63–80.

Björkman, A. and P.A. Phillips-Howard. "Drug-Resistant Malaria: Mechanisms of Development and Inferences for Malaria Control," *Transactions of the Royal Society of Tropical Medicine and Hygiene*, vol. 84 (1990), 323–324.

Bødker, René, Hamisi A. Msangeni, William Kisinza, and Steve W. Lindsay. "Relationship between the Intensity of Exposure to Malaria Parasites and Infection in the Usambara Mountains, Tanzania," *American Journal of Tropical Medicine and Hygiene*, vol. 74, no. 5 (2006), 716–723.

Bollet, Alfred Jay. *Civil War Medicine: Challenges and Triumphs* (Tucson, AZ: Galen Press, 2002).

Boucher de la Ville Jossy, Paul. *Quelques réflexions sur l'action physiologique du sulfate de quinine à haute dose en general; et en particulier dans le traitement de la fièvre typhoïde* (Paris: Faculté de médicine de Paris, 1846).

Bouma, Menno and Mark Rowland. "Failure of Passive Zooprophylaxis: Cattle Ownership in Pakistan is Associated with a Higher Prevalence of Malaria," *Transactions of the Royal Society of Tropical Medicine and Hygiene*, vol. 89 (1995), 351–353.

Bower, B. "African Finds Revise Cultural Roots," *Science News*, vol. 147, no. 17 (April 29, 1995), 260.

Boyce, Rubert W. *Health, Progress, and Administration in the West Indies* (London: J. Murray, 1910).

Boyd, Mark F. "An Historical Sketch of the Prevalence of Malaria in North America," *American Journal of Tropical Medicine*, vol. 21 (1941), 223–244.

Boyd, Mark, ed. *Malariology: A Comprehensive Survey of All Aspects of this Group of Disease from a Global Standpoint* (Philadelphia: Saunders, 1949).

Boyd, M.F. and S.F. Kitchen. "Simultaneous Inoculation with *Plasmodium Vivax* and *Plasmodium Falciparum*," *American Journal of Tropical Medicine*, vol. 17 (1937), 855–859.

Boyd, M.F. and W.K. Stratman-Thomas. "Studies on Benign Tertian Malaria. IV. On the Refractoriness of Negroes to Inoculation with *Plasmodium Vivax*," *American Journal of Hygiene*, vol. 18 (1933), 485–489.

Bradley, D.J. "Malaria: Old Infections, Changing Epidemiology," *Health Transition Review*, vol. 2, suppl. (1992), 137–153.

———. "Watson, Swellengrebel and Species Sanitation: Environmental and Ecological Aspects," *Parassitologia*, vol. 36, nos. 1–2 (1994), 137–148.

Braslow, Joel T. "The Influence of a Biological Therapy on Physicians' Narratives and Interrogations: The Case of General Paralysis of the Insane and Malaria Fever Therapy, 1910–1950," *Bulletin of the History of Medicine*, vol. 70, no. 4 (1996), 577–608.

Briercliffe, R. "Discussion on the Malaria Epidemic in Ceylon," *Proceedings of the Royal Society of Medicine*, vol. 29 (1935), 537–562.

Briquet, Pierre. *Traité thérapeutique du quinquina et de ses préparations* (Paris: V. Masson, 1853).

Brock, Thomas D. *Robert Koch: A Life in Medicine and Bacteriology* (Washington, DC: ASM Press, 1988).

Brooks, Alison S. and Peter Robertshaw. "The Glacial Maximum in Tropical Africa: 22000–12000 BP," in ed. Clive Gamble and Olga Soffer, *The World at 18000 BP* (London: Unwin Hyman, 1990), 120–169.

Brooks, George E. *Eurafricans in Western Africa* (Athens: Ohio University Press, 2003).

Brown, Peter J. "Culture and the Global Resurgence of Malaria," in ed. M.C. Inhorn and Peter J. Brown, *Anthropology of Infectious Disease* (Australia: Gordon and Breach, 1997), 119–141.

———. "Malaria, Miseria, and Underdevelopment in Sardinia: The 'Malaria Blocks Development' Cultural Model," *Medical Anthropology*, vol. 17 (1997), 239–254.

———. "Failure-As-Success: Multiple Meanings of Eradication in the Rockefeller Foundation Sardinia Project," *Parassitologia*, vol. 40 (1998), 117–130.

Bruce-Chwatt, L.J. "Malaria and Its Prevention in Military Campaigns," *Zeitschrift fur Tropenmedizin und Parasitologie*, vol. 22 (1971), 370–390.

———. "Qinghaosu: A New Antimalarial," *British Medical Journal*, vol. 284 (March 13, 1982), 767–768.

———. "Lessons Learned from Applied Field Research Activities in Africa during the Malaria Eradication Era," *Bulletin of the World Health Organization*, vol. 62, suppl. (1984), 19–29.

Bruce-Chwatt, Leonard Jan and Julian de Zulueta. *The Rise and Fall of Malaria in Europe: A Historico-Epidemiological Study* (Oxford: Oxford University Press, 1980).

Brun, Charles-Vital. *Du sulfate de cinchonine, et de son emploi dans les fièvres intermittentes*. Thèse pour le doctorat en médecine. (Paris: Faculté de médecine de Paris, 1860).

Bryson, Alexander. *Report on the Climate and Principal Diseases of the African Station* (London: W. Clowes, 1847).

———. "On the Prophylactic Influence of Quinine," *The Medical Times and Gazette*, new series, vol. 8 (January 7–June 24, 1854), 6–7.

Buchanan, W.J. "The Value of Prophylactic Issue of Cinchona Preparations. An Experiment in Indian Jails," *Journal of Tropical Medicine*, vol. 1 (1899), 201–203.

Bullock, Lloyd. "On Amorphous Quinine," in ed. Edward Latham Ormerod, *On the Pathology and Treatment of Valvular Disease of the Heart and Its Secondary Affections: Being the Gulstonian Lectures Delivered at the Royal College of Physicians in February 1851* (London: Wilson and Ogilvy, 1851).

[Bureau for Increasing the Use of Quinine]. *Malaria and Quinine* (Amsterdam: Bureau for Increasing the Use of Quinine, 1927).

Burnet, Sir Frank Macfarlane. *Natural History of Infectious Disease*, 3rd ed. (Cambridge: Cambridge University Press, 1962).

Busvine, James R. *Disease Transmission by Insects* (Berlin: Springer-Verlag, 1993).

Butler, F.A. and J.J. Sapero. "Pacific Vivax Malaria in the American Negro," *American Journal of Tropical Medicine*, vol. 27 (1947), 111–115.

Byam, W. and R.G. Archibald, eds. *The Practice of Medicine in the Tropics*, 3 vols. (London: H. Frowde and Hodder and Stoughton, 1921–1923).

Bynum, W.F. "An Experiment That Failed: Malaria Control at Mian Mir," *Parassitologia*, vol. 36 (1994), 107–120.

———. "'Reasons for Contentment': Malaria in India, 1900–1920," *Parassitologia*, vol. 40, nos. 1–2 (1998), 19–27.

———. "Malaria in Interwar British India," *Parassitologia*, vol. 42, nos. 1–2 (2000), 25–31.

Caldas de Castro, Marcia and Burton H. Singer. "Was Malaria Present in the Amazon before European Conquest? Available Evidence and Future Research Agenda?" *Journal of Archaeological Science*, vol. 32 (2005), 337–340.

Carlson, Dennis G. *African Fever: A Study of British Science, Technology, and Politics in West Africa, 1787–1864* (Canton, MA: Science History Publications, 1984).

Carney, Judith A. *Black Rice: The African Origins of Rice Cultivation in the Americas* (Cambridge, MA: Harvard University Press, 2001).

Carson, Rachel. *Silent Spring* (Boston: Houghton Mifflin, 1962).

Carter, R. and K.N. Mendis. "Evolutionary and Historical Aspects of the Burden of Malaria," *Clinical Microbiology Review*, vol. 15 (2002), 564–594.

Carter, Richard. "Speculations on the Origins of *Plasmodium Vivax* Malaria," *Trends in Parasitology*, vol. 19, no. 5 (2003), 214–219.

Cartwright, S.A. "Report on the Diseases and Physical Peculiarities of the Negro Race," *The New Orleans Medical and Surgical Journal* (May 1851), 691–715.

Casas Orrego, A.L. "Comercio, Quina y Piretología: Prolongaciones en la Explotación y el Uso de la Quina en el Siglo XIX," in ed. Javier Guerrero Baron, *Medicina y Salud en la Historia de Colombia* (Tunja, Colombia: Universidad Pedagógica y Tecnológica de Colombia, 1997), 96–108.

Cavalli-Sforza, L.L., Paolo Menozzi, and Alberto Paizzo. *The History and Geography of Human Genes* (Princeton: Princeton University Press, 1994).

Cell, John W. "Anglo-Indian Medical Theory and the Origins of Segregation in West Africa," *American Historical Review*, vol. 91, no. 2 (1986), 307–335.

Childs, St. Julien Ravenel. *Malaria and Colonization in the Carolina Low Country 1526–1696* (Baltimore: Johns Hopkins University Press, 1940).

Chomel, A. "Sur L'emploi de la quinine et de la cinchonine dans les fièvres intermittentes," *Journal de pharmacie et des sciences accessoires*, vol. 7 (1821), 134–137, 226–231.

Chopra, Ananda S. "Ayurveda," in ed. Helaine Selin, *Medicine across Cultures: History and Practice of Medicine in Non-Western Cultures* (Dordrecht, Holland: Kluwer Academic Publishers, 2003), 75–83.

Chopra, R.N. "Present Position of Anti-Malarial Drug Therapy in India," *Indian Medical Gazette* (July 1938), 418–423.

Chow, C.Y. and M.C. Balfour. "The Natural Infection and Seasonal Prevalence of Anopheles Mosquitoes in Chefang and Vicinity, Yunnan-Burma Border," *Chinese Medical Journal*, vol. 67, no. 8 (1949), 405–413.

Christian, David. *Maps of Time: An Introduction to Big History* (Berkeley: University of California Press, 2005).

Christopher, Emma. *Slave Ship Sailors and Their Captive Cargoes* (New York: Cambridge University Press, 2006).

Christophers, Major S.R. *Malaria in the Punjab* (Calcutta: Superintendent Government Printing, 1911).

Christophers, S.R. "The Mechanisms of Immunity against Malaria in Communities Living under Hyperendemic Conditions," *Indian Journal of Medical Research*, vol. 12 (1924), 273–294.

Christophers, S.R. and J.W.W. Stephens, "The Malaria of Expeditionary Forces and the Means of Its Prevention," in *Further Reports to the Malaria Committee of the Royal Society* (London, 1900), 20–22.

———. "The Native as the Prime Agent in the Malarial Infection of Europeans (with Map)," in *Further Reports to the Malaria Committee of the Royal Society* (London, 1900), 3–19.

———. "The Segregation of Europeans," in *Reports to the Malaria Committee of the Royal Society, third series.* (London: Harrison and Sons, 1900), 21–24.

Churchman, J.W. "The Use of Quinine during the Civil War," *Johns Hopkins Hospital Bulletin*, vol. 17 (1906), 175–181.

Cinchona Products Institute. *Influenza and Quinine: A Review of Modern Clinical Practice* (New York: Cinchona Products Institute, 1938).

Cloëtta, Antoine. *Le problème économique et social de la quinine* (Bâle: Impr. Kreis, 1928).

Clyde, David F. *History of the Medical Services of Tanganyika* (Dar es Salaam, Tanzania: Government Press, 1962).

———. *Malaria in Tanzania* (London: Oxford University Press, 1967).

Coatney, G. Robert, William E. Collins, McWilson Warren, and Peter G. Contacos. *The Primate Malarias* (Atlanta: Centers for Disease Control, 2003).

Coelho, Philip R. P. and Robert A. McGuire. "African and European Bound Labor in the British New World: The Biological Consequences of Economic Choices," *Journal of Economic History*, vol. 57, no. 1 (1997), 83–115.

Cohen, Mark Nathan. *The Food Crisis in Prehistory: Overpopulation and the Origins of Agriculture* (New Haven: Yale University Press, 1977).

———. *Health and the Rise of Civilization* (New Haven: Yale University Press, 1989).

Cohn Jr., Samuel K. "The Black Death: The End of a Paradigm," *American Historical Review*, vol. 107, no. 3 (2002), 703–738.

Colbourne, Michael. *Malaria in Africa* (London: Oxford University Press, 1966).

Collins, William E. and Geoffrey M. Jeffrey. "*Plasmodium Ovale*: Parasite and Disease," *Clinical Microbiology Reviews*, vol. 18, no. 3 (2005), 570–581.

Coluzzi, M. "The Clay Feet of the Malaria Giant and Its African Roots: Hypotheses and Influences about Origin, Spread, and Control of *Plasmodium Falciparum*," *Parassitologia*, vol. 41 (1999), 277–283.

————. "Plasmodium falciparum en Afrique subsaharienne. Spéciation recente des vecteurs, transmissibilité, evolution de la pathogenèse/contrôle de la maladie, et capacité vectorielle," *Annales de l'Institut Pasteur. Actualités,* no. 13 (2002), 81–99.

Coluzzi, M., A. Sabatini, V. Petrarca, and M.A. Di Deco, "Chromosomal Differentiation and Adaptation to Human Environments in the *Anopheles Gambiae* Complex," *Transactions of the Royal Society for Tropical Medicine and Hygiene,* vol. 73 (1979), 483–497.

Connolly, Bob and Robin Anderson. *First Contact* (New York: Viking Press, 1987).

Conroy, Mary Schaeffer. "Malaria in Late Tsarist Russia," *Bulletin of the History of Medicine,* vol. 56, no. 1 (1982), 41–55.

Conte, Christopher A. *Highland Sanctuary: Environmental History in Tanzania's Usambara Mountains* (Athens: Ohio University Press, 2004).

Conway, D.J., C. Fanello, J.M. Lloyd, M.A.-S. Ban, A.H. Baloch, S.D. Somanath, C. Roper, A.M.J. Oduola, B. Mulder, M.M. Povoa, B. Singh, and A.W. Thomas. "Origin of *Plasmodium Falciparum* Malaria Is Traced by Mitochondrial DNA," *Molecular Biochemical Parasitology,* vol. 111 (2000), 163–171.

Conway, David J. "Tracing the Dawn of *Plasmodium Falciparum* with Mitochondrial Genome Sequences," *Trends in Genetics,* vol. 19, no. 12 (2003), 671–674.

Conway, David J. and Jake Baum. "In the Blood – The Remarkable Ancestry of *Plasmodium Falciparum,*" *Trends in Parasitology,* vol. 18, no. 8 (2002), 351–355.

Coolidge, R.H. "On the Medical Topography of Fort Gibson, Arkansas," *Southern Medical Reports,* vol. 2 (1850), 440–452.

Coolidge, R.H. and T.R. Lawson. *Statistical Report on the Sickness and Mortality of the Army of the United States Jan. 1839 to Jan. 1855* (Washington, DC: A.O.P. Nicholson, 1856).

Cooper, Donald B. and Kenneth F. Kiple. "Yellow Fever," in ed. Kenneth F. Kiple, *The Cambridge World History of Human Disease* (New York: Cambridge University Press, 1993), 1100–1107.

Cooper, Richard S., Babatunde Osotimehin, Jay S. Kaufman, and Terrence Forrester. "Disease Burden in Sub-Saharan Africa: What Should We Conclude in the Absence of Data?" *The Lancet,* vol. 351 (January 17, 1998), 208–210.

Corbellini, G. "Acquired Immunity against Malaria as a Tool for the Control of the Disease: The Strategy Proposed by the Malaria Commission of the League of Nations in 1933," *Parassitologia,* vol. 40 (1998), 109–115.

Coursey, D.G. *Yams: An Account of the Nature, Origins, Cultivation, and Utilisation of the Useful Members of the Dioscoreaceae* (London: Longmans, 1967).

————. "The Origins and Domestication of Yams in Africa," in ed. J.R. Harlan, J.M.J. de Wet, and A.B.L. Stemler, *Origins of African Plant Domestication* (The Hague, The Netherlands: Mouton, 1975), 383–408.

Courtwright, David T. *Forces of Habit: Drugs and the Making of the Modern World* (Cambridge, MA: Harvard University Press, 2001).

Courvisier, Jean-Nicolas. "Eau, paludisme et démographie en Grèce péninsulaire," in ed. René Ginouvès, Anne-Marie Guimier-Sorbets, Jacques Jouanna, and Laurence Villard, *L'eau, la santé et la maladie dans le monde grec* (Athens: École française d'Athènes, 1994), 297–319.

Covell, Gordon. *Malaria in Bombay* (Bombay: Government Press, 1928).

———. *Malaria Control by Anti-Mosquito Measures*, 2nd ed. (Calcutta and Simla: Thacker, Spink, and Co., 1941).

Cowan, J.M. "Cinchona in the Empire," *Empire Forestry Journal*, vol. 8, no. 1 (1929), 45–53.

Craig, M.H., R.W. Snow, and D. le Sueur. "A Climate-based Distribution Model of Malaria Transmission in Sub-Saharan Africa," *Parasitology Today*, vol. 15, no. 3 (1999), 105–111.

Crosby, Alfred W. *The Columbian Exchange: The Biological and Cultural Consequences of 1492* (Westport, CT: Greenwood Publishing, 1972).

———. *Ecological Imperialism: The Biological Expansion of Europe, 900–1900*, 2nd ed. (New York: Cambridge University Press, 2004).

Cross, Samuel H. "Quinine Production and Marketing," Supplement to Commerce Reports, *U.S. Department of Commerce Trade Information Bulletin*, no. 273 (October 1924), 1–50.

Cueto, Marcos. *El Regreso de las Epidemias; Salud y Sociedad en el Perú del Siglo XX* (Lima, Peru: Instituto de Estudios Peruanos, 1997).

———. "The Meanings of Control and Eradication of Malaria in the Andes," *Parassitologia*, vol. 40 (1998), 177–182.

Curtin, Philip D. "Epidemiology and the Slave Trade," *Political Science Quarterly*, vol. 83 (1968), 190–216.

———. *Cross-Cultural Trade in World History* (New York: Cambridge University Press, 1984).

———. "Medical Knowledge and Urban Planning in Colonial Tropical Africa," *American Historical Review*, vol. 90, no. 3 (1985), 594–613.

———. *Death by Migration* (New York: Cambridge University Press, 1989).

———. *The Rise and Fall of the Plantation Complex* (New York: Cambridge University Press, 1990).

———. "Disease Exchange across the Tropical Atlantic," *History and Philosophy of the Life Sciences*, vol. 15 (1993), 329–356.

———. "Malarial Immunities in Nineteenth-Century West Africa and the Caribbean," *Parassitologia*, vol. 36 (1994), 69–82.

———. *Disease and Empire* (New York: Cambridge University Press, 1998).

D'Alessandro, U. and H. Buttiëns, "History and Importance of Antimalarial Drug Resistance," *Tropical Medicine and International Health*, vol. 6, no. 11 (2001), 845–848.

Daniels, C.W. "Prophylaxis," in *Reports to the Malaria Committee of the Royal Society*, 3rd series (London: Harrison and Sons, 1900), 37–43.

Das, Aparup, Ruchi Bajaj, Sujata Mohanty, and Vijaylakshmi Swain. "Genetic Diversity and Evolutionary History of Plasmodium Falciparum and P. Vivax," *Current Science*, vol. 92, no. 11 (2007), 1516–1524.

Davis, Mike. *Late Victorian Holocausts: El Niño Famines and the Making of the Third World* (London: Verso Press, 2001).

Dawson, Ray F. "Quinine and Quinidine Production in the Americas," *Horticultural Technology*, vol. 1, no. 1 (1991), 17–21.

Dawson, W.T. "Cinchona Alkaloids and Bark in Malaria," *International Clinics*, vol. II, series 40 (1930), 121–149.

De Langhe, E., R. Swennen, and D. Vuylsteke. "Plantain in the Early Bantu World," *Azania*, vols. 29–30 (1994–1995), 147–160.

De La Warr, Thomas West. *The Relation of the Right Honourable the Lord De-La-Warre, Lord Governour and Capitaine Generall of the Colonie, Planted in Virginea* (London: W. Hall for W. Welbie, 1611).

de Zulueta, J. "Changes in the Geographical Distribution of Malaria throughout History," *Parassitologia*, vol. 29 (1987), 193–205.

———. "Malaria and Ecosystems: From Prehistory to Posteradication," *Parassitologia*, vol. 36 (1994), 7–15.

Dean, Warren. *With Broadax and Firebrand: The Destruction of the Brazilian Atlantic Forest* (Berkeley: University of California Press, 1995).

Dempster, T.E. "Notes on the Application of the Test of Organic Disease of the Spleen as an Easy and Certain Method of Detecting Malarious Localities in Hot Climates [1848]," in ed. J.A. Sinton, *Records of the Malaria Survey of India*, vol. 1, 1929–1930 (Calcutta: Thacker, Spink, and Co., n.d.), 69–85.

Denevan, William M. "The Aboriginal Population of Amazonia," in ed. William M. Denevan, *The Native Population of the Americas in 1492*, 2nd ed. (Madison: University of Wisconsin Press, 1992), 205–234.

Denham, T.P., S.G. Haberle, C. Lentfer, R. Fullagar, J. Field, M. Therin, N. Porch, and B. Winsborough. "Origins of Agriculture at Kuk Swamp in the Highlands of New Guinea," *Science*, vol. 301, no. 5630 (July 11, 2003), 189–193.

Denham, Tim, Simon Haberle, and Carol Lentfer. "New Evidence and Revised Interpretations of Early Agriculture in Highland New Guinea," *Antiquity*, vol. 78, no. 4 (2004), 839–857.

DeSaussure, H.W. "Quinine, a Prophylactic of Intermittent and Remittent Fevers," *American Journal of the Medical Sciences* (January 1861), 296–297.

Desowitz, R.S. "The Malaria Vaccine: Seventy Years of the Great Immune Hope," *Parassitologia*, vol. 42 (2000), 173–182.

Desowitz, Robert S. *The Malaria Capers* (New York: W.W. Norton, 1993).

Diamond, Jared. *Guns, Germs, and Steel: The Fates of Human Societies* (New York: W.W. Norton, 1997).

Dobson, Mary J. "Marsh Fever – The Geography of Malaria in England," *Journal of Historical Geography*, vol. 6 (1980), 357–389.

———. "Mortality Gradients and Disease Exchanges: Comparisons from Old England and Colonial America," *Social History of Medicine*, vol. 2 (1989), 259–297.

———. "Malaria in England: A Geographical and Historical Perspective," *Parassitologia*, vol. 36 (1994), 35–60.

———. *Contours of Death and Disease in Early Modern England* (New York: Cambridge University Press, 1997).

———. "Bitter-Sweet Solutions for Malaria: Exploring Natural Remedies from the Past," *Parassitologia*, vol. 40 (1998), 69–81.

Dobson, M.J., M. Malowany, and R.W. Snow. "Malaria Control in East Africa: The Kampala Conference and the Pare-Taveta Scheme: A Meeting of Common and High Ground," *Parassitologia*, vol. 42 (2000), 149–166.

Doby, Jean-Marie. "Histoire du traitement du paludisme depuis l'Antiquité jusqu'à la preparation de la quinine," *Bulletin de la Société française de parasitologie*, vol. 10, fasc. 1 (1992), 133–159.

Dominguez, Camilo and Augusto Gómez. *La Economia Extractiva en la Amazonia Colombiana 1850–1930* (Colombia: TROPENBOS; Araracuara: Corporación Colombiana para la Amazonia, 1990).

Dougall, Joseph. "The Febrifuge Properties of the Cinchona Alkaloids – Cinchonia, Quinidia, and Cinchonidia," *Edinburgh Medical Journal*, vol. 19, no. 3 (1873), 193–209.

Douglas, John. *A Short Account of the Mortifications, and of the Surprising Effect of the Bark* (London: John Nourse, 1732).

Dounias, Edmond. "The Management of Wild Yam Tubers by the Baka Pygmies in Southern Cameroon," *African Study Monographs*, suppl. 26 (March 2001), 135–156.

Drake, Daniel. *A Systematic Treatise, Historical, Etiological, and Practical, of the Principal Diseases of the Interior Valley of North America* (Cincinnati: W.B. Smith and Co., 1850).

Duffy, John. "Medical Practice in the Ante Bellum South," *Journal of Southern History*, vol. 25, no. 1 (1959), 53–72.

———. *Epidemics in Colonial America* (Port Washington, NY: Kennicat Press, 1972).

Dumett, Raymond. "The Campaign against Malaria and the Expansion of Scientific Medical and Sanitary Services in British West Africa, 1898–1910," *African Historical Studies*, vol. 1, no. 2 (1968), 153–197.

Duncan, Louis C. "A Medical History of General Zachary Taylor's Army of Occupation in Texas and Mexico, 1845–1847," *Military Surgeon*, vol. 48 (1921), 76–104.

———. "Medical History of General Scott's Campaign to the City of Mexico in 1847," *Military Surgeon*, vol. 47 (1920), 436–470, 596–609.

Dunlap, Thomas R. *DDT: Scientists, Citizens, and Public Policy* (Princeton: Princeton University Press, 1981).

Dunn, Richard S. *Sugar and Slaves* (Chapel Hill: University of North Carolina Press, 1972).

Duran-Reynals, M.L. *The Fever Bark Tree* (Garden City, NY: Doubleday, 1946).

Durham, J.E. "Testing the Malaria Hypothesis in West Africa," in ed. J.E. Bowman, *Distribution and Evolution of Hemoglobin and Globin Loci* (New York: Elsevier, 1983), 45–76.

Dutta, Hiran M. and Ashok K. Dutt. "Malarial Ecology: A Global Perspective," *Social Science and Medicine*, vol. 12 (1978), 69–84.

Ebisawa, I. "Malaria in China and the Equatorial Pacific Area from 1937 to 1943," *Yale Journal of Biology and Medicine*, vol. 46 (1973), 94–101.

Eckart, W.U. "Malaria and Colonialism in the German Colonies New Guinea and the Cameroons. Research, Control, Thoughts of Eradication," *Parassitologia*, vol. 40 (1998), 83–90.

Edelstein, Stuart J. *The Sickled Cell: From Myths to Molecules* (Cambridge, MA: Harvard University Press, 1986).

Ehret, Christopher. "Historical/Linguistic Evidence for Early African Food Production," in ed. J.D. Clark and S.A. Brandt, *From Hunters to Farmers* (Berkeley: University of California Press, 1984), 26–39.

———. "Bantu Expansions: Re-Envisioning A Central Problem of Early African History," *International Journal of African Historical Studies*, vol. 34, no. 1 (2001), 5–41.

———. *The Civilizations of Africa* (Charlottesville: University of Virginia Press, 2002).

Ellingwood, Finley. *The American Materia Medica, Therapeutics, and Pharmacognosy* (Chicago: Ellingwoods Therapeutist, 1919).

Elliotson, John. "Illustrations of the Medical Properties of Quinine," *Medico-Chirugical Transactions*, vol. 12 (1821–1823), 543–564.

———. *The Principles and Practice of Medicine* (Philadelphia: Carey and Hart, 1844).

Elvin, Mark. *The Retreat of the Elephants: An Environmental History of China* (New Haven: Yale University Press, 2004).

England, Joseph W. "The American Manufacture of Quinine Sulphate," *Alumni Report, Philadelphia College of Pharmacy* (March 1898), 57–64.

———. "Pioneer Drug Milling in the United States," *American Journal of Pharmacy*, vol. 103 (1931), 389–398.

Escalante, A.A. and F.J. Ayala. "Phylogeny of the Malarial Genus *Plasmodium*, Derived from rRNA Gene Sequences," *Proceedings of the National Academy of Sciences USA*, vol. 91 (1994), 11373–11377.

Escalante, A.A., Omar E. Cornejo, Denise E. Freeland, Amanda C. Poe, Ester Durrego, William E. Collins, and Altaf A. Lal. "A Monkey's Tale: The Origin of *Plasmodium Vivax* as a Human Malaria Parasite," *Proceedings of the National Academy of Sciences*, vol. 102, no. 6 (2005), 1980–1985.

Etkin, Nina L. "Plants as Antimalarial Drugs: Relation to G6PD Deficiency and Evolutionary Implications," in ed. L.S. Greene and M.E. Danubio, *Adaptation to Malaria: The Interaction of Biology and Culture* (Amsterdam: Gordon and Breach, 1997), 139–176.

———. "The Co-Evolution of People, Plants, and Parasites: Biological and Cultural Adaptations to Malaria," *Proceedings of the Nutrition Society*, vol. 62 (2003), 311–317.

Evans, Hughes. "European Malaria Policy in the 1920s and 1930s: The Epidemiology of Minutiae," *Isis*, vol. 80 (1989), 40–59.

Ewald, Paul W. *Evolution of Infectious Disease* (New York: Oxford University Press, 1994).

———. "The Evolution of Virulence: A Unifying Link between Parasitology and Ecology," *Journal of Parasitology*, vol. 81, no. 5 (1995), 659–669.

———. "Evolution of Virulence," *Infectious Disease Clinics of North America*, vol. 18, no. 1 (2004), 1–15.

Fantini, B. "Anophelism without Malaria," *Parassitologia*, vol. 36 (1994), 83–106.

———. "Unum Facere et Alterum Non Omittere: Antimalarial Strategies in Italy, 1880–1930," *Parassitologia*, vol. 40 (1998), 91–101.

Farid, M.A. "The Malaria Programme – From Euphoria to Anarchy," *World Health Forum*, vol. I, nos. 1–2 (1980), 8–33.

Farley, J. "Mosquitoes or Malaria? Rockefeller Campaigns in the American South and Sardinia," *Parassitologia*, vol. 36 (1994), 165–173.

Farr, John. "On Extract of Quinia," *Journal of the Philadelphia College of Pharmacy*, vol. 1, no. 2 (1826), 43–45.

Farriss, Nancy M. *Maya Society under Colonial Rule: The Collective Enterprise of Survival* (Princeton: Princeton University Press, 1984).

Faust, Ernest. "The Distribution of Malaria in North America, Central America and the West Indies," in ed. Forest Ray Moulton, *A Symposium on Human Malaria* (Washington, DC: American Association for the Advancement of Science, 1941), 8–18.

———. "Clinical and Public Health Aspects of Malaria in the United States from an Historical Perspective," *American Journal of Tropical Medicine*, vol. 25 (1945), 185–201.

———. "Malaria Incidence in North America," in ed. Mark Boyd, *Malariology* (Philadelphia: Saunders, 1949), 749–763.

———. "The History of Malaria in the United States," *American Scientist*, vol. 39 (1951), 121–130.

Fayrer, Sir Joseph. *On the Climate and Fevers of India* (London: Churchill, 1882).

Fenn, Elizabeth A. *Pox Americana: The Great Smallpox Epidemic of 1775–1782* (New York: Hill and Wang, 2001).

Ferguson, Heather M. and Andrew F. Reid, "Why Is the Effect of Malaria Parasites on Mosquito Survival Still Unresolved?," *Trends in Parasitology*, vol. 18, no. 6 (2002), 256–261.

Field, J.W. *Notes on the Chemotherapy of Malaria* (Kuala Lumpur: Federated Malay States Government Press, 1938).

Findley, Thomas. "Sappington's Anti-Fever Pills and the Westward Migration," *Transactions of the Clinical and Climatological Association*, vol. 79 (1967), 34–44.

Flannery, Michael A. *Civil War Pharmacy* (New York: Pharmaceutical Products Press, 2004).

Flory, James H. and Philip Kitcher. "Global Health and the Scientific Research Agenda," *Philosophy and Public Affairs*, vol. 32, no. 1 (2004), 36–65.

Flückiger, Friedrich August. *The Cinchona Barks, Pharmacognostically Considered* (London: Churchill, 1884).

Fonfría Díaz, José. "La utilizacíon de la quina en las epidemias de la segunda mitad des siglo XVIII," in ed. Juan Luis García Hourcade, Juna M. Moreno Yuste, and Gloria Ruiz Hernández, *Estudios de histoira de las técnicas, la arqueología industrial y las ciencias: actas del VI Congreso de la Sociedad Española de Historia de la Ciencias y de las Técnicas* (Salamanca, Spain: Junta de Castilla y León, Consejería de Educación y Cultura, 1998), 919–934.

Fontaine, Russell E., Abdallah E. Najjar, and Julius S. Prince. "The 1958 Malaria Epidemic in Ethiopia," *American Journal of Tropical Medicine and Hygiene*, vol. 10, no. 1 (1961), 795–803.

Ford, John. *The Role of the Trypanosomiases in African Ecology* (Oxford: Clarendon Press, 1971).

Foster, Susan D.F. "The Distribution and Use of Antimalarial Drugs – Not a Pretty Picture," in ed. G.A. Targett, *Malaria – Waiting for the Vaccine* (Chichester and New York: Wiley, 1991), 123–139.

Frances, Carmen, Jerónimo Garcia, Antonia Olivares, and Fernando Adan. "Le quinquina: son commerce et son emploi en Espagne au cours de l'histoire," in *Acts of the International Congress for the History of Pharmacy* (Padova, Italy: Accademia italiana di storia della farmacia, 1989), 51–58.

Frenkel, Stephen and John Western. "Pretext or Prophylaxis: Racial Segregation and Malarial Mosquitos in a British Tropical Colony: Sierra Leone," *Annals of the Association of American Geographers*, vol. 78, no. 2 (1988), 211–228.

Gadelha, P. "From 'Forest Malaria' to 'Bromeliad Malaria': A Case-Study of Scientific Controversy and Malaria Control," *Parassitologia*, vol. 36 (1994), 175–195.

Gage, Lt.-Col. A.T. *Report on the Extension of Cinchona Cultivation in India* (Calcutta: Government Printer, 1918).

Gagnon, Alexandre S., Karen E. Smoyer-Tomic, and Andrew B.G. Bush. "El Niño Southern Oscillation and Malaria Epidemics in South America," *International Journal of Biometeorology*, vol. 46, no. 2 (2002), 81–89.

Galvani, Alison P. "Epidemiology Meets Evolutionary Ecology," *Trends in Ecology and Evolution*, vol. 18, no. 3 (2003), 132–139.

Gathorne-Hardy, F.J. and W.E.H. Harcourt-Smith, "The Super-Eruption of Toba, Did It Cause a Human Bottleneck?," *Journal of Human Evolution*, vol. 45 (2003), 227–230.

Geggus, David. "Yellow Fever in the 1790s: The British Army in Occupied Saint Domingue," *Medical History*, vol. 23 (1979), 38–58.

Gelfand, Michael. *Rivers of Death in Africa* (London: Oxford University Press, 1964).

Gemery, Henry A. "Emigration from the British Isles to the New World, 1630–1700: Inferences from Colonial Populations," *Research in Economic History*, vol. 5 (1980), 179–231.

Gernet, Jacques. *Daily Life in China on the Eve of the Mongol Invasion, 1250–1279* (Stanford: Stanford University Press, 1962).

Getting, Vlado A. "Malaria in Massachusetts," *New England Journal of Medicine*, vol. 230, no. 12 (1944), 350–357.

Gifford-Gonzalez, Diane. "Pastoralism and Its Consequences," in ed. Ann Brower Stahl, *African Archaeology* (Malden, MA: Blackwell Publishing, 2005), 187–224.

Gillet, M.C. *The Army Medical Department 1818–1865* (Washington, DC: Center for Military History, United States Army, 1987).

Gomes, Melba. "Economic and Demographic Research on Malaria: A Review of the Evidence," *Social Science Medicine*, vol. 37, no. 9 (1993), 1093–1108.

Goudsblom, Johan. *Fire and Civilization* (London: Allen Lane, 1994).

[Government of British India]. *Proceedings of the Imperial Malaria Conference* (Simla, India: Government Central Branch Press, 1910).

Gracner, Gordana Greguric and Vesna Vucevac Bajt. "History of Eradication of Malaria in Croatia," *Orvostörténeti közlemények*, vols. 178–181 (2002), 145–155.

Gramiccia, Gabriele. *The Life of Charles Ledger (1808–1905): Alpacas and Quinine* (Basingstoke, UK: Macmillan, 1988).

Gramiccia, G. and P.F. Beales. "The Recent History of Malaria Control and Eradication," in ed. Walther H. Wernsdorfer and Sir Ian McGregor, *Malaria. Principles and Practice of Malariology*, vol. I (Edinburgh: Churchill Livingstone, 1988), 1335–1378.

Gramont, J.L. "Le Paludisme," *Marchés Tropicaux* (November 1947), 1679–1683.

Gray, R.H. "The Decline of Mortality in Ceylon and the Demographic Effects of Malaria Control," *Population Studies*, vol. 28, no. 2 (1974), 205–228.

[Great Britain]. "Cinchona Plant in India: Correspondence, 1852–1863," *Parliamentary Papers*, House of Commons, 1863, vol. 45, paper 118.

———. "Cinchona Plant: (Introduction into India): Correspondence," *Parliamentary Papers*, House of Commons, 1866, vol. 53, paper 353.

———. "Cultivation of Cinchona Plant: Correspondence 1866–1870," *Parliamentary Papers*, House of Commons, 1870, vol. 51, paper 432.

———. "Cinchona Cultivation: Correspondence from August 1870 to July 1875," *Parliamentary Papers*, House of Commons, 1876, vol. 55, paper 120.

———. "Cinchona Cultivation: Correspondence from 1870 to 1875," *Parliamentary Papers*, House of Commons, 1877, vol. 63, paper 279.

Greenwood, David. "The Quinine Connection," *Journal of Antimicrobial Chemotherapy*, vol. 30 (1992), 417–427.

———. "Conflicts of Interest: The Genesis of Synthetic Antimalarial Agents in Peace and War," *Journal of Antimicrobial Chemotherapy*, vol. 36 (1995), 857–872.

Groussin, Lucien-Joseph. *Des fièvres intermittentes simples, considérées principalement sous le rapport de leur traitement par le quinquina et le sulfate de quinine à hautes doses* (Paris: Impr. Didot le jeune, 1831).

Grove, Richard H. *Green Imperialism: Colonial Expansion, Tropical Island Edens, and the Origins of Environmentalism, 1600–1860* (New York: Cambridge University Press, 1995).

Guerra, C.A., R.W. Snow, and S.I. Hay. "A Global Assessment of Closed Forests, Deforestation, and Malaria Risk," *Annals of Tropical Medicine and Parasitology*, vol. 100, no. 3 (2006), 189–204.

Guerra, Francisco. *Epidemiología Americana y Filipina, 1492–1898* (Madrid: Ministerio de sanidad y consumo, 1999).

Hackett, L.W. *Malaria in Europe: An Ecological Study* (London: Oxford University Press, 1937).

———. "The Malaria of the Andean Region of South America," *Revista del Instituto de Salubridad y Enfermedades Tropicales*, vol. 6, no. 4 (1945), 239–252.

Hagen, Joel B. *An Entangled Bank: The Origins of Ecosystem Ecology* (New Brunswick, NJ: Rutgers University Press, 1992).

Haggett, Peter. "Sauer's 'Origins and Dispersals': Its Implications for the Geography of Disease," *Transactions of the Institute of British Geography*, new series, vol. 17 (1992), 387–398.

Haggis, A.W. "Fundamental Errors in the Early History of Cinchona," *Bulletin of the History of Medicine*, vol. 10, no. 3 (1941), 417–459, 568–592.

Hall, Thomas B. "John Sappington," *Missouri Historical Review*, vol. 24 (1930), 177–199.

Hall, Jr. Thomas B. and Thomas B. Hall III. *Dr. John Sappington of Saline County, Missouri 1776–1856* (Arrow Rock, MO: The Friends of Arrow Rock, 1975).

Hamblin, Martha T. and Anna Di Rienzo. "Detection of the Signature of Natural Selection in Humans: Evidence from the Duffy Blood Group Locus," *American Journal of Human Genetics*, vol. 66 (2000), 1669–1679.

Hamblin, Martha T., Emma E. Thompson, and Anna Di Rienzo. "Complex Signatures of Natural Selection at the Duffy Blood Group Locus," *American Journal of Human Genetics*, vol. 70 (2002), 369–383.

Hamilton, John. *Notes and Statistics of Cinchona Bark* (London: J.W. Collings, 1883).

Handler, A.M. "An Introduction to the History and Methodology of Insect Gene Transformation," in ed. A.M. Handler and A.A. James, *Insect Transgenesis: Methods and Applications* (Boca Raton, FL: CRC Press, 2000), 3–26.

Harper, P.A., E.T. Lisansky, and B.E. Sasse. "Malaria and Other Insect-Borne Diseases in the South Pacific Campaign, 1942–1945; I. General Aspects and Control Measures," *American Journal of Tropical Medicine*, vol. 27, suppl. (1947), 1–67.

Harrison, Gordon. *Mosquitoes, Malaria and Man: A History of the Hostilities since 1880* (New York: E.P. Dutton, 1978).

Harrison, Mark. *Public Health in British India: Anglo-Indian Preventive Medicine, 1859–1914* (New York: Cambridge University Press, 1994).

———. "Medicine and the Culture of Command: The Case of Malaria Control in the British Army during the Two World Wars," *Medical History*, vol. 40, no. 4 (1996), 437–452.

———. "'Hot Beds of Disease': Malaria and Civilization in Nineteenth-Century British India," *Parassitologia*, vol. 40 (1998), 11–18.

———. *Climates and Constitutions: Health, Race, Environment, and British Imperialism in India, 1600–1850* (New Delhi: Oxford University Press, 1999).

———. *Medicine and Victory: British Military Medicine in the Second World War* (Oxford: Oxford University Press, 2004).

Hartl, Daniel L. "The Origin of Malaria: Mixed Messages from Genetic Diversity," *Nature Reviews Microbiology*, vol. 2, no. 1 (2004), 15–22.

Hastings, Ian M. "Malaria Control and the Evolution of Drug Resistance: An Intriguing Link," *Trends in Parasitology*, vol. 19, no. 2 (2003), 70–73.

———. "The Origins of Antimalarial Drug Resistance," *Trends in Parasitology*, vol. 20, no. 11 (2004), 512–518.

Hay, Simon I., Carlos A. Guerra, Andrew J. Tatem, Abdisalan M. Noor, and Robert W. Snow. "The Global Distribution and Population at Risk of Malaria: Past, Present, and Future," *Lancet Infectious Diseases*, vol. 4, no. 6 (2004), 327–336.

Hays, C.W. "The United States Army and Malaria Control in World War II," *Parassitologia*, vol. 42 (2000), 47–52.

Hays, J.N. *The Burdens of Disease: Epidemics and Human Response in Western History* (New Brunswick, NJ: Rutgers University Press, 2000).

Hehir, Major-General Sir Patrick. *Malaria in India* (London: Oxford University Press, 1927).

Henige, David. *Numbers from Nowhere: The American Indian Contact Population Debate* (Norman: University of Oklahoma Press, 1998).

Henry, Maud, Sandrine Alibert, Eve Oralndi-Pradines, Hervé Bogreau, Theirry Fusai, Christophe Rogier, Jacques Narbe, and Bruno Pradines, "Chloroquine Resistance Reversal Agents as Promising Antimalarial Drugs," *Current Drug Targets*, vol. 7 (2006), 935–948.

Hicks, E.P. and Diwan Chand, "The Relative Clinical Efficacy of Totaquina and Quinine," *Records of the Malarial Survey of India*, vol. 5, no. 1 (March 1935), 39–50.

Hildreth, S.P. "Notes on the Epidemic Fever, As It Appeared at Marietta, in the State of Ohio, and Its Vicinity, in the Years 1822 and 1823," *Philadelphia Journal of the Medical and Physical Sciences*, vol. 9 (1824), 105–116.

Hill, Jenny, Jo Lines, and Mark Rowland, "Insecticide-Treated Nets," *Advances in Parasitology*, vol. 61 (2006), 77–128.

Hirsch, August. *Handbook of Geographical and Historical Pathology*, vol. I: *Acute Infective Diseases* (London: New Sydenham Society, 1883).

Hoeppli, R. "Malaria in Chinese Medicine," *Sinologica*, vol. 4, no. 2 (1955), 91–101.

Hoffman, Frederick L. *The Malaria Problem in Peace and War* (Newark, NJ: Prudential Press, 1918).

———. *Malaria Problems* (Wellesley Hills, MA: Prudential Press, 1928).

Holmes, Oliver Wendell. "Dissertation on Intermittent Fevers in New England," *Boylston Prize Dissertations for the Years 1836 and 1837* (Boston: C.C. Little and J. Brown, 1838).

Holmes, R.H. "Remarks on the Use of Quinine in Florida, and on Malaria and Its influence in that State; Being the Substance of a Report Made to the Surgeon-General U.S. Army," *American Journal of the Medical Sciences*, no. 24 (October 1846), 297–309.

Honig, Pieter and Frans Verdoorn, eds. *Science and Scientists in the Netherlands Indies* (New York: Board for the Netherlands Indies, Surinam, and Curaçao, 1945).

Honigsbaum, Mark. *The Fever Trail: In Search of the Cure for Malaria* (New York: Farrar, Straus, and Giroux, 2001).

Hooker, William Dawson. *Inaugural Dissertation upon the Cinchonas, Their Uses, History, and Effects* (Glasgow: Khull, 1839).

Howard, Bernard F. *Some Notes on the Cinchona Industry*. Streatfield Memorial Lecture, 1930 (London: Institute of Chemistry of Great Britain and Ireland, 1931).

———. *Howards 1797–1947* (Plaistow, UK: Howards and Sons, 1947).

Howard, David Lloyd. "The History and Development of the British Fine Chemical Industry," *Pharmaceutical Journal and Pharmacist* (August 7, 1926), 8–9.

Hsu, Elisabeth. "The History of Qing Hao in the Chinese Materia Medica," *Transactions of the Royal Society of Tropical Medicine and Hygiene*, vol. 100 (2006), 505–508.

———. "Reflections on the 'Discovery' of the Antimalarial Qinghao," *British Journal of Clinical Pharmacology*, vol. 61, no. 6 (2006), 666–670.

Huddleston, W.E. "An Analysis of Our Present Position with Regard to the Prevention and Cure of Malarial Infections," *Journal of the Royal Army Medical Corps*, vol. 21 (1913), 320–328.

Hughes, A.L. and F. Verra, "Extensive Polymorphism and Ancient Origin of *Plasmodium Falciparum*," *Trends in Parasitology*, vol. 18 (2003), 348–351.

Hughes, Robert. *The Fatal Shore: The Epic Story of Australia's Founding* (New York: Knopf, 1987).

Huldén, Lena, Larry Huldén, and Kari Heliövaara. "Endemic Malaria: An 'Indoor' Disease in Northern Europe: Historical Data Analysed," *Malaria Journal*, no. 19, vol. 4 (2005). This article can be found online at http://www.malariajournal.com/content/4/1/19.

Hume, J.C.C., J. Lyons, and K.P. Day. "Human Migration, Mosquitoes and the Evolution of *Plasmodium Falciparum*," *Trends in Parasitology*, vol. 19, no. 3 (2003), 144–149.

Humphreys, Margaret. "Kicking a Dying Dog: DDT and the Demise of Malaria in the American South, 1942–1950," *Isis*, vol. 87, no. 1 (1996), 1–17.

———. "Water Won't Run Uphill: The New Deal and Malaria Control in the American South, 1933–1940," *Parassitologia*, vol. 40 (1998), 183–191.

———. *Malaria: Poverty, Race, and Public Health in the United States* (Baltimore: Johns Hopkins University Press, 2001).

Hutchinson, T.J. *Narrative of the Niger, Tshadda, and Binuë Exploration* (London: Longman, Brown, Green, and Longmans, 1855; reprint: London: Cass, 1966).

Imperial Institute (Great Britain). "The World's Cinchona Bark Industry – I," *Bulletin of the Imperial Institute*, vol. 27, no. 1 (1939), 18–31.

———. "The World's Cinchona Bark Industry – II," *Bulletin of the Imperial Institute*, vol. 27, no. 2 (1939), 183–196.

Irving, Ralph. *Experiments on the red and quill Peruvian bark : with observations on its history, mode of operation, and uses ; and on some other subjects connected with the phænomena and doctrines of vegetable astringents. Being a dissertation which gained the first prize given by the Harveian Society of Edinburgh for the year 1784* (Edinburgh: C. Elliot, 1785).

Irwin, Graham W. *Africans Abroad* (New York: Columbia University Press, 1977).

Ivey, T. N. "Medicine in the Pioneer West, 1850–1900," *North Carolina Medical Journal*, vol. 26 (1965), 161–165.

Iwu, Maurice M. *Handbook of African Medicinal Plants* (Boca Raton: CRC Press, 1993).

Jackson, Fatimah. "Ecological Modeling of Human-Plant-Parasite Coevolutionary Triads: Theoretical Perspectives on the Interrelationships of Human HbßS, G6PD, *Manihot esculenta, Vicia faba*, and *Plasmodium falciparum*," in ed. Lawrence S. Greene and Maria Enrica Danubio, *Adaptation to Malaria: The Interaction of Biology and Culture* (Amsterdam: Gordon and Breach, 1997), 177–207.

Jackson, J. "Cognition and the Global Malaria Eradication Programme," *Parassitologia*, vol. 40 (1998), 193–216.

Jackson, J.B.S. "Diseases of the Island of Barbadoes," *Boston Medical and Surgical Journal*, vol. 76, no. 22 (July 4, 1867), 445–448.

Jackson, Robert, *An Outline of the History and Cure of Fever* (Edinburgh: Printed for Mundell, 1798).

James, S.P. "A Report of the Anti-Malarial Operations at Mian Mir (1901–1902)," in *Reports to the Malarial Committee of the Royal Society*, 8th series (London: Harrison and Sons, 1903), 27–77.

———. *Malarial Fevers* (Calcutta: Superintendent Government Printing, 1908).

———. "A Note on Some of the Measures That Have Been Taken to Make Quinine Available to the Poor in India," in ed. S.P. James and S.R. Christophers, *Paludism, Being the Transactions of the Committee for the Study of Malaria in India* (Simla, India: Government Central Branch Press, 1911), 10–14.

———. "Advances in Knowledge of Malaria since the War," *Transactions of the Royal Society of Tropical Medicine and Hygiene*, vol. 31, no. 3 (1937), 263–280.

James, S.P. and S.R. Christophers, "Malaria: Synonyms; Definition; Geographical Distribution," in ed. W. Byam and R.G. Archibald, *The Practice of Medicine in the Tropics*, vol. 2 (London: H. Frowde and Hodder and Stoughton, 1922), 1500–1507.

Jaramillo-Arango, Jaime. "A Critical Review of the Basic Facts in the History of Cinchona," *Journal of the Linnean Society*, vol. 53, no. 351 (1949), 272–309.

Jarco, Saul. "A Cartographic and Literary Study of the Word Malaria," *Journal of the History of Medicine and Allied Sciences*, vol. 25 (1970), 31–39.

———. *Quinine's Predecessor* (Baltimore: Johns Hopkins University Press, 1993).

Jaspers, Karl. *The Origin and Goal of History* (New Haven: Yale University Press, 1953).

Jingfeng, Cai and Zhen Yan, "Medicine in Ancient China," in ed. Helaine Selin, *Medicine across Cultures: History and Practice of Medicine in Non-Western Cultures* (Dordrecht, Holland: Kluwer Academic Publishers, 2003), 49–73.

Jobling, M.A., M.E. Hurles, and C. Tyler-Smith. *Human Evolutionary Genetics: Origins, Peoples and Disease* (New York: Garland Science, 2004).

Johnson, James. *The Influence of Tropical Climates, More Especially the Climate of India, on the Constitutions of Europeans* (London: J.J. Stockdale, 1813).

Jones, Joseph. "Sulphate of Quinia in Small Doses during Health, the Best Means of Preventing Chill and Fever, and Bilious Fever, and Congestive Fever, in Those Exposed to the Unhealthy Climate of the Rich Low Lands and Swamps of the Southern Confederacy," *Southern Medical and Surgical Journal*, vol. 17, no. 8 (August 1861), 593–614.

———. *Quinine as a Prophylactic against Malarial Fever: Being an Appendix to the Third Report on Typhoid and Malarial Fevers, Delivered to the Surgeon General of the Late C.S.A., August, 1864* (Nashville: University Medical Press, 1867).

Jones, Margaret. *Health Policy in Britain's Model Colony: Ceylon (1900–1948)* (New Delhi: Orient Longman, 2004).

Jongwutiwes, Somchai, Chaturong Putaporntip, Takuya Iwasaki, Marcelo U. Ferreira, Hiroji Kanbara, and Austin L. Hughes. "Mitochondrial Genome Sequences Support Ancient Population Expansion in *Plasmodium Vivax*," *Molecular Biology and Evolution*, vol. 8, no. 22 (2005), 1733–1739.

Joy, Robert J.T. "Malaria in American Troops in the South and Southwest Pacific in World War II," *Medical History*, vol. 43, no. 2 (1999), 192–208.

Karafet, Tatiana, Liping Xu, Ruofu Du, William Wang, Shi Feng, R.S. Wells, Alan J. Redd, Stephen L. Zegura, and Michael F. Hammer. "Paternal Population History of East Asia: Sources, Patterns, and Microevolutionary Processes," *American Journal of Human Genetics*, vol. 69 (2001), 614–628.

Kaufman, Teodoro S. and Edmundo A. Rúveda. "The Quest for Quinine: Those Who Won the Battles and Those Who Won the War," *Angewandte Chemie-International Edition*, vol. 44, no. 6 (2005), 854–885.

Karunaweera, Nadira D., Subadra K. Wijesekera, Deepani Wanadekera, Kamini N. Mendis, and Richard Carter, "The Paroxysm of *Plasmodium Vivax*," *Trends in Parasitology*, vol. 19, no. 4 (2003), 188–193.

Katz, S. H. "Fava Bean Consumption: A Case for the Evolution of Genes and Culture," in ed. Marvin Harris and Eric B. Ross, *Food and Evolution* (Philadelphia: Temple University Press, 1987), 139–159.

Kean, B.H., Kenneth E. Mott, and Adair J. Russell, eds. *Tropical Medicine and Parasitology: Classic Investigations*, vol. I (Ithaca, NY: Cornell University Press, 1978).

Keiser, Jennifer, Burton H. Singer, and Jürg Utzinger. "Reducing the Burden of Malaria in Different Eco-Epidemiological Settings with Environmental Management: A Systematic Review," *Lancet Infectious Diseases*, vol. 5 (2005), 695–708.

Keiser, Jennifer, Marcia Caldas de Castro, Michael F. Maltese, Robert Bos, Marcel Tanner, Burtohn H. Singer, and Jürg Utzinger. "Effect of Irrigation and Large Dams on the Burden of Malaria on a Global and Regional Scale," *American Journal of Tropical Medicine*, vol. 72, no. 4 (2005), 392–406.

Kennedy, Dale. *The Magic Mountains: Hill Stations and the British Raj* (Berkeley: University of California Press, 1996).

Kentish, Richard. *Experiments and Observations on a New Species of Bark* (London: J. Johnson, 1784).

Kerbosch, M. "Some Notes on Cinchona Culture and the World Consumption of Quinine," *Bulletin of the Colonial Institute of Amsterdam*, vol. 3, no. 1 (1939), 36–51.

Kerner, G. "On the Examination of Commercial Sulphate of Quinine for Other Alkaloids Found in the Cinchona Barks," *Pharmaceutical Journal and Transactions*, vol. 4, 2nd series (1862–1863), 19–26.

Khazanov, Anatoly M. *Nomads and the Outside World*, 2nd ed. (Madison: University of Wisconsin Press, 1994).

Kidson, C. and K. Indaratna. "Ecology, Economics and Political Will: The Vicissitudes of Malaria Strategies in Asia," *Parassitologia*, vol. 40 (1998), 39–46.

Kinds, R. *Introduction des quinquinas au Congo Belge* (Bruxelles, Belgium: Impr. industrielle et financière, 1926).

King, George. *A Manual of Cinchona Cultivation in India* (Calcutta: Office of the Superintendent of Government Printing, 1880).

Kiple, Kenneth F. "Response to Sheldon Watts," *Journal of Social History*, vol. 34, no. 4 (2001), 969–974.

———. *The Caribbean Slave: A Biological History* (New York: Cambridge University Press, 2002).

Kiple, Kenneth F. and Virginia Himmelsteib King. *Another Dimension to the Black Diaspora: Diet, Disease, and Racism* (New York: Cambridge University Press, 1981).

Kiszewski, Anthony, Andrew Mellinger, Andrew Spielman, Pia Malaney, Sonia Ehrlich Sachs, and Jeffrey Sachs. "A Global Index Representing the Stability of Malaria Transmission," *American Journal of Tropical Medicine and Hygiene*, vol. 70, no. 5 (2004), 486–498.

Kitron, Uriel. "Malaria, Agriculture, and Development: Lessons from Past Campaigns," *International Journal of Health Services*, vol. 17, no. 2 (1987), 295–326.

Klayman, Daniel L. "Qinghaosu (Artemisinin): An Antimalarial Drug from China," *Science*, new series, vol. 228, no. 4703 (May 13, 1985), 1049.

Klein, I. "Death in India, 1871–1921," *Journal of Asian Studies*, vol. 32 (1972–1973), 639–659.

Klieman, Kairn. *"The Pygmies Were Our Compass": Bantu and Batwa in the History of West Central Africa, Early Times to c. 1900 C.E.* (Portsmouth, NH: Heinemann, 2003).

Kligler, Israel J. *The Epidemiology and Control of Malaria in Palestine* (Chicago: University of Chicago Press, 1930).

Knowles, Robert and Ronald Senior-White. *Malaria. Its Investigation and Control with Special Reference to Indian Conditions* (Calcutta: Thacker, Spink, and Co., 1927).

Korenromp, E.L., Brian G. Williams, Sake J. de Vlas, Eleanor Gouws, Charles F. Gilks, Peter D. Ghys, and Bernard L. Nahlen. "Malaria Attributable to the HIV-1 Epidemic, Sub-Saharan Africa," *Emerging Infectious Diseases*, vol. 11, no. 9 (2005), 1410–1419.

Krettli, Antoniana U., Valter F. Andrade-Neto, Maria des Graças L. Brandão, and Wanêssa M.S. Ferrari. "The Search for New Antimalarial Drugs from Plants Used to Treat Fever and Malaria or Plants Randomly Selected: A Review," *Memórias do Instituto Oswaldo Cruz*, vol. 96, no. 8 (2001), 1033–1042.

Kropp Dakubu, M.E. "The Peopling of Southern Ghana: A Linguistic Viewpoint," in ed. Christopher Ehret and Merrick Posnansky, *The Archaeological and Linguistic Reconstruction of African History* (Berkeley: University of California Press, 1982), 245–255.

———. "Linguistics and History in West Africa," in ed. Emmanuel Akyeampong, *Major Themes in West Africa's History* (London: James Currey, 2005), 52–72.

Kukla, Jon. "Kentish Agues and American Distempers: The Transmission of Malaria from England to Virginia in the Seventeenth Century," *Southern Studies*, vol. 25 (1986), 135–147.

Kwiatkowski, Dominic P. "How Malaria Has Affected the Human Genome and What Human Genetics Can Teach Us About Malaria," *American Journal of Human Genetics*, vol. 77 (2005), 171–192.

Lacroix, Renaud, Wolfgang R. Mukabana, Louis Clement Gouagna, and Jacob C. Koella. "Malaria Infection Increases Attractiveness of Humans to Mosquitoes," *PLoS Biology*, vol. 3, no. 9 (2005), 1590–1593.

Laderman, Carol. "Malaria and Progress: Some Historical and Ecological Considerations," *Social Science and Medicine*, vol. 9 (1975), 587–594.

Lambert, Aylmer Bourke. *A description of the genus Cinchona, comprehending the various species of vegetables from which the Peruvian and other barks of a similar quality are taken. Illustrated by figures of all the species hitherto discovered. To which is prefixed Professor Vahl's dissertation on this genus, read before the Society of natural history at Copenhagen. Also a description, accompanied by figures, of a new genus named Hyænanche: or hyæna poison* (London: Printed for B. and J. White, 1797).

———. *An illustration of the genus Cinchona: comprising descriptions of all the officinal Peruvian barks including several new species. Baron de Humboldt's Account of the Cinchona forests of South America, and Laubert's Memoir on the different species of Quinquina. To which are added several dissertations of Don Hippolito Ruiz on various medicinal plants of South America . . . And a short account of the spikenard of the ancients* (London: Printed for J. Searle, 1821).

Laufer, Miriam K., Phillip C. Thesing, Nicole D. Eddington, Rhoda Mosonga, Fraction K. Dzinjalamala, Shannon L. Takala, Terrie E. Taylor, and Christopher V. Plowe. "Return of Chloroquine Antimalarial Efficacy in Malawi," *New England Journal of Medicine*, vol. 355, no. 19 (November 9, 2006), 1959–1966.

Le Lannou, Maurice. "Le role géographique de la malaria," *Annales de géographie*, no. 254 (March 15, 1936), 113–135.

Le Sueur, David, Brian L. Sharp, and Chris. C. Appleton, "Historical Perspective of the Malaria Problem in Natal with Emphasis on the Period 1928–1932," *South African Journal of Science*, vol. 89 (1993), 232–239.

Lebret, Jean Maxime. *L'organisation du marché du quinquina et de la quinine* (Paris: Impr. A. Lapied, 1942).

Lebot, V. "Biomolecular Evidence for Plant Domestication in Sahul," *Genetic Resources and Crop Evolution*, vol. 46, no. 6 (1999), 619–628.

Leclerc, M.C., P. Durand, C. Gauthier, S. Patot, N. Bilotte, M. Menegon, C. Severini, F.J. Ayala, and F. Renaud. "Meager Genetic Variability of the Human Malaria Agent *Plasmodium Vivax*," *Proceedings of the National Academy of Sciences*, vol. 101, no. 40 (2004), 14455–14460.

Lelean, P.S. "Quinine as a Malarial Prophylactic: A Criticism," *Journal of the Royal Army Medical Corps*, vol. 17 (1911), 463–480.

Lengeler, Christian, Jacqueline Cattani, and Don de Savigny, eds. *Net Gain: A New Method for Preventing Malaria Deaths* (Ottawa, ON: International Development Research Centre/World Health Organization, 1997).

Levin, Bruce R. "The Evolution and Maintenance of Virulence in Microparasites," *Emerging Infectious Diseases*, vol. 2, no. 2 (1996), 93–102.

Lin-Hua, Tang, Qian Lui-Lin, and Xu Shu-hui. "Malaria and Its Control in the People's Republic of China," *Southeast Asian Journal of Tropical Medicine and Public Health*, vol. 22 (1991), 467–476.

Litsios, Socrates. *The Tomorrow of Malaria* (Karori, NZ: Pacific Press, 1996).

———. "Malaria Control, the Cold War, and the Postwar Reorganization of International Assistance," *Medical Anthropology*, vol. 17 (1997), 255–278.

———. "Criticism of WHO's Revised Malaria Eradication Strategy," *Parassitologia*, vol. 42 (2000), 167–172.

Livadas, Gregory A. and John C. Sphangos. *Malaria in Greece (1930–1940)* (Athens: Pyrsos Press, 1941).

Livingstone, F.B. "Anthropological Implications of Sickle Cell Gene Distribution in West Africa," *American Anthropologist*, vol. 60 (1958), 533–562.

———. "Malaria and Human Polymorphisms," *Annual Review of Genetics*, vol. 5 (1971), 33–64.

———. "The Duffy Blood Groups, Vivax Malaria, and Malaria Selection in Human Populations: A Review," *Human Biology*, vol. 56 (1984), 413–425.

———. "Who Gave Whom Hemoglobin S: The Use of Restricted Haplotype Variation for the Interpretation of the Evolution of the B–globin Gene," *American Journal of Human Biology*, vol. 1, no. 3 (1989), 289–302.

Lloyd, John Uri. *Origin and History of All the Pharmacopeial Vegetable Drugs, Chemicals and Preparations with Bibliography* (Cincinnati: Caxton Press, 1921).

Mabaso, Musawenkosi L.H., Brian Sharp, and Christian Lengeler. "Historical Review of Malarial Control in Southern Africa with Emphasis on the Use of Indoor Residual Spraying," *Tropical Medicine and International Health*, vol. 9, no. 8 (2004), 846–856.

Mabberley, D.J. "William Roxburgh's 'Botanical Description of a New Species of *Swietenia* (Mahogany)' and Other Overlooked Binomials in 36 Vascular Plant Families," *Taxon*, vol. 31, no. 1 (1982), 65–73.

MacCulloch, J. *An Essay on the Remittent and Intermittent Diseases* (Philadelphia: Carey and Lea, 1830).

MacDonald, George. *The Epidemiology and Control of Malaria* (London: Oxford University Press, 1957).

———. *The Dynamics of Tropical Disease* (London: Oxford University Press, 1973).

MacKinnon, Aran S. "Of Oxford Bags and Twirling Canes: The State, Popular Responses, and Zulu Antimalaria Assistants in the Early-Twentieth Century Zululand Malaria Campaigns," *Radical History Review*, vol. 80 (spring 2001), 76–100.

Mackinnon, Margaret J. and Andrew F. Read. "Virulence in Malaria: An Evolutionary View Point," *Philosophical Transactions of the Royal Society of London, Series B, Biological Sciences*, vol. 359, no. 14466 (2004), 965–986.

———. "Immunity Promotes Virulence Evolution in a Malaria Model," *PLoS Biology*, vol. 2, no. 9 (2004), 1286–1292.

MacLeod, Murdo J. *Spanish Central America: A Socioeconomic History, 1520–1720* (Berkeley: University of California Press, 1973).

Magendie, François. "Fièvre intermittente pernicieuse guérie par une faible dose de sulfate de quinine," *Journal de physiologie expérimentale et pathologique*, vol. 1 (1821), 393–395.

———. *Formulary for the Preparation and Mode of Employing Several New Remedies*. Trans. from the French of the 3rd ed. of Magendie's "Formulaire" by Robley Dunglison (Philadelphia: J. Webster, 1824).

Maillot, François Clement. *Traité des fièvres* (Paris: J.B. Baillière, 1836).

Maley, Jean with the collaboration of Alex Chepstow-Lusty. "*Elaeis guineensis* Jacq. (Oil Palm) Fluctuations in Central Africa during the Late Holocene:

Climate or Human Driving Forces for This Pioneering Species," *Vegetation History and Archaeobotany*, vol. 10 (2001), 117–120.

Malowany, Maureen. "Unfinished Agendas: Writing the History of Medicine of Sub-Saharan Africa," *African Affairs*, vol. 99 (2000), 325–349.

Mann, Charles C. and Mark L. Plummer. *The Aspirin Wars: Money Medicine, and 100 Years of Rampant Competition* (Boston, MA: Harvard Business School Press, 1991).

———. *1491. New Revelations of the Americas before Columbus* (New York: Vintage, 2005).

Manson, Otis F. *A Treatise on the Physiological and Therapeutic Action of the Sulphate of Quinine* (Philadelphia: J.B. Lippincott and Co., 1882).

Marcilío, Maria Luiza. "The Population of Colonial Brazil," in ed. Leslie Bethell, *The Cambridge History of Latin America*, vol. 2 (Cambridge: Cambridge University Press, 1984), 37–63.

Marelli, Mauro T., Chaoyang Li, Jason L. Rasgon, and Marcelo Jacobs-Lorena. "Transgenic Malaria-Resistant Mosquitoes Have a Fitness Advantage When Feeding on Plasmodium-Infected Blood," *Proceedings of the National Academy of Sciences*, vol. 104, no. 13 (March 27, 2007), 5580–5583.

Marin, A., N. Cerutti, and E. Rabino Massa. "Use of the Amplification Refractory Mutation System (ARMS) in the Study of HBS in Predynastic Egyptian Remains," *Bolletino della Società Italiana di Biologia Sperimentale*, vol. 75, nos. 5–6 (1999), 27–30.

Markham, Clements R. "On the Supply of Quinine and the Cultivation of Chinchona Plants in India," *Journal of the Society of Arts*, vol. 11 (1862–1863), 325–337.

———. *Peruvian Bark: An Account of the Introduction of Chinchona Cultivation into British India* (London: John Murray, 1880).

Martenet, Pierre-Joseph-Eugène. *Sur les fièvres miasmatiques de marais, dans le nord d'Afrique, et l'emploi du sulfate de quinine à hautes doses dans leur traitement* (Montpellier, France: J. Martel aîné, 1837).

Mason, John and Philippe Cavalie. "Malaria Epidemic in Haiti Following a Hurricane," *American Journal of Tropical Medicine and Hygiene*, vol. 14, no. 4 (1965), 533–539.

Matthewson, Tim. "Napoleon's Haitian Guerilla War," *Military History*, vol. 18, no. 6 (2002), 30–36.

May, Jacques M. "Map of the World Distribution of Malaria Vectors," *Geographical Review*, vol. 41, no. 4 (1951), 638–639.

———. "The Ecology of Malaria," in ed. Jacques M. May, *Studies in Disease Ecology* (New York: Hafner Publishing, 1961), 161–229.

Mbida, Christophe M. "Evidence for Banana Cultivation and Animal Husbandry during the First Millennium BC in the Forest of Southern Cameroon," *Journal of Archaeological Science*, vol. 27 (2000), 151–162.

Mbida, Christophe M., Hughes Doutrelepont, Luc Vrydaghs, Rony L. Swennen, Rudy J. Swennen, Hans Beeckman, Edmond de Langhe, and Pierre de Maret. "First Archaeological Evidence of Banana Cultivation in Central Africa during the Third Millennium before Present," *Vegetation History and Archaeobotany*, vol. 10 (2001), 1–6.

McBrearty, Sally and Alison S. Brooks. "The Revolution That Wasn't: A New Interpretation of the Origin of Modern Human Behavior," *Journal of Human Evolution*, vol. 39 (2000), 453–563.

McCann, James C. *Maize and Grace: Africa's Encounter with a New World Crop* (Cambridge, MA: Harvard University Press, 2005).

McGown, Thompson. *A Practical Treatise on the Most Common Diseases of the South* (Philadelphia: Grigg, Elliot, 1849).

McIntosh, Roderick J. *The Peoples of the Middle Niger* (Malden, MA: Blackwell Publishers, 1998).

———. *Ancient Middle Niger: Urbanism and the Self-Organizing Landscape* (New York: Cambridge University Press, 2003).

McKenzie, F.E., J. Kevin Baird, John C. Beier, Altaf A. Lal, and William H. Bossert. "A Biologic Basis for Integrated Malaria Control," *American Journal of Tropical Medicine and Hygiene*, vol. 67, no. 6 (2002), 751–577.

McNeill, John R. and William H. McNeill. *The Human Web: A Bird's-Eye View of World History* (New York: W.W. Norton, 2003).

McNeill, William H. *Plagues and Peoples* (Garden City, NY: Anchor Press, 1976).

MacPherson, John. *On Bengal Dysentery and Its Statistics; With a Notice of the Use of Large Enemata in that Disease, and of Quinine in Remittent Fever* (Calcutta: Thacker, 1850).

———. *Quinine and Antiperiodics in Their Therapeutic Relations* (Calcutta: Lepage, 1856).

Mendelsohn, J. Andrew. "From Eradication to Equilibrium: How Epidemics Became Complex After World War I," in ed. Christopher Lawrence and George Weisz, *Greater Than the Parts: Holism in Biomedicine, 1920–1950* (New York: Oxford University Press, 1998), 303–331.

Mendis, Kamini, Barbara J. Sina, Paola Marchesini, and Richard Carter. "The Neglected Burden of *Plasmodium Vivax* Malaria," *American Journal of Tropical Medicine and Hygiene*, vol. 64, nos. 1–2, suppl. (2001), 97–106.

Metcalf, John T. "Miasmatic Fevers," in ed. William A. Hammond, *Military Medical and Surgical Essays* (Philadelphia: J.B. Lippincott and Co., 1864), 207–236.

Miller, Louis H. "Impact of Malaria on Genetic Polymorphism and Genetic Diseases in African and African Americans," in ed. Bernard Roizman, *Infectious Diseases in an Age of Change: The Impact of Human Ecology and Behavior on Disease Transmission* (Washington, DC: National Academy Press, 1995), 99–112.

Mitman, Gregg. "In Search of Health: Landscape and Disease in American Environmental History," *Environmental History*, vol. 10, no. 2 (2005), 184–210.

Miyasita, Saburo. "Malaria (*yao*) in Chinese Medicine during the Chin and Yuan Periods," *Acta Asiatica*, vol. 36 (1979), 90–112.

Molineaux, L. and G. Gramiccia. *The Garki Project: Research on the Epidemiology and Control of Malaria in the Sudan Savanna of West Africa* (Geneva: World Health Organization, 1980).

Monginot, François. *A New Mystery in Physick Discovered, by Curing of Fevers and Agues by Quinquina or Jesuites Powder* (London: Printed for Will. Crook, 1681).

Moreau, R.E. *An Annotated Bibliography of Cinchona-growing from 1883–1943* (Nairobi, Kenya: Government Printer, 1945).

Morse, Richard M. "Introduction: The Historical Role of the Bandeirantes," in ed. Richard M. Morse, *The Bandeirantes: The Historical Role of the Brazilian Pathfinders* (New York: Knopf, 1964), 3–36.

Morton, Jeremy M. *Morton's Medical Bibliography*, 5th ed. (Brookfield, VT: Gower, 1991).

Mouchet, Jean, Sylvie Manguin, Jacques Sircoulon, Stéphane Laventure, Ousmane Faye, Ambrose W. Onapa, Pierre Carnevale, Jean Julvez, and Didier Fontenille. "Evolution of Malaria in Africa for the Past 40 Years: Impact of Climatic and Human Factors," *Journal of the American Mosquito Control Association*, vol. 14, no. 2 (1998), 121–130.

Moya, Alba. *Auge y Crisis de la Cascarilla en la Audencia de Quito, siglo XVIII* (Quito, Euador: Facultad Latinoamericano de Ciencias Sociales, Sede Ecuador, 1994).

Muirhead-Thomson, R.C. "Where Do Most Mosquitoes Acquire Their Malarial (*Plasmodium Falciparum*) Infection? From Adults or From Children?," *Annals of Tropical Medicine and Parasitology*, vol. 92, no. 8 (1998), 891–893.

Muraleedharan, V.R. "Quinine (Cinchona) and the Incurable Malaria: India c. 1900–1930s," *Parassitologia*, vol. 42 (2000), 91–100.

Muraleedharan, V.R. and D. Veeraraghavan. "Anti-Malarial Policy in the Madras Presidency: An Overview of the Early Decades of the Twentieth Century," *Medical History*, vol. 36, no. 3 (1992), 290–305.

Nájera, J.A. "Malaria Control: Present Situation and Need for Historical Research," *Parassitologia*, vol. 32 (1990), 215–229.

———. "Tropical Diseases and Socioeconomic Development," *Parassitologia*, vol. 36 (1994), 17–33.

———. "Malaria Control: Achievements, Problems, and Strategies," *Parassitologia*, vol. 43, no. 1–2 (2001), 1–89.

Nash, Linda. *Inescapable Ecologies: A History of Environment, Disease, and Knowledge* (Berkeley: University of California Press, 2007).

Nelson, William. *Observations on the Management of Peruvian Bark* (Philadelphia: Printed by John Geyser, 1802).

Newman, R.K. "Opium Smoking in Late Imperial China: A Reconsideration," *Modern Asian Studies*, vol. 29, no. 4 (1995), 765–794.

Norcom, William A.B. *Haemorrhagic Malarial Fever: An Address Delivered before the Medical Society of North Carolina at its 21st Annual Meeting* (Raleigh, NC: Edwards, Broughton, 1874).

Norman Howard-Jones, *International Public Health between the Two World Wars – The Organizational Problems* (Geneva: World Health Organization, 1978).

Numbers, Ronald L. and Todd L. Savitt, eds. *Science and Medicine in the Old South* (Baton Rouge: Louisiana State University Press, 1989).

O'Brien, Patricia J. "Sweet Potatoes and Yams," in ed. Kenneth F. Kiple and Kriemheld Coneè Ornelas, *The Cambridge World History of Food*, vol. 1 (New York: Cambridge University Press, 2000), 207–218.

O'Connell, J.F. and J. Allen, "Dating the Colonization of Sahul (Pleistocene Australia–New Guinea): A Review of Recent Research," *Journal of Archaeological Science*, vol. 31 (2004), 835–853.

Ocampo, José Antonio. *Colombia y la Economia Mundial, 1830–1910* (Mexico City: Siglo Veintiuno Editores, 1984).

Oliver, Roland, Thomas Spear, Kairn Klieman, Jan Vansina, Scott MacEachern, David Schoenbrun, James Denbow, Yvonne Bastin, H.M. Batibo, and Bernd Heine. "Comments on Christopher Ehret, 'Bantu History: Re-Envisioning the Evidence of Language'," *International Journal of African Historical Studies*, vol. 34, no. 1 (2001), 43–87.

Ortiz Crespo, Fernando I. "Fragoso, Monardes and pre-Chinchonian Knowledge of Cinchona," *Archives of Natural History*, vol. 22, no. 2 (1995), 169–181.

———. *La Corteza del Árbol Sin Nombre* (Quito, Ecuador: Fundación Fernando Ortiz Crespo, 2002).

Owen, David Edward. *British Opium Policy in China and India* (New Haven: Yale University Press, 1934).

Packard, Randall M. "Malaria Dreams: Postwar Visions of Health and Development in the Third World," *Medical Anthropology*, vol. 17 (1997), 279–296.

———. "'No Other Logical Choice': Global Malaria Eradication and the Politics of International Health in the Post-War Era," *Parassitologia*, vol. 40 (1998), 217–229.

———. "'Malaria Blocks Development': The Role of Disease in the History of Agricultural Development in the Eastern and Northern Transvaal Lowveld, 1890–1960," *Journal of Southern African Studies*, vol. 27, no. 3 (2001), 591–612.

———. *The Making of a Tropical Disease: A Short History of Malaria* (Baltimore: Johns Hopkins University Press, 2007).

Packard, Randall M. and Paulo Gadehla. "A Land Filled with Mosquitoes: Fred L. Soper, the Rockefeller Foundation, and the *Anopheles Gambiae* Invasion of Brazil," *Parassitologia*, vol. 36, nos. 1–2 (1994), 197–214.

Pampana, Emilio J. "Changing Strategy in Malaria Control," *Bulletin of the World Health Organization*, vol. 11 (1954), 513–520.

———. *A Textbook of Malaria Eradication* (London: Oxford University Press, 1963).

Pardo Valle, Nazario. *Cinchona Versus Malaria: Historia, Economía, Ciencía* (La Paz, Bolivia: Portada de Rene Norieza, 1951).

Parent, Anthony. *Foul Means: The Formation of a Slave Society in Virginia, 1660–1740* (Chapel Hill: University of North Carolina Press, 2003).

Parrot, Dr. "La quininisation préventive dans les écoles primaries d'Algérie," *La malariologia*, vol. 8, nos. 1 and 2 (1915), 1–6.

Parrot, L., A. Catanei, and R. Ambialet. "Comparative Experiments in Mass Prophylaxis by Means of Quinine and of Synthetic Drugs (Quinacrine and Praequine)," *Bulletin of the Health Organisation* [League of Nations], vol. 6, no. 5 (1937), 683–765.

Paul, Richard E.L., Mawlouth Diallo, and Paul T. Brey. "Mosquitoes and Transmission of Malaria Parasites – Not Just Vectors," *Malaria Journal*, vol. 3, no. 1 (2004). Online at http://www.malariajournal.com/content/3/1/39.

Paz Soldán, Carlos Enrique. "La Vida Aventura de Abel Victorino Brandin, el Introductor del Sulfato de Quinina en la América Meridional," *Anales de la Sociedad Peruana de Historia de la Medicina*, vol. 2 (1940), 10–29.

Pelletier, J. and J. Caventou. *Analyse chimique des quinquina par MM. Pelletier et Caventou* (Paris: Colas, 1821).

Pérez Moreda, Vincente. "El Paludismo en Espana a Fines des Siglo XVIII: La Epidemia de 1786," *Asclepio*, vol. 34 (1982), 295–316.

———. "Crisis Demográficos y Crisis Agrarias: Paludismo y Agricultura en Espana a Fines del Siglo XVIII," in *Congreso de Historia Rural, Siglos VV al XIX*. U.C.M. (Madrid: Casa de la Velázquez, 1984), 333–354.

Perrine, H. "Fever Treated with Large Doses of Sulphate of Quinine in Adams County near Natchez, Miss.," *Philadelphia Journal of the Medical and Physical Sciences*, vol. 13 (November 1826 and February 1827), 36–41.

Perrot, Emile. *Quinquina et quinine* (Paris: Presses universitaires de France, 1926).

Peters, W. *Chemotherapy and Drug Resistance in Malaria* (London: Academic Press, 1970).

Pinel, Thénard, and Hallé. "Rapport fait à l'Académie des Sciences par MM. Pinel, Thénard, et Hallé, Sur un Mémoire de M. Chomel, intitulé: Observations sur l'emploi des sulfates de quinine et de cinchonine dans les fièvres intermittentes," *Journal de pharmacie et des sciences accessoires*, vol. 7 (1821), 226–231.

Pitman, Henry. *A Relation of the Great Sufferings and Strange Adventures of Henry Pitman, Chyrurgion to the Late Duke of Monmouth* (London: Andrew Sowle, 1689).

Pizer, I. H. "Medical Aspects of the Westward Migrations, 1830–1860," *Bulletin of the Medical Library Association*, vol. 53 (1965), 1–14.

Pollack, Nancy J. "Taro," in ed. Kenneth F. Kiple and Kriemheld Coneè Ornelas, *The Cambridge World History of Food* (New York: Cambridge University Press, 2000), vol. 1, 218–230.

Poser, Charles M. and George W. Bruyn, *An Illustrated History of Malaria* (New York: Parthenon Publishing Group, 1999).

Potier, A.J. *Dissertation sur l'emploi du sulfate de quinine et du sulfate de cinchonine dans le traitement des fièvres intermittentes*. Thèse pour le doctorat en médecine. Faculté de médecine de Paris (Paris, 1821).

Prain, Sir David. "History in Botanical Study," *Essex Naturalist*, vol. 23, pt. 3 (1931), 101–116.

Prothero, R. Mansell. *Migrants and Malaria* (London: Longmans, 1965).

———. "Disease and Mobility: A Neglected Factor in Epidemiology," *International Journal of Epidemiology*, vol. 6, no. 3 (1977), 259–267.

———. "Malaria in Latin America: Environmental and Human Factors," *Bulletin of Latin American Research*, vol. 14, no. 3 (1995), 357–365.

———. "Migration and Malaria risk," *Health Risk and Society*, vol. 3, no. 1 (2001), 19–38.

Prudhomme, Émile. *Le quinquina: culture, préparation, commerce* (Paris: Challamel, 1902).

Puri, I.M. "Anophelines of the Oriental Region," in ed. Mark Boyd, *Malariology: A Comprehensive Survey of All Aspects of this Group of Disease from a Global Standpoint* (Philadelphia: Saunders, 1949), 483–505.

Quinn, Milton J. "Malaria in New England," *Boston Medical and Surgical Journal*, no. 194 (1926), 244–247.

Raina, B.L. *Introduction to the Malaria Problem in India*, 2nd ed. (New Delhi: Commonwealth Publishers, 1991).

Ramasubban, Radhika. *Public Health and Medical Research in India. Their Origins under the Impact of British Colonial Policy* (Stockholm: Swedish Agency for Research Cooperation with Developing Countries, 1982).

———. "Imperial Health in British India, 1857–1900," in ed. Roy Macleod and Milton Lewis, *Disease, Medicine, and Empire* (London: Routledge, 1988), 38–60.

Rambo, A.T. "Primitive Man's Impact on the Genetic Resources of the Malaysian Tropical Rainforest," *Malaysian Applied Biology Journal*, vol. 8 (1979), 59–65.

Rampino, Michael R. and Stanley H. Ambrose, "Volcanic Winter in the Garden of Eden: The Toba Supereruption and the Late Pleistocene Human Population Crash," in ed. F.W. McCoy and G. Heiken, *Volcanic Hazards and Disasters in Human Antiquity* (Boulder, CO: Geological Society of America, 2000), 71–82.

Ramsdale, C.D. and M. Coluzzi. "Studies on the Infectivity of Tropical African Strains of Plasmodium Falciparum to Some Southern European Vectors of Malaria," *Parassitologia*, vol. 17, nos. 1–3 (1975), 39–48.

Ransford, Oliver. *"Bid the Sickness Cease": Disease in the History of Black Africa* (London: J. Murray, 1983).

Relph, John. *An Inquiry into the Medical Efficacy of a New Species of Peruvian Bark* (London: J. Phillips, 1794).

Rich, Stephen M. "The Unpredictable Past of *Plasmodium Vivax* Revealed in Its Genome," *Proceedings of the National Academy of Sciences*, vol. 101, no. 44 (2004), 15547–15548.

Richards, John F. "The Opium Industry in British India," *Indian Economic and Social History Review*, vol. 39, no. 2 (2002), 149–180.

———. *The Unending Frontier: An Environmental History of the Modern World* (Berkeley: University of California Press, 2003).

Riera Palmero, J. "Quina in Spain in the XVIIIth Century," *Acts of the International Congress for the History of Pharmacy* (Padova, Italy: Accademia italiana di storia della farmacia, 1989), 184–187.

Risso, Patricia. *Merchants and Faith: Muslim Commerce and Culture in the Indian Ocean* (Boulder, CO: Westview Press, 1995).

Robbins, D.C. *The Tariff on Quinine. Remarks of D.C. Robbins on the Petition of the Manufacturers for the Retention of the Present Duty of 20 Per Cent, with a Counter Petition and Argument for Free Quinine. New York. March 25th, 1876* (New York: Thitchener and Glastaeter, 1876).

———. *Quinine and Our Tariff Policy. Quinine in its Commercial Relations. Its Value Past and Present* (New York: Press of Drug Topics and Medical Abstract, 1888).

Roberts, D.R., S. Manguin, and J. Mouchet. "DDT House Spraying and Re-Emerging Malaria," *The Lancet*, vol. 356, no. 9226 (July 22, 2000), 330–332.

Roberts, D.R., L.L. Laughlin, P. Hsheih, and L. Legters. "DDT, Global Strategies, and a Malaria Control Crisis in South America," *Emerging Infectious Diseases*, vol. 3, no. 3 (1997), 295–302.

Robertson, R. "Malaria in Western Yunnan with Reference to the China-Burma Highway," *Chinese Medical Journal*, vol. 57 (1940), 57–73.

Rocco, Fiammetta. *The Miraculous Fever-Tree: Malaria and the Quest for a Cure That Changed the World* (New York: Harper Collins, 2003).

Rogier, C., T. Fusai, B. Pradines, and J.-F. Trape. "Comment évaluer la morbidité attribuable au paludisme en zone d'endémie?" *Revue d'épidémiologie et de santé publique*, vol. 53, no. 3 (2005), 299–309.

Rosenberg, Tina. "What the World Needs Now Is DDT," *New York Times*, April 11, 2004.

Rosengarten and Sons. *Reply to a Pamphlet Entitled "The Tariff on Quinine," Published by D.C. Robbins, Wholesale Druggist and Importer, Manufacturer of Quinine Pills, and other Specialities, New York, Dated March 25th, 1876, Addressed to the Honorable Senate and the House of Representatives, at Washington, and to Dealers in Drugs, Chemicals, and Throughout the United States* (Philadelphia, 1876).

Ross, Ronald. *Malarial Fever: Its Cause, Prevention and Treatment* (London: For the University Press of Liverpool by Longmans, Green, and Co., 1902).

———. "The Logical Basis of the Sanitary Policy of Mosquito Reduction," *Science*, new series, vol. 22, no. 570 (December 1, 1905), 689–699.

———. "The Best Antimalarial Organization for the Tropics," *Separat-Abdruck aus Malaria*, Band I, Heft 2, (Leipzig, 1909), 89–94.

———. ed. *Observations on Malaria* (London: H.M.S.O., 1919).

Rowe, Alexander K., Samantha Rowe, Robert W. Snow, Eline L. Korenromp, Joanna R.M. Armstrong Schellenberg, Claudia Stein, Bernard L. Nahlen, Jennifer Bryce, Robert E. Black, and Richard W. Steketee. "The Burden of Malaria Mortality among African Children in the Year 2000," *International Journal of Epidemiology*, vol. 35 (2006), 691–704.

Rusby, H.H. "The Cultivation of Cinchona in Bolivia," *Pharmaceutical Record* (October 1, 1887), 305–308.

Russell, A.J.H. "Quinine Supplies in India," *Records of the Malaria Survey of India*, vol. 7, no. 4 (1937), 233–244.

Russell, Edmund. *War and Nature: Fighting Humans and Insects with Chemicals from World War I to Silent Spring* (New York: Cambridge University Press, 2001).

Russell, Paul F. "Lessons in Malariology from World War II," *American Journal of Tropical Medicine*, vol. 26 (1946), 5–13.

———. *Man's Mastery of Malaria* (London: Oxford University Press, 1955).

Rutman, Darrett B. and Anita H. Rutman. "Of Agues and Fevers: Malaria in the Early Chesapeake," *William and Mary Quarterly*, vol. 33, no. 1 (1976), 31–60.

Rutten, A.M.G. *Dutch Transatlantic Medicine Trade in the Eighteenth Century under the Cover of the West India Company* (Rotterdam, The Netherlands: Erasmus Pub., 2000).

Sallares, R., A. Bouwman, and C. Anderung. "The Spread of Malaria to Southern Europe in Antiquity: New Approaches to Old Problems," *Medical History*, vol. 48 (2005), 311–328.

Sallares, Robert. *Malaria and Rome: A History of Malaria in Ancient Italy* (Oxford: Oxford University Press, 2002).

————. "Pathocoenoses Ancient and Modern," *History and Philosophy of the Life Sciences*, vol. 27 (2005), 210–220.

Sanchez-Albornoz, Nicholás. "The Population of Colonial Spanish America," in ed. Leslie Bethell, *The Cambridge History of Latin America, vol. 2, Colonial Latin America* (Cambridge: Cambridge University Press, 1984), 3–35.

Sappington, John. *The Theory and Treatment of Fevers* (Arrow Rock, MO: Published by the author, 1844).

Saul, Allan. "Zooprophylaxis or Zoopotentiation: The Outcome of Introducing Animals on Vector Transmission is Highly Dependent on the Mosquito Mortality While Searching," *Malaria Journal*, vol. 2 (2003). Online at http://www.malariajournal.com/content/2/1/32.

Saunders, William. *Observations on the Superior Efficacy of the Red Peruvian Bark in the Cure of Agues and other Fevers* (London: Robert Hodge, for William Green, 1782).

Sauer, Carl O. *Agricultural Origins and Dispersals* (Cambridge, MA: M.I.T. Press, 1969).

Scholtens, R.G., R.L. Kaiser, and A.D. Langmuir. "An Epidemiologic Examination of the Strategy of Malaria Eradication," *International Journal of Epidemiology*, vol. 1, no. 1 (1972), 15–24.

Scott, Susan and Christopher J. Duncan. *Biology of Plagues: Evidence from Historical Populations* (New York: Cambridge University Press, 2001).

Service, Mike W. and Harold Townson. "The Anopheles Vector," in ed. David A. Warrell and Herbert M. Gilles, *Essential Malariology*, 4th ed. (London: Arnold Press, 2002), 59–84.

Shapiro, Judith. *Mao's War Against Nature: Politics and the Environment in Revolutionary China* (New York: Cambridge University Press, 2001).

Shaw, George Elliott. *Quinine Manufacture in India* (London: Institute of Chemistry of Great Britain and Ireland, 1935).

Shiffman, Jeremy, Tanya Beer, and Yonghong Wu. "The Emergence of Global Disease Control Priorities," *Health Policy and Planning*, vol. 17, no. 3 (2002), 225–234.

Shulman, Caroline and Edgar Dorman. "Clinical Features of Malaria in Pregnancy," in ed. David A. Warrell and Herbert M. Gilles, *Essential Malariology*, 4th ed. (London: Arnold Press, 2002), 219–235.

Sigerist, Henry E. *Medicine and Health in the Soviet Union* (New York: Citadel Press, 1947).

Silva, Kalinga Tudor. "Malaria Eradication as a Legacy of Colonial Discourse: The Case of Sri Lanka," *Parassitologia*, vol. 36 (1994), 149–163.

————. "'Public Health' for Whose Benefit? Multiple Discourses on Malaria in Sri Lanka," *Medical Anthropology*, vol. 17 (1997), 195–214.

Silvy, Félix-Célestin. *Dissertation sur l'emploi du sulfate de quinine dans le traitement des fièvres intermittentes*. Thèse pour le doctorat en médecine. Faculté de médecine de Paris (Paris: Didot, Jnr., 1828).

Simmons, James Stevens. "The Malaria Control Program of the United States Army during World War II," *Proceedings of the Fourth International Congresses on Tropical Medicine and Malaria*, vol. I (Washington, DC: Department of State, 1948), 827–840.

Sinden, Robert E. and Herbert M Gilles. "The Malaria Parasites," in ed. David A. Warrell and Herbert M. Gilles, *Essential Malariology*, 4th ed. (London: Arnold Press, 2002), 8–34.

Skeete, Thomas. *Experiments and Observations on Quilled and Red Bark* (London: J. Murray, 1786).

Slater, Leo B. "Malaria Chemotherapy and the 'Kaleidoscopic' Organisation of Biomedical Research during World War II," *Ambix*, vol. 51, no. 2 (2004), 107–134.

———. "Malarial Birds: Modeling Infectious Human Disease in Animals," *Bulletin of the History of Medicine*, vol. 79 (2005), 261–294.

Small, Jennifer, Scott J. Goetz, and Simon I. Hay. "Climatic Suitability for Malaria Transmission in Africa, 1911–1995," *Proceedings of the National Academy of Sciences*, vol. 100, no. 26 (2003), 15341–15345.

Smart, Charles. "On the Paroxysmal Fevers," in *Medical and Surgical History of the War of the Rebellion (1861–65)*, vol. 5 (Washington, DC: Government Printing Office, 1870–1888; repr.: [*Medical and Surgical History of the Civil War*], Wilmington, NC: Broadfoot Publishing Co., 1990), 77–190.

Smil, Vaclav. *Energy in World History* (Boulder, CO: Westview Press, 1994).

———. "Eating Meat: Evolution, Patterns, and Consequences," *Population and Development Review*, vol. 28, no. 4 (2002), 599–639.

Smith, Andrew B. "Origins and Spread of Pastoralism in Africa," *Annual Review of Anthropology*, vol. 21 (1991), 125–141.

Smith, Bruce D. "Low-Level Food Production," *Journal of Archaeological Research*, vol. 9, no. 1 (2001), 1–43.

Smith, Dale C. "Quinine and Fever: The Development of the Effective Dosage," *Journal of the History of Medicine and Allied Sciences*, vol. 31 (1976), 343–367.

Smith, Daniel B. *On the Cheaper Alkaloids of the Cinchonas* (Philadelphia: Powers and Weightman, 1855).

Snewin, V.A., S. Longacre, and P.H. David. "*Plasmodium Vivax*: Older and Wiser?," *Research in Immunology*, vol. 142 (1991), 631–636.

Snow, Robert W. and Herbert M. Gilles. "The Epidemiology of Malaria," in ed. David A. Warrell and Herbert M. Gilles, *Essential Malariology*, 4th ed. (London: Arnold Press, 2002), 85–106.

Snow, Robert W., Jean-François Trape, and Kevin Marsh. "The Past, Present, and Future of Childhood Malaria Mortality in Africa," *Trends in Parasitology*, vol. 17, no. 12 (2001), 593–597.

Snow, Robert W., Carlos A. Guerra, Abdisalan M. Noor, Hla Y, Myint, and Simon I. Hay. "The Global Distribution of Clinical Episodes of *Plasmodium Falciparum* Malaria," *Nature*, vol. 434 (March 10, 2005), 214–217.

Snowden, Frank M. *The Conquest of Malaria: Italy, 1900–1962* (New Haven: Yale University Press, 2006).

Sota, T. and M. Mogi. "Effectiveness of Zooprophylaxis in Malaria Control: A Theoretical Inquiry, with a Model for Mosquito Populations with Two Bloodmeal Hosts," *Medical and Veterinary Entomology*, vol. 3 (1989), 337–345.

Sowunmi, M. Adebisi. "The Significance of the Oil Palm (*Elaeis guineensis* Jacq.) in the Late Holocene Environments of West and West Central Africa: A

Further Consideration," *Vegetation History and Archaeobotany*, vol. 8 (1999), 199–210.

Spence, Jonathan. "Opium Smoking in Ch'ing China," in ed. Frederic Wakeman Jr. and Carolyn Grant, *Conflict and Control in Late Imperial China* (Berkeley: University of California Press, 1975), 143–173.

———. *The Search for Modern China* (New York: W.W. Norton, 1990).

Spencer, J.E. *Shifting Cultivation in Southeast Asia* (Berkeley: University of California Press, 1966).

Spencer, Margaret. *Malaria: The Australian Experience 1843–1991* (Townsville, Australia: Australasian College of Tropical Medicine, 1994).

Spielman, Andrew, Uriel Kitron, and Richard J. Pollack. "Time Limitation and the Role of Research in the Worldwide Attempt to Eradicate Malaria," *Journal of Medical Entomology*, vol. 30 (1993), 6–19.

Stapleton, Darwin H. "The Dawn of DDT and Its Experimental Use by the Rockefeller Foundation in Mexico, 1943–1952," *Parassitologia*, vol. 40 (1998), 149–158.

———. "Technology and Malaria Control, 1930–1960: The Career of Rockefeller Foundation Engineer Frederick W. Knipe," *Parassitologia*, vol. 42 (2000), 59–68.

———. "Internationalism and Nationalism: The Rockefeller Foundation, Public Health, and Malaria in Italy, 1923–1951," *Parassitologia*, vol. 42 (2000), 127–134.

———. "Lessons of History? Anti-Malarial Strategies of the International Health Board and the Rockefeller Foundation from the 1920s to the Era of DDT," *Public Health Reports*, vol. 119 (March–April 2004), 206–215.

Steckel, Richard H. and Jerome C. Rose, eds. *The Backbone of History: Health and Nutrition n the Western Hemisphere* (New York: Cambridge University Press, 2005).

Steiner, Paul E. *Disease in the Civil War* (Springfield, IL: C.C. Thomas, 1968).

Stepan, Nancy Leys. "'The Only Serious Terror in These Regions,' Malaria Control in the Brazilian Amazon," in ed. Diego Armus, *Disease in the History of Modern Latin America* (Durham, NC: Duke University Press, 2003), 25–50.

Stephens, J.W.W. "Pâtes Médicinales and Quinquina. The Treatment of K'ang Hsi, Emperor of China (1662–1723)," *The Journal of Tropical Medicine and Hygiene*, vol. 40, no. 16 (August 16, 1937), 187–188.

Strickland, W.A. "Quinine Pills Manufactured on the Missouri Frontier (1832–1862)," *Pharmaceutical History*, vol. 25 (1983), 61–68.

Stringer, Christopher and Robin McKie. *African Exodus: The Origins of Modern Humanity* (New York: Henry Holt, 1996).

Su, B., J. Xiao, P. Underhill, R. Deka, W. Zhang, J. Akey, W. Huang, D. Shen, D. Lu, J. Luo, J. Chu, J. Tan, P. Shen, R. Davis, L. Cavalli-Sforza, R. Chakraborty, M. Xiong, R. Du, P. Oefner, Z. Chen, and L. Jin. "Y-Chromosome Evidence for a Northward Migration of Modern Humans into Eastern Asia during the Last Ice Age," *American Journal of Human Genetics*, vol. 65, no. 6 (1999), 1718–1724.

Su, Xin-zhuan, Jianbing Mu, and Dierdre Joy. "The 'Malaria's Eve' Hypothesis and the Debate Concerning the Origin of the Human Malaria Parasite Plasmodium Falciparum," *Microbes and Infection*, vol. 5 (2003), 891–896.

Suppan, L. "Three Centuries of Cinchona," in *Proceedings of the Celebration of the Three Hundredth Anniversary of the First Recognized Use of Cinchona* (St. Louis: Missouri Botanical Garden, 1931), 29–138.

Sutherst, Robert W. "Global Change and Human Vulnerability to Vector-Borne Diseases," *Clinical Microbiology Reviews*, vol. 17, no. 1 (2004), 136–173.

Swellengrebel, N.H. "The Parasite-Host Relationship in Malaria," *Annals of Tropical Medicine and Parasitology*, vol. 44 (April–December 1950), 84–92.

———. "Reflections à propos de la Conference sur le paludisme de Kampala (1950)," *Annales de la Société Belge de Médicine Tropicale*, vol. 31 (1950), 111–119.

Swellengrebel, N.H. and A. de Buck. *Malaria in the Netherlands* (Amsterdam: Scheliema and Holkema, 1938).

Talisuna, Ambrose A., Peter Bloland, and Umberto D'Alessandro. "History, Dynamics, and Public Health Importance of Malaria Parasite Resistance," *Clinical Microbiology Reviews*, vol. 17, no. 1 (2004), 235–254.

Tarassevich, L. "Expansion pandémique de la malaria en Russie," *Bulletin de la Société de Pathologie Exotique*, vol. 16 (1923), 71–74.

Taylor, Frank O. "Forty-Five Years of Manufacturing Pharmacy," *Journal of the American Pharmaceutical Association*, vol. 4 (April 1915), 468–481.

Taylor, Norman. *Cinchona in Java: The Story of Quinine* (New York: Greenberg, 1945).

———. *Quinine: The Story of Cinchona* (New York: Cinchona Products Institute, 1952).

Taylor, S.A.G. *The Western Design: An Account of Cromwell's Expedition to the Caribbean*, 2nd ed. (London: Solstice Productions, 1969).

Taylor-Robinson, A.W. "A Model of Development of Acquired Immunity to Malaria in Humans Living under Endemic Conditions," *Medical Hypotheses*, vol. 58 (2002), 148–156.

Tchesnova, L. "Socio-economic and Scientific Premises for Forming the Strategies against Malaria in Russia under Soviet Power," *Parassitologia*, vol. 40 (1998), 103–108.

Thapar, Romila. *Early India: From the Origins to AD 1300* (Berkeley: University of California Press, 2002).

Thompson, H.N. "The Prophylactic Use of Quinine," *Journal of the Royal Army Medical Corps*, vol. 21 (1913), 587–589.

Thomson, James W. "An Inquiry into the Medical Topography and Epidemic Fevers of the Valley of Virginia," *Philadelphia Journal of the Medical and Physical Sciences*, vol. 1, new series (1825), 96–114.

Thornton, John. *Africa and Africans in the Making of the Atlantic World, 1400–1800* (New York: Cambridge University Press, 1998).

Tishkoff, Sarah A. et al. "Haplotype Diversity and Linkage Disequilibrium at Human G6PD: Recent Origin of Alleles That Confer Malarial Resistance," *Science*, vol. 293 (2001), 455–462.

Trape, Jean-François. "The Public Health Impact of Choloroquine Resistance in Africa," *American Journal of Tropical Medicine and Hygiene*, vol. 64, nos. 1–2 (2001), 12–17.

Trung, H.D., W. Van Bortel, T. Sochantha, K. Keokenchanh, N.T. Quang, L.D. Cong, and M. Coosemans. "Malaria Transmission and Major Malaria

Vectors in Different Geographical Areas of Southeast Asia," *Tropical Medicine and International Health*, vol. 9, no. 2 (2004), 230–237.

Tschirch, Alexandre. *Handbuch der Pharmakognosie* (Leipzig, Germany: C.H. Tauchnitz, 1933), 3 vols.

Unschuld, Paul U. *Medicine in China: A History of Pharmaceutics* (Berkeley: University of California Press, 1986).

Urban, Michael A. "An Uninhabited Waste: Transforming the Grand Prairie in Nineteenth Century Illinois, USA," *Journal of Historical Geography*, vol. 31 (2005), 647–665.

Valencius, Conevery Bolton. *The Health of the Country: How American Settlers Understood Themselves and Their Land* (New York: Basic Books, 2002).

Van Buren, William H. "Quinine as a Prophylactic Against Malarious Diseases," in ed. William A. Hammond MD, *Military, Medical and Surgical Essays Prepared for the United States Sanitary Commission* (Philadelphia: J.B. Lippincott and Co., 1864), 93–115.

Van Gorkom. K.W. "II. The Introduction of Cinchona into Java," in ed. Pieter Honig and Frans Verdoorn, *Science and Scientists in the Netherlands Indies* (New York: Board for the Netherlands Indies, Surinam, and Curaçao, 1945), 182–190.

Van Gorkom, Karel Wessel. *A Handbook of Cinchona Culture*, trans. Benjamin Daydon Jackson (London: Trübner and Co., 1883).

Vansina, Jan. "New Linguistic Evidence and 'The Bantu Expansion'," *Journal of African History*, vol. 36, no. 2 (1995), 173–195.

———. *Paths in the Rainforests* (Madison: University of Wisconsin Press, 1999).

Vaughan, J.G. and C.A. Geissler. *The New Oxford Book of Food Plants* (Oxford: Oxford University Press, 1999).

Vaughan, Walter. *The Evidence of the Superior Efficacy of the Cinchona Flava, or Yellow Peruvian Bark* (London: Printed for T. Cox, Borough, 1795).

Vaughn, Megan. "Healing and Curing: Issues in the Social History and Anthropology of Medicine in Africa," *Social History of Medicine*, vol. 7, no. 2 (1994), 283–295.

Verhave, Jan Peter. "The Dutch School of Malaria Research," *Parassitologia*, vol. 29 (1987), 263–274.

———. "Malaria: Epidemiology and Immunity in the Malay Archipelago," in ed. G.M. van Heteren, A. de Knecht-van Eekelen, and M.J.D. Poulissen, *Dutch Medicine in the Malay Archipelago* (Amsterdam: Rodopi, 1989), 87–104.

———. "The Use of Quinine for Treatment and Control of Malaria in The Netherlands," *Tropical and Geographical Medicine*, vol. 47, no. 6 (1995), 252–258.

Vinkhuysen, H. "On Quinetum and Its Therapeutic Value," *The Practitioner*, vol. 20, no. 11 (February 1878), 81–84.

Wade, Nicholas. *Before the Dawn: Recovering the Lost History of Our Ancestors* (New York: Penguin, 2006).

Wafer, Lionel. *A New Voyage and Description of the Isthmus of America* (London: Printed for James Knapton, 1699).

Walker, Kathleen R., Marie D. Ricciardone, and Janice Jensen. "Developing an International Consensus on DDT: A Balance of Environmental Protection and Disease Control," *International Journal of Hygiene and Environmental Health*, 206 (2003), 423–435.

Waring, Edward John. *Bibliotheca Therapeutica*, vol. I (London: New Sydenham Society, 1878).

Warrell, David A. "Clinical Features of Malaria," in ed. David A. Warrell and Herbert M. Gilles, *Essential Malariology*, 4th ed. (London: Arnold Press, 2002), 191–205.

Warrell, David A. and Herbert M. Gilles, eds. *Essential Malariology*, 4th ed. (London: Arnold Press, 2002).

Warren, Christian. "Northern Chills, Southern Fevers: Race Specific Mortality in American Cities, 1730–1900," *Journal of Southern History*, vol. 63, no. 1 (1997), 23–56.

Watson, Robert, and Briggs and Redginal Hewitt. "Topographical and Related Factors in the Epidemiology of Malaria in North America, Central America, and the West Indies," in ed. Forest Ray Moulton, *A Symposium on Human Malaria* (Washington, DC: American Association for the Advancement of Science, 1941), 135–147.

Watson, Sir Malcolm. *African Highway: The Battle for Health in Central Africa* (London: J. Murray, 1953).

Watt, Sir George. *The Commercial Products of India* (London: J. Murray, 1908).

Watts, David. *The West Indies: Patterns of Development, Culture, and Environmental Change since 1492* (New York: Cambridge University Press, 1987).

Watts, Sheldon. *Epidemics and History: Disease, Power, and Imperialism* (New Haven: Yale University Press, 1997).

———. "British Development Policies and Malaria in India 1897 – c. 1929," *Past and Present*, vol. 165, no. 1 (1999), 141–181.

———. "Yellow Fever Immunities in West Africa and the Americas in the Age of Slavery and Beyond: A Reappraisal," *Journal of Social History*, vol. 34, no. 4 (2001), 955–967.

———. "Reply to Kenneth Kiple," *Journal of Social History*, vol. 34, no. 4 (2001), 975–976.

———. *Disease and Medicine in World History* (New York: Routledge, 2003).

Webb Jr., James L.A. *Desert Frontier: Ecological and Economic Change along the Western Sahel, 1600–1850* (Madison: University of Wisconsin Press, 1995).

———. *Tropical Pioneers: Human Agency and Ecological Change in the Highlands of Sri Lanka, 1800–1900* (Athens: Ohio University Press, 2002).

———. "Ecology and Society in West Africa," in ed. Emmanuel Akyeampong, *Major Themes in West Africa's History* (London: James Currey, 2005), 33–51.

———. "Malaria and the Peopling of Early Tropical Africa," *Journal of World History*, vol. 16, no. 3 (2005), 269–291.

Weddell, H. *Histoire naturelle des quinquinas* (Paris: V. Masson, 1849).

Wenyon, C.M. "Malaria. Aetiology, Incidence and Distribution," in ed. W.G. MacPherson, W.P. Herringham, T.R. Elliott, and A. Balfour, *History of the Great War Based on Official Documents. Medical Services. Diseases of the War.* vol. 1 (London: H.M.S.O., n.d.), 227–263.

Wernsdorfer, Walther H. and Sir Ian McGregor, eds. *Malaria: Principles and Practice of Malariology*, 2 vols. (Edinburgh: Churchill Livingstone, 1988).

Willcox, Merlin L. and Gerard Bodeker. "Traditional Herbal Medicines for Malaria," *Clinical Research*, vol. 329, no. 7475 (2004), 1156–1159.

Willcox, Merlin, Gerard Bodeker, and Philippe Rasoanaivo, eds. *Traditional Medicinal Plants and Malaria* (Boca Raton: CRC Press, 2004).

Willoughby, W.G. and Louis Cassidy. *Anti-Malarial Work in Macedonia among British Troops* (London: H.K. Lewis, 1918).

Wilson, Bagster D. "Implications of Malarial Endemicity in East Africa," *Transactions of the Royal Society of Tropical Medicine and Hygiene*, vol. 32, no. 4 (1939), 435–465.

———. "Malarial Infectivity in African Soldiers in a Hyper-Endemic Area," *East African Medical Journal*, vol. 22 (1945), 295–296.

———. "Susceptibility to Malaria in East Africans," *Proceedings of the Fourth International Congresses on Tropical Medicine and Malaria* (Washington, DC: Department of State, 1948), 783–792.

———. "A Review of Hyperendemic Malaria," *Tropical Diseases Bulletin*, vol. 47, no. 8 (1950), 677–698.

———. "Construction, Irrigation, and Malaria," *East African Medical Journal*, vol. 34, no. 9 (1957), 479–485.

Wilson, Charles Morrow. *Quinine – Reborn in Our Hemisphere* (New York, 1943).

Wilson, Leonard G. "Fevers and Science in Early Nineteenth Century Medicine," *Journal of the History of Medicine and Allied Sciences*, vol. 33, no. 3 (1978), 386–407.

Wilson, Thomas. *An Enquiry into the Origin and Intimate Cause of Malaria* (London: Renshaw, 1858).

Winther, Paul C. *Anglo-European Science and the Rhetoric of Empire: Malaria, Opium, and British Rule in India, 1756–1895* (Lanham, MD: Lexington Books, 2003).

Wood, Peter H. *Black Majority: Negroes in Colonial South Carolina from 1670 through the Stono Rebellion* (New York: Knopf, 1974).

Worboys, Michael. "From Miasmas to Germs: Malaria, 1850–1879," *Parassitologia*, vol. 36 (1994), 61–68.

World Health Organization. *WHO Expert Committee on Malaria: Twentieth Report* (Geneva: World Health Organization, 2000).

Worster, Donald. *Nature's Economy: A History of Ecological Ideas* (New York: Cambridge University Press, 1994).

———. "The Ecology of Order and Chaos," in ed. Char Miller and Hal Rothman, *Out of the Woods: Essays in Environmental History* (Pittsburgh: University of Pittsburgh Press, 1997), 3–17.

Worthen, Dennis B. "The National Quinine Pool: When Quinine Went to War," *Pharmacy in History*, vol. 38, no. 3 (1996), 143–147.

Wright, Angus. *The Death of Ramón González: The Modern Agricultural Dilemma* (Austin: University of Texas Press, 1990).

Yarnell, Eric and Kathy Abascal. "Botanical Treatment and Prevention of Malaria. Part 2 – Selected Botanicals," *Alternative and Complementary Therapies*, vol. 10, no. 5 (2004), 277–284.

Yao, Y.T., L.C. Ling, and K.B. Liu. "Studies on the So-called Changch'i: Part I: Changch'i in Kweichow and the Kwangsi border," *Chinese Medical Journal*, vol. 50 (1936), 726–738.

———. "Studies on the So-called Changch'i: Part II: Changch'i in Yunnan," *Chinese Medical Journal*, vol. 50 (1936), 1815–1828.

Yellen, John E., Alison S. Brooks, Els Cornelissen, Michael J. Mehlman, and Kathlyn Stewart. "A Middle Stone Age Worked Bone Industry from Katanda, Upper Semliki Valley, Zaire," *Science*, vol. 268, no. 5210 (April 28, 1995), 553–556.

Yip, K. "Antimalarial Work in China: A Historical Perspective," *Parassitologia*, vol. 40 (1998), 29–38.

———. "Malaria Eradication in Taiwan," *Parassitologia*, vol. 42 (2000), 117–126.

Young, Martin D., Don E. Eyles, Robert W. Burgess, and Geoffrey M. Jeffrey. "Experimental Testing of the Immunity of Negroes to *Plasmodium Vivax*," *Journal of Parasitology*, vol. 41 (1955), 315–319.

Zárate Botía, Carlos Gilberto. *Extracción de Quina: La Configuración del Espacio Andino-Amazónico de Fines des Siglo XIX* (Bogotá: Universidad Nacional de Colombia, Sede Leticia, Instituto Amazónico de Investigaciones, 2001).

Zurbrigg, Sheila. "Re-Thinking the 'Human Factor' in Malaria Mortality: The Case of the Punjab, 1868–1940," *Parassitologia*, vol. 36 (1994), 121–135.

———. "Did Starvation Protect From Malaria?," *Social Science History*, vol. 21, no. 1 (1997), 27–58.

Index